Introduction to Mental Retardation

DAVID L. WESTLING

Florida State University

Prentice-Hall, Inc., Englewood Cliffs, New Jersey 07632

Library of Congress Cataloging in Publication Data

Westling, David L.
  Introduction to mental retardation.

  Bibliography: p.
  Includes index.
  1. Mental retardation.   I. Title.
RC570.W524 1986   616.85′88   85-6477
ISBN 0-13-487927-9

© 1986 by Prentice-Hall, Inc., Englewood Cliffs, New Jersey 07632

Printed in the United States of America

10 9 8 7 6 5 4 3 2 1

Editorial/production supervision: Virginia Cavanagh Neri
Cover design: Ben Santora
Manufacturing buyer: Barbara Kelly Kittle

ISBN 0-13-487927-9 01

Prentice-Hall International (UK) Limited, *London*
Prentice-Hall of Australia Pty. Limited, *Sydney*
Editora Prentice-Hall do Brasil, Ltda., *Rio de Janeiro*
Prentice-Hall Canada Inc., *Toronto*
Prentice-Hall Hispanoamericana, S. A., *Mexico*
Prentice-Hall of India Private Limited, *New Delhi*
Prentice-Hall of Japan, Inc., *Tokyo*
Prentice-Hall of Southeast Asia Pte. Ltd., *Singapore*
Whitehall Books Limited, *Wellington, New Zealand*

To Wendy and our children,
Jennifer, Jessica, and Meredith

Contents

3   Identification Procedures   42

PART II   WHY DOES MENTAL RETARDATION OCCUR?

4   Physiological Causes of Mental Retardation   67

PART IV   HOW DO WE ASSIST RETARDED INDIVIDUALS?

PART V   SPECIAL TOPICS

Preface

For many reasons, the present is a good time for mentally retarded people. It is also an exciting time for professional involvement with these individuals. Consider the following:

A free and appropriate public school education based on an individual educational plan is guaranteed by law for all mentally retarded and other handicapped children.

More time and careful planning is being committed to diagnosing and arranging services than ever before.

More mentally retarded people are residing in community facilities today than in large residential facilities.

Research in applied behavior analysis and educational technology is beginning to tap into the previously undetected learning potential of many of these persons. The contribution of the computer age for this process can only be imagined.

In the medical field, better health care and preventative technology is rapidly developing.

The formulation of many preschool programs and postschool services is broadening the public role in providing necessary assistance to these individuals.

The civil and legal rights of retarded individuals have been guaranteed and strongly asserted in several court cases.

The parents of retarded children have the right and are being given the opportunity to become involved in the education and treatment of their children.

With little effort the list could be expanded. The most important thing about each of the above statements is that they have only become true within the last fifteen or twenty years, many probably being realized in the lifetime of most readers of this text.

Of course, much remains to be done. For example:

Some educational programs are appropriate and individualized more according to the letter of the law than its spirit.

Many environmental and physiological conditions still exist that contribute to the mentally retarded population.

Various necessary services are sometimes difficult to access.

We have yet to realize the full learning potential of most retarded individuals.

Society still shows a degree of immaturity by not completely accepting those who are retarded into its system.

Such conditions as these lay the foundation of work, the challenge of the future, for professionals who will serve the needs of retarded persons in the next several years. It is the purpose of this text to provide a broad yet basic level of information for these professionals-to-be.

Of course, no single book can be enough. The field moves too fast to be covered simply or cursorily. Even as this book goes into production, changes are occurring. Most importantly, Congress has just passed PL 98–199 which continues the benefits brought forth in 1975 by PL 94–142, the Education for All Handicapped Children Act. PL 98–199 also focuses on the development of preschool programs, secondary and postsecondary programs, continuing education, personnel preparation programs, parent training and information, and the improvement of educational technology.

It is hoped that readers of this book will approach it with a great desire for information about retarded individuals and related issues. The writing has been presented in a fashion that was intended to be orderly, factual, and readable. It attempts to address four major questions about mental retardation:

Who are the mentally retarded?
(Part I, Chapters 1, 2, and 3)

Why does mental retardation occur?
(Part II, Chapters 4 and 5)

What are mentally retarded individuals like?
(Part III, Chapters 6, 7, and 8)

How do we assist retarded individuals?
(Part IV, Chapters 9, 10, and 11)

In addition, Part V addresses two special topics: the mentally retarded adult (Chapter 12) and parents of retarded children (Chapter 13). It is believed that the breadth and degree of information provided will adequately serve undergraduate or graduate students in an introductory course on the subject.

In the preparation of this book many students, colleagues, and friends offered different kinds of support and advice. In all instances I sincerely appreciated their consideration and help. In fairness, however, I cannot hold any of them responsible for any shortcomings that may appear because, in the end, it was my work. Still, I would like to mention and express sincere gratitude to the following people who reviewed and reacted to different parts of the manuscript during various stages of its development: Terry Cronis, Donna Fletcher, Chuck Forgnone, Bob Fowler, Joe Justin, Mark Koorland, John Langone, Julie Lee, Elliott Lessen, Doris Mattraw, Andy Oseroff, Lou Schwartz, Pearl Tait, Ron Taylor, Pattee Tobik, John Venn, Tom Whitten, and Jim Whorton. Additionally, I am especially grateful to Mrs. Mary Hafner, an excellent typist, who waded through many drafts of this product and finally brought it all together. Too, I thank Prentice-Hall, Ms. Susan Katz Willig, its Education Editor, and Ms. Ginny Neri, the production editor for this project, for their continuous support and encouragement.

Finally, I will spend the rest of my life trying to pay back my wife, Wendy, for doing double duty in managing our home and children while I worked on this project. For so many days, so many nights, so many weekends she held things together so I could write. And even though this did not particularly strain this superperson, I remain devotionally indebted. To my children, Jennifer, Jessica, and Meredith, I also say thanks. Thanks for the hugs and kisses when I was too busy to respond, thanks for trusting me and hanging in there, and thanks for trying to understand why sometimes I couldn't go to the ball games and swimming pool.

It is hoped that the readers of this book will gain insight into the population of mentally retarded individuals and the many issues related to them and their needs. An effort was made throughout the text to provide information in an objective fashion without too much editorializing. Virtually every chapter contains at least one issue on which complete agreement cannot be found. My goal was to present positions in an unbiased fashion and relate the ramifications of each as clearly as possible. From this foundation, readers may further pursue the necessary depth to develop their own personal and professional opinions.

D. L. W.

1

Concepts and Definitions

DEFINING MENTAL RETARDATION

We attempt to define a condition such as mental retardation in order to clearly communicate with each other its existence and related information. In any social science a certain degree of ambiguity will always be found. Mental retardation is no exception. By having a clear definition, we try to reduce the ambiguity and promote more definitive communication about the population of concern.

A definition of mental retardation should provide the criteria used to judge whether a person is mentally retarded or not. If the definition is clear and the criteria are explicit, everyone should be able to reach the same conclusion about a group of people or an individual person; that is, they are retarded or they are not. A high degree of consensus would be most desirable. Unfortunately this is not always the case.

In the social sciences we deal with definitions and concepts created by humans. It is not that conditions such as mental retardation (or mental illness, or intellectual giftedness) do not exist. Certainly they do. It is simply that the definitions and commensurate criteria for these conditions are subjectively decided upon. In short, mental retardation is what professional consensus says it is. When the condition is most apparent, most people will agree upon its existence; when it is closer to normalcy, fewer will agree.

What people consider to be mental retardation has been influenced by various factors. Definitions have been based on perceptions of intelligence, behavior, and physical characteristics. Criteria and decisions regarding these factors have in turn been influenced by the personal, social, moral, and political values of the definers.

Although professionals in the field of mental retardation have not fully acknowledged a universal definition of mental retardation, the one most commonly used is that provided by the American Association on Mental Deficiency (AAMD, Grossman, 1973, 1977, 1983). Even this definition, however, lacks total acceptance. This lack of harmony, however, should not be surprising or dismaying. This is the nature of the social sciences. At best we can only speak in terms of probabilities because in the study of humans, there are few absolute truths.

THE 1973/1977/1983 AAMD DEFINITION OF MENTAL RETARDATION

The most often used definition of mental retardation today is that provided by the AAMD in its "Classification in Mental Retardation"

(Grossman, 1983), which is identical to earlier definitions published by AAMD (Grossman, 1973, 1977). It reads:

> Mental retardation refers to significantly subaverage general intellectual functioning existing concurrrently with deficits in adaptive behavior and manifested during the developmental period. (p. 1.)

Three elements or criteria necessary for a person to be considered mentally retarded appear in the definition. First, the person must have "significantly subaverage general intellectual functioning." Second, this limited level of intelligence must be associated with or occur "concurrently with deficits in adaptive behavior." Third, the condition must arise initially during the developmental period; that is, between conception and eighteen years. The first two components of the definition are its essence.

"Significantly Subaverage General Intellectual Functioning"

According to the AAMD definition, a person may be judged as mentally retarded only if there is evidence of below average intellectual ability. As operationalized by the AAMD, this means that one must score approximately 70 points or lower on a standardized intelligence test (Grossman, 1983).

The use of a single IQ score indicates a unitary concept of intelligence. In other words, overall intelligence is seen to be reflected in the one score. This theoretical assumption of intelligence as a general factor is a widely held belief but not the only position accepted. Various theorists and researchers have offered contrasting views of intelligence; some support the general intellectual ability theory while others argue for several ability factors. The latter position suggests that several types of intelligence exist. Guilford's (1967) Structure of the Intellect Model (see Figure 1–1) is a noteworthy model of factorial intelligence. Readers wishing detailed discussion on various theories of intelligence can refer to several sources (e.g., Boring, 1950; Fancher, 1979; Herrnstein & Boring, 1965; Matarazzo, 1972; Sattler, 1982).

The IQ standard for retardation presented by the AAMD is meant as a guideline. Standard errors of measurement on intelligence tests (the inclination for the score to vary a few points from one time of testing to another) and adaptive behavior performance must be considered by practitioners when making a judgment about the retardation of an individual. A person with an IQ somewhat above the criterion may be judged as mentally retarded if their adaptive behavior is limited severely enough to warrant such a decision (Grossman, 1977; 1983).

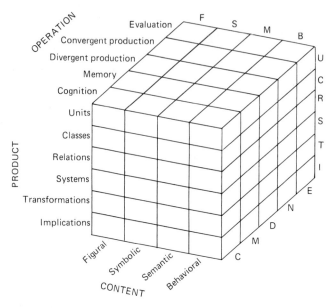

FIGURE 1–1   Guilford's Structure of the Intellect

J. P. Guilford, *The Nature of Human Intelligence* (New York: McGraw-Hill, 1967). Reproduced by permission.

"Deficits in Adaptive Behavior"

Adaptive behavior is considered the individual's ability to function normally in the environment in accordance with standards appropriate for a given chronological age. During the preschool years, this may mean the child demonstrates the common milestones of development within a reasonable period of time; for example, sitting, standing, crawling, walking, and talking. An older child might be expected to acquire knowledge and skills through experience. This usually is taken to mean the child can learn academic matter in the school but may also include the ability to function adequately in the home or neighborhood. As an adult, adaptive behavior is usually judged by the individual's social interactions. Successful employment and getting along with peers is often considered an important indication.

Adaptive behavior is not as easy to quantify as intelligence is. There are a number of instruments available to measure adaptive behavior (e.g., the AAMD Adaptive Behavior Scale; Nihira, Foster Shellhaas & Leland, 1971) but operationalizing the concept has not been as readily achieved as operationalizing intelligence has. Because of this, adaptive behavior judgments are often subjective. In making a clinical judgment, one professional may judge a deficiency while another may not. Some professionals may look at one situation as being the most indicative aspect of adaptive behavior (e.g., school learning), while others may consider other types of behavior more important (e.g., functioning in the community). Because there is relatively less consistency in defining adaptive behavior, there is often conflict, particularly in higher functioning subaverage IQ individuals, about whether or not "mental retardation" is an appropriate label.

Generally speaking, lower IQ level retarded persons, those with IQs below about 50 or 55, will clearly demonstrate deficits in adaptive behavior. The lower the IQ, the more obvious the behavioral limitations will be. These individuals will always meet the criteria for retardation.

What Is Not Required by the AAMD Definition

Some earlier definitions of mental retardation and even some contemporary concepts (particularly those held by lay persons) often would affix certain conditions to mental retardation not required by the AAMD definition. As a student of mental retardation, the reader should be aware of what the AAMD definition does not imply as well as what it does.

Some earlier theorists felt that mental retardation was primarily a polygenetically inherited condition or a result of a physiological disorder. While these sources may result in mental retardation, the AAMD definition does not state that a *particular* etiology (cause) is necessary for a person to be classified as retarded. In other words, we do not have to show evidence of "brain damage" or any other condition in judging the existence of mental retardation.

The AAMD also does not state that mental retardation is necessarily a permanent condition. Often people may think "once retarded, always retarded." Certainly this has been a position taken by previous writers (e.g., Doll, 1941). Essentially, however, the AAMD statement is a "here and now" definition. In short, it is possible (and for many mildly retarded persons, probable) that a person can be judged as mentally retarded at one point in life but not at another. The concept of the "six-hour retarded child" (President's Committee on Mental Retardation, 1970) conveys this notion. These children, mostly of low socioeconomic backgrounds, are often classified as mentally retarded while at school, but not at home or in their adult years. The AAMD definition allows such flexibility to exist.

Finally, we must realize that the current predominant concept of mental retardation does not depict a homogeneous group of individuals. In fact, the population of retarded persons is extremely heterogeneous. There is at least as much diversity among them as there is in the nonretarded population. While we must attempt to find a common point of reference for the reasons discussed earlier, we should not lose sight of the fact that we are speaking of individuals who vary greatly in many human characteristics.

EARLIER CONCEPTS AND DEFINITIONS

In order to gain greater understanding of and appreciation for the 1973/1977/1983 AAMD definition, it might be useful to briefly trace some earlier concepts of retardation.

Preintelligence Tests

Before the development of intelligence tests in the early 1900s, mental retardation was primarily considered a medical disorder (Matarazzo, 1972). Individuals whose behavior and appearance were not considered normal were often judged to be retarded. Clinical descriptions were used to distinguish various levels of retardation and sometimes to designate etiology. The lower the level the more readily apparent the condition. Incompetence in living and learning were primary criteria along with distinguishing physical characteristics. According to Sheerenberger (1983), prior to the development of intelligence tests, most mentally retarded persons were judged by five standards:

1. Physiognomy ("You need only to look at him to see that he is bright [or stupid]")
2. Use of age ("She acts like a two-year-old")
3. Quality of school work
4. Physical coordination ("He's slow and clumsy")
5. Physical signs, such as premature aging (or, "She's a funny looking kid"). (p. 65.)

Intelligence Tests and Social Adaption

In 1905, Alfred Binet and Theodore Simon of France published the first mental test that would ultimately become known as an intelligence test. Earlier work in the field, primarily that of Sir Francis Galton, had attempted to measure intelligence through human sensory and physical abilities. Binet's test examined more complex human activity such as arithmetic, language, and memory.

During the time Binet was conducting his research on the measurement of intelligence, people were becoming concerned about the quality of public education in France and elsewhere. The government of Paris asked Binet to help determine which children would and would not benefit from public education. It was this impetus that moved Binet away from the theoretical issue of intelligence and toward a more "practical" concept. In other words, Binet had to devise a test that would *predict* whether or not a child would benefit from the normal schooling procedures.

Binet's test was truly a landmark in the field of intelligence testing. The content of this instrument consisted of thirty items. Binet considered the 1905 scale to be very crude. However, it adequately served to predict and objectively classify a child as being a moron (mildly retarded), an imbecile (moderately retarded), or an idiot (severely/profoundly retarded).

The second Binet scale was produced in 1908 and introduced the concept of "mental age." There were three to eight items for each age of a child between three and thirteen years. Thus by passing the items at a certain level, a child was considered to have a certain mental age. In 1911, the third scale was published. This test included a number of content revisions. It was considered to be quite thorough and extended the age level upward to include adults. Since 1905, every test of intelligence has had basically the same purpose as the first scale by Binet and Simon: *to predict school achievement.*

In the United States during the early years of the twentieth century, Lewis Terman of Stanford University and H. H. Goddard of the Vineland Training School translated the Binet test into English. Terman (1916) standardized it in this country and began to use it to identify individuals with various levels of intelligence. It was called the Stanford-Binet Intelligence Test. Terman was the first to use the measure we call the Intelligence Quotient (IQ) that was developed in Germany by Stern (1912).

Terman and Goddard advanced the notion that the test was a complete measure of intelligence, that intelligence was a general ability, that it was hereditary and fixed, and that a low IQ (generally below 70) constituted a sufficient criterion for retardation. Terman and Goddard's conceptualization of mental retardation became very dominant in the United States from about 1910 to 1950.

There were some, however, who did not accept a low IQ as being the sole criterion for mental retardation. In England, Tredgold (1908, 1937) took the position that *social inadequacy* (which we now refer to as adaptive behavior) was also a necessary condition for mental retardation. Tredgold (1937) wrote:

> Mental deficiency or amentia is a state of incomplete mental development of such a kind and degree that the individual is *incapable of adapting himself to the normal environment of his fellows* in such a way as to maintain existence independently of supervision, control, or external support. [Italics added]

Clearly, Tredgold felt that environmental adaption was equally as important as measured intelligence was.

The significance of social inadequacy in the conceptualization of mental retardation eventually became stronger. Edgar A. Doll, who some years later followed Goddard at the Vineland Training School, like Tredgold, supported the notion that social incompetence was a necessary criterion for a person to be considered mentally retarded. Doll (1941) specified six elements that he felt should be included in the concept of mental deficiency. He said: "The mentally deficient person is (1) socially incompetent; that is, socially inadequate and occupationally incompetent and unable to manage his own affairs; (2) mentally subnormal; (3) retarded intellectually from birth or early age; (4) retarded at maturity; (5) mentally deficient as a result of constitutional origin through heredity or disease; and (6) essentially incurable" (Doll, 1941, p. 215).

In an attempt to objectively measure social competence, Doll developed the Vineland Social Maturity Scale (1936, 1964) and the Preschool Attainment Record (1966). These scales, unlike the Binet/Terman tests, allowed the clinician or teacher to assess the day-to-day functioning of an individual and thus, by comparison, to judge the individual's social competence. Only if this ability was low *and* measured IQ was low would Doll have considered someone to be mentally retarded.

The 1959/1961 AAMD Definition

The AAMD has been a primary definer of mental retardation for over one hundred years. Wilmarth (1906, as cited in Scheerenberger [1983]) stated that the first definition "formulated and endorsed" by the Association appeared in 1877. It stated that "idiocy and imbecility" were conditions in which there was a "want of natural or harmonious development of the mental, active, and moral powers of the individual . . . usually associated with some visible defect . . . expressed in various forms and degrees of disordered vital action . . ." (Scheerenberger, 1983, p. 110). Of greater pertinence to the present discussion, however, was the definition published for the Association in 1959 by Heber. It read:

> Mental retardation refers to subaverage general intellectual functioning which originates during the developmental period and is associated with impairment in one or more of the following: (1) maturation, (2) learning, and (3) social adjustment. (Heber, 1959, p. 3)

Two years later, there was a slight revision which read:

> Mental retardation refers to subaverage general intellectual functioning which originates during the developmental period and is associated with impairment in adaptive behavior. (Heber, 1961, p. 499)

In presenting this definition, the AAMD acknowledged the significance of the lack of social competence or adaptive behavior as a criterion for mental retardation. The term "subaverage general intellectual functioning" meant that a person needed only to score − 1 standard deviation (S.D.) below the mean on an intelligence test, about 84 or 85 points, in order to satisfy the subaverage intelligence criterion. It is very important to note that this is about 14 or 15 points higher than required in the most current definition (1983). Individuals who scored between − 1 S.D. and − 2 S.D. (or about 70 to 85 IQ) were referred to as the "borderline" mentally retarded in the earlier (1959/1961) AAMD definition. This early definition thus broadened the concept of retardation from the traditional criterion of about a 70 or 75 IQ used by most professionals in that period.

Besides the difference in the IQ criterion, another important difference between the earlier (1959 and 1961) and later (1973, 1977, and 1983) AAMD definitions is that the later manuals allowed, and in fact encouraged, the use of clinical judgment in determining the existence of mental retardation. In doing so, they realized the difficulty in judging mental retardation, particularly at higher levels, based on an intelligence test score. The "standard error of measurement" on a particular test must be considered, as must the person's level of adaptive behavior. In the latest AAMD manual, Grossman (1983) wrote:

> This upper limit (an IQ of 70) is intended as a guideline; it could be extended upward through 75 or more, depending on the reliability of the intelligence test used. This particularly applies in schools and similar settings if behavior is impaired and clinically determined to be due to deficits in reasoning and judgment. (p. 11)

CRITICISM OF THE AAMD DEFINITIONS

As stated previously, arriving at a consensus on definitions and the corresponding criteria for mental retardation has not been fully achieved. While the AAMD definitions were accepted by many, others contested their requirements.

Criticism of the IQ Criterion

When the 1959/1961 criteria were published, many practitioners had historically placed the upper IQ level for mental retardation at about 70 or 75. Most states, local school districts, and professionals of various backgrounds had used this IQ level (albeit with flexibility) as a cutoff point. Most IQ test constructors had also adhered to this lower cutoff point (Wechsler, 1958).

Garfield and Wittson (1960) pointed out that the more liberal IQ criterion (e.g. up to 84 or 85 points) could result in two problems. These included:

> A significant increase in the number of persons considered mentally retarded; that is, four times the number of those existing under the below-70 IQ criterion.
> "Too wide a latitude" for judging a person to be retarded.

Garfield and Wittson therefore suggested that the borderline group (IQ 70–84) be excluded from the concept of mental retardation.

This suggestion was evidently taken when the later definitions and criteria of mental retardation were published (Grossman, 1973; 1977; 1983). In these writings, the borderline group was dropped as the IQ criterion was lowered first to -2 standard deviations (S.D.) from the mean (Grossman, 1973; 1977) and then to about 70 points (Grossman, 1983).[1] Officially, the AAMD no longer considered "borderline" persons as retarded.

Ironically, this change in position again generated criticism. This time some professionals took the position that the IQ criterion should *not* have been lowered in the later definitions and the borderline category should have been maintained. Their rationale was that those in the borderline group needed services which they could not receive if they were not classified as borderline. In commenting on the 1973 AAMD definition, Kidd (1977) suggested that the -2 S.D. was too low and that a borderline or "slow-learner" group *should* be included. In a later publication, Kidd and his colleagues (Kidd, Bartlett, Forgnone, Goldstein, Gorton, Moreno-Milne, Roseboro & White, 1979) wrote:

> Since the 1973 *Manual* appeared, not only have eleven states adopted the 68 IQ 'ceiling' but another approximately 25 have abandoned the IQ 75 'ceiling' for unstated IQ criteria. Thus only some fifteen states now use the 'ceiling' of IQ 75 or so for eligibility for special education and other services for the mentally retarded. (p. 74)

Kidd et al. suggested it would have been better for the AAMD to have set a higher cut-off point (e.g., IQ 80) and have said that some cases *below* this point may not warrant being considered mentally retarded instead of setting a lower IQ and saying some cases *above* this cut-off point may be considered mentally retarded.

---

[1]In the 1983 manual, the AAMD set the criterion for mental retardation at 70 IQ. In the 1973 and 1977 manuals, the criterion was set at -2 standard deviations which for most intelligence tests is about 68 or 69 points. The difference is obviously small, but it was incorporated to indicate that precision of IQ is not as important as is clinical judgment.

Kidd et al. (1979) offered an alternate definition of mental retardation. It read:

> Mental retardation refers to subaverage general human cognitive functioning, irrespective of etiology(ies), typically manifested during the developmental period, which is of such severity as to markedly limit one's ability to (a) learn, and consequently, to (b) make logical decisions, choices, and judgments, and (c) cope with one's self and one's environment. (p. 76)

From this definition it may be realized that Kidd's concern is really not so much with IQ per se, but with the potential effect it may have on limiting those who should be validly considered mentally retarded for the purpose of receiving appropriate schooling.

Additional criticism of the 1973 AAMD definition was expressed by Baumeister and Muma (1975). Their criticism went beyond the IQ scores and instead criticized the general use of intelligence tests as the basis for the concept of mental retardation. According to Baumeister and Muma, the AAMD was advocating a general ability theory of intelligence by defining intelligence as what is tested by intelligence tests and simultaneously committing itself to a unitary concept of mental retardation. Their position was that much important, socially relevant behavior results from dynamic and complex systems and a unitary psychometric concept of intelligence inadequately described this process. They stated that the AAMD definition "does not adequately provide for measures that meaningfully reflect the interactive effects of psychological and social systems" (p. 297). Furthermore, they said that "the IQ score is the most trivial bit of information we have about an individual" (p. 301).

What Baumeister and Muma (1975) were saying was that human behavioral adaption is far too complex to place a very heterogeneous group of individuals in the same group based on a single score that itself may be derived in many ways. However, they could not offer a simple alternative to the IQ criterion. Instead, they wrote:

> . . . it seems to us that the obvious diversity and variability of human behavior precludes the statement of a small set of relatively static variables as sufficient to render individually useful a unitary conception of MR. We advocate instead a theory-guided approach to the definition of human adjustment that focuses upon the developing organism and its interactions with a dynamic environment. . .In such a system there would not be "MR" but rather a complex and continually changing profile of an individual's adjustment to the constantly changing exigencies of his environment. All of us would have a place in such a system. (p. 305)

Criticism of the Adaptive Behavior Criterion

Some writers strongly opposed the inclusion of adaptive behavior in the AAMD definitions. Clausen (1967, 1972) argued strongly for a strictly *psychometric* definition of mental retardation. That is, he wanted to define mental retardation only in terms of IQ level and disregard attempts to measure adaptive behavior. A similar position was taken by Nagler (1972) and Penrose (1972). Clausen's basic position was that adaptive behavior tended to destabilize the concept of mental retardation since it could not be as reliably measured as could intelligence. Clausen felt that the concept of adaptive behavior and its measurement would require unique standards for different environments. On the other hand, tests of intelligence could be used validly and reliably without regard to a person's particular daily living situation. Clausen (1972) wrote:

> To tie a diagnosis of mental deficiency to the particular community in which a person is living would be like giving up the universality of the metric system for a personal system of fathoms and feet. (p. 54)

While he felt that educational and training programs should focus on improving adaptive behavior, Clausen suggested that attempts to define and accurately measure the concept were elusive and added only confusion. Therefore, he thought it best not to include it as a criterion for defining mental retardation.

Despite the criticism by Clausen (1967, 1972) and others regarding the use of adaptive behavior, it has continued to be included by the AAMD as part of its definition. Grossman (1973) stated that the "pluralistic norms which characterize every highly developed society greatly complicate the assessment of social competence" (p. xi). He maintained, however, that the limitations in measurement systems did not nullify the significance of the concept or its inclusion in the definition of mental retardation.

ALTERNATIVE CONCEPTS AND DEFINITIONS

While the AAMD definition is the one most often cited and used, others have been written. Some that are more notable are presented in this section. In studying them the reader should note how they diverge from the dominant definition offered by the AAMD.

Mercer's Sociological Perspective

Mercer (1970, 1971, 1973a, b) viewed mental retardation from a social perspective rather than from a psychological or educational viewpoint. Mercer opposed the definition of mental retardation from a clinical perspective as offered by the AAMD. She reasoned that mental retardation was a socially assigned condition and that its definition should be sociologically based. Mercer (1973b) stated: "According to our sociological definition, mental retardation is an achieved social status in a social system. Like any social status, the status of mental retardate is associated with a role which persons occupying that status are expected to play" (p. 3). To Mercer, the "visibility" of the person in the community is the most important criterion for determining whether a person is mentally retarded. Thus "adaptive behavior" was considered to be determined by people in the community. Even though Mercer (1973a) found that adaptive behavior correlated highly with IQ when IQ was below 50, the IQ per se could not be used to adequately determine mental retardation when it was above 50.

Mercer's greatest concern was that too many minority children from low socioeconomic homes were being classified as "educable mentally retarded" or "borderline" retarded by the public school system. She reasoned that if such individuals were not socially identified in their community as being retarded, why should a clinical diagnosis of retardation be placed upon them by agencies such as public schools.

Mercer posited that intelligence tests were inadequate for identifying individuals from minority backgrounds because the tests contained cultural biases. In order to take the individual's cultural background into consideration, she developed the System of Multicultural Pluralistic Assessment (SOMPA, Mercer & Lewis, 1978). This system was intended to avoid the identification of persons who might be clinically diagnosed as retarded by intelligence tests, but not considered as such in their home or neighborhood.

Dunn's General Learning Disability Concept

Like Mercer, Dunn (1968) expressed concern about the number of minority individuals placed in special classes. While he recognized the need for special education for many of these children, he also believed that the label "mental retardation" carried an unwarranted stigma. In its place, he suggested schools use the term "mild general learning disabilities" instead of "educable mentally retarded" (Dunn, 1973). He offered the following criteria:

> To be classified as having a mild general learning disability for purposes of receiving special education services, a pupil (1) must have reached the age of six years; (2) must score no higher than the second percentile for his ethnic subgroup based on local school district norms on both verbal and performance types of individual intelligence tests administered in his most facile language, yet not in the lower one-half of one percent; and (3) must be achieving in all basic school subjects, as measured by age norms on an individual, nationally standardized test of school attainment administered in the language of instruction, no higher than his capacity as determined by the average mental age expectancy score derived from his scores on both the verbal and performance types of nationally standardized intelligence tests administered in the language of instruction. (p. 128)

The most important part of Dunn's definition was clearly a social element. He proposed that, instead of national norms being used in the assessment of intelligence of minority children, local ethnic norms be used. Only from this data could minority children be judged as being mildly generally learning disabled.

Bijou's Natural Science Definition

While Mercer and Dunn were concerned about the social issues related to the concept of mental retardation, Bijou (1963), a behaviorist, expressed concern about the commonly perceived internality of the condition. To him terms like "mental" development, "intellectual processes" and "mental retardation" are merely inferences made about an individual based on observation of the person's behavior. The use of such assuming terms does nothing to add to the understanding of the condition and, in fact, may hinder it. Bijou (1963) explained that "defective intellect" or "mentality" is a hypothetical construct assumed to cause the behavioral phenomenon we refer to as mental retardation. In this sense it is an "intervening variable"; that is, it has no direct cause-effect relationship to the retarded behavior except what many assume to exist. Figure 1–2 depicts the relationship proposed by Bijou (1963) of stimulational, hypothetical, and behavioral variables typically occurring.

On the right side of the figure we see the behavioral variables; for example, retarded behavior. We all know that this exists because many children and adults demonstrate retarded *behavior*. Looking at the left side of the figure we see what Bijou refers to as the stimulational variables. These variables, faulty heredity, and/or deleterious environment, are in fact often documented as being the source of retarded behavior. If we were to disregard the hypothetical variables in the center of the figure (defective intellect or mentality), we could draw our arrows directly from the left side of the figure to the right side. We could, in other words, com-

FIGURE 1–2   The Relationships Among Stimulational, Hypothetical, and Behavioral Variables

S. W. Bijou, "Theory and research in mental [developmental] retardation," *The Psychological Record*, 1963, *13*, 95–110. Reprinted by permission.

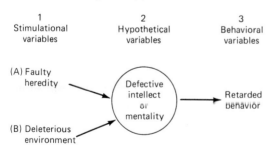

pletely account for the behavioral variables by looking only at the stimulational variables. In this way, all observable variables would be present and accounted for. What traditional concepts do, however, is say that the stimulational variables result in the hypothetical variables (i.e., "mental retardation") and then, use the hypothetical variables (which cannot be directly observed) to explain the behavioral variables. Bijou (1963) argued against such inferential reasoning. He wrote:

> A sequence of behavior is observed, measured, or described, then a verbal statement is made, giving the estimated level of intelligence that must be present to account for the observed behavior. *Nothing is gained.* An additional word or phrase is attached to a description of behavior. (p. 97, italics added)

Bijou implied that such a conceptualization results in much effort being spent trying to find the "true meaning" of intelligence or retardation, and that while the behavior is generally considered to be a "symptom," "more fundamental" aspects of the condition are assumed to exist within the individual. Instead of building theories about unobservable hypothetical variables and "extending the system of hypothetical terms," Bijou suggests a "natural science" approach to understanding retarded behavior. This approach would focus on various minute aspects of the stimulational variables such as the effects of "biological, physical, and social interactions past and current" (Bijou, 1963, p. 101). From a natural science perspective, Bijou (1963) wrote the following:

> It is suggested that retardation be conceptualized in observable, functionally defined relationships without appealing to hypothetical constructs. . .In other words, a retarded individual is one who has a limited repertoire of behavior evolving from interactions of the individual with environmental contacts which constitute his history. (pp. 100–101)

Kolstoe's Developmental/Neurophysiological Definition

In great contrast to Bijou, Kolstoe (1972) considered mental retardation to be an arrested state of cognitive development that is concomitantly rooted to inadequate neurophysiological development. Kolstoe's conceptualization was based on a combination of Jean Piaget's theory of qualitative changes in cognitive processes (c.f. Flavell, 1963; Ginsburg & Opper, 1969) and Hebb's (1949) theory of neurological organization. Kolstoe felt that mental ability and thus mental retardation could be explained by linking neurocellular activity to cognitive processes.

Kolstoe cited various studies, pointing out that the mentally retarded subjects of the studies had not been able to achieve Piaget's level of formal operations. He suggested that this might indicate an important generalization about the population. As such, he offered the following definition:

> . . .mental retardation can now be defined as a condition of intellectual arrest at some level below Piaget's level of formal thought. (p. 23)

Additionally, he wrote that:

> . . .mental retardation would appear from a neurophysiological viewpoint to be a "diminished efficiency of the central nervous system" which results in a limited capacity for the formation of cell assemblies, intercellular, and superordinate associations, and a consequent reduced ability for perceptual and conceptual integration. (p. 23)

In regard to IQ scores, Kolstoe did not completely disregard their utility for identifying mentally retarded individuals, but maintained that such a quantitative concept did not define mental retardation. Instead, he suggested that low IQ scores might serve as a warning that restricted, lesser developed mental abilities were present. Having secured a low IQ score, a more precise determination of mental retardation could be based on determining the Piagetian level of development attained. The major drawback to his definition as Kolstoe pointed out was that, for the higher levels of mental retardation, an ultimate determination of mental retardation could not be made until the person reached chronological maturity and still had not attained formal thought processes.

Public Concepts of Mental Retardation

As can be seen, professionals have offered different views of what they have considered mental retardation to be. They have had much opportunity to study the phenomenon and the significance of such criteria as measured intelligence and adaptive behavior. Most lay persons are not so knowledgeable. To them, mental retardation may present a vague image or an undesirable condition. The student of mental retardation must not only be aware of professional views but also of the public's view. Such information will be useful when one attempts to bridge the gap between professional knowledge and public understanding.

One of the most extensive studies of public knowledge about mental retardation was conducted by Gottwald (1970). In this study, a national sample of 1,515 people were asked, among other things, what the phrase "mentally retarded" meant to them. A variety of responses resulted. While many of the respondents (45%) said that mental retardation meant some degree of mental deficiency existed (e.g. mentally retarded people had below normal levels of intelligence), some (14%) said it was a result of birth injuries, defects, or brain damage. Eighteen percent of the people equated mental retardation with being a slow learner or not having the ability to learn. Almost 14% said that such people were mentally ill or in some way sick, and about 1% said that mentally retarded persons lacked judgment, maturity, and/or responsibility. A little over 8% of the people said that the mentally retarded person was unable to support himself while about 6.5% said that they needed care, help, and treatment. In another study reported by Gottlieb and Corman (1975), 86.3% of the 336 people who answered the questions described the mentally retarded child as a slow learner. In this same group, only 13.4% said that mentally retarded children exhibited some deficits in adaptive behavior.

In yet another study on this topic, Budoff, Siperstein, and Conant (1979) asked 1,142 grade school children, junior high schoolers, and high school adolescents what they knew (or thought they knew) about mentally retarded people. The most common response was that mentally retarded people were slow thinkers. Other commonly cited characteristics included abnormal physical appearance and brain impairment. Only a few of the students mentioned anything at all about deficits in adaptive behavior. Budoff et al. concluded that none of the students had much information about mental retardation as professionals perceive it to be.

These studies reveal that most people think of mental retardation in very stereotypical terms—slow learners, physically deformed, injured before or during birth, sick, and so on. They do not have a clearly defined concept of mental retardation. Probably most of their ideas have been drawn from personal experience, myths, or misunderstandings. While this is understandable, it may also lead to undesirable public opinion or biases.

STATES' CRITERIA FOR CLASSIFICATION AS MENTALLY RETARDED

In the different states, each state department of education is usually charged with providing a definition of mental retardation to be used as a guideline by its various school districts. To what degree do the different states use the AAMD definition? What additional or different criteria are used? Huberty, Koller, and Ten Brink (1980) attempted to answer such questions by surveying the different state departments of education.

Questionnaires were sent to all fifty state departments of education and to the District of Columbia. From the fifty-one requests, forty-one responses were received. Of these forty-one, eight used the AAMD definition and six used the definition with only some slight modifications. Another twenty-seven of the states used their own definitions, all twenty-seven being different. With the exception of Alaska, all states included the "concept of deficient intellectual ability" as a prime characteristic of mental retardation (Huberty et al., 1980, p. 257). Table 1–1 summarizes the findings of the study.

As can be seen, fifteen of the states did not specify a particular IQ cut-off score, thirteen stated cut-offs in terms of standard deviations, thirteen used IQs of 80 or less. Although twenty-six of the states replying referred to adaptive behavior in their definition, only eight of the states indicated the adaptive behavior criteria and/or the measure to be used in assessing adaptive behavior.

From this study by Huberty et al., we can see that while the concept of adaptive behavior may be advocated by the AAMD (Heber, 1959, 1961; Grossman, 1973, 1977, 1983); in actuality, the IQ score has dominated the operational definition of mental retardation in state educational systems.

TABLE 1–1   Summary of States' Guidelines Concerning IQ and Adaptive Behavior in the Mentally Retarded

STATE	DATE OF GUIDELINES	TYPE OF DEFINITION	INTELLIGENCE CRITERIA	INCLUDE ADAPTIVE BEHAVIOR IN DEFINITION	ADAPTIVE BEHAVIOR CRITERIA INDICATED	ADAPTIVE BEHAVIOR MEASURES INDICATED
Alabama	1973	Other	30-80-IQ	No	No	No
Alaska	1975	Other	Not specified	Yes	No	No
Arizona	1977	Other	Not specified	No	No	No
Arkansas	1977	Other	≤ − 2.0 S.D.	Yes	No	Yes
Colorado	1976	Similar	≤ − 1.75 S.D.	Yes	No	No
Connecticut	1976	Other	Not specified	No	No	No
Delaware	1974	Other	Not specified	No	No	No
District of Columbia	Not specified	AAMD & BEH	≤ − 2.0 S.D.	Yes	No	No
Florida	1976	AAMD	≤ − 2.0 S.D.	Yes	Yes	Yes
Georgia	1975	Similar	≤ − 2.0 S.D.	Yes	No	No
Hawaii	1966	Other	Not specified	No	No	No
Idaho	1975	Similar	≤75 IQ	Yes	No	No
Illinois	1976	Other	Not specified	Yes	No	No
Indiana	1973	Other	≤75 IQ	No	No	No
Iowa	1974	Other	≤1.0 S.D.	Yes	No	No
Kansas	1976	Other	Not specified	Yes	No	No
Kentucky	1975	Other	Not specified	No	No	No
Maine	Draft	Other	Not specified	No	No	No
Michigan	1973	Other	Not specified	Yes	No	Yes
Missouri	1976	AAMD	≤ − 2.0 S.D.	Yes	No	No
Montana	Not specified	Similar	≤75 IQ ≤ − 1.6 S.D.	Yes	No	No
Nebraska	1975	Other	Not specified	Yes	No	No
Nevada	1976	Other	≤75 IQ	No	No	No

TABLE 1–1 *Continued*

STATE	DATE OF GUIDE- LINES	TYPE OF DEFINI- TION	INTELLIGENCE CRITERIA	INCLUDE ADAPTIVE BEHAVIOR IN DEFINITION	ADAPTIVE BEHAVIOR CRITERIA INDICATED	ADAPTIVE BEHAVIOR MEASURES INDICATED
New Hampshire	1976	Other	Not specified	No	No	No
New Jersey	1976	Other	≤ − 1.5 S.D.	Yes	No	No
New York	1975	Other	≤ − 1.5 S.D.	No	No	No
North Dakota	1976	Other	≤75 IQ	No	No	No
Ohio	1973	Other	≤80 IQ	No	No	No
Oklahoma	1976	Other	≤75 IQ	No	No	No
Oregon	1976	AAMD	≤ − 2.0 S.D.	Yes	No	Yes
Pennsylvania	1976	Similar	≤80 IQ	Yes	No	No
Rhode Island	1963	Other	Not specified	Yes	No	No
South Carolina	1972	Other	≤70 IQ	Yes	No	Yes
South Dakota	1974	Similar	Not specified	Yes	No	No
Tennessee	1976-77	Other	Not specified	Yes	No	No
Utah	1975	AAMD	≤75 IQ	Yes	No	Yes
Virginia	1972	Other	≤ − 2.0 S.D.	No	No	No
Washington	1976	Other	≤75 IQ	Yes	Yes	No
West Virginia	1974	AAMD	≤75 IQ	Yes	No	Yes
Wisconsin	Not specified	AAMD	≤ − 2.0 S.D.	Yes	No	No
Wyoming	1975	AAMD	≤ − 2.0 S.D.	Yes	No	No

Key to abbreviations:
AAMD = American Association on Mental Deficiency
BEH = Bureau of Education for the Handicapped
Other = definition other than AAMD & BEH
S.D. = standard deviation(s)
Similar = similar to AAMD definition, with only minor variations
≤ = less than or equal to

SOME FINAL THOUGHTS: RETARDED PERSONS' VIEWS OF MENTAL RETARDATION

What does it mean to a mentally retarded person to be mentally retarded? Some insights into this issue have been provided by Edgerton (1967), Edgerton and Bercovici (1976), Bogdan and Taylor (1976), and Bogdan (1980), among others. These researchers sought to answer this question by talking to mentally retarded, formerly institutionalized persons. Their basic finding was this: Mentally retarded people do not want to be mentally retarded or considered mentally retarded. They want to be normal; they want to work; and they want to have friends. In other words, they want to be like others.

Edgerton (1967 and in a follow-up in 1976 with Bercovici) reported on the lives of forty-nine ex-residents of a state institution. He reported many interesting findings. But the most important was that the mentally retarded persons generally attempted to deny their former status and project themselves as "normal" people. Bogdan and Taylor (1976) reported an interview they had with a man named Ed Murphy. At the time, the man was twenty-six years old. He had been out of the state institution for about three years. Some of his remarks warrant our attention:

> It's funny. You hear so many people talking about IQ. The first time I ever heard the expression was when I was at Empire State School. I didn't know what it was or anything, but some people were talking and they brought the subject up. It was on the ward, and I went and asked one of the staff what mine was. They told me 49. Forty-nine isn't 50, but I was pretty happy about it. I mean I figured that it wasn't a low grade. I really didn't know what it meant but it sounded pretty high. Hell, I was born in 1948 and 49 didn't seem too bad. Forty-nine didn't sound hopeless. I didn't know anything about the highs and the lows, but I knew I was better than most of them. What is retardation? It's hard to say. I guess it's having problems thinking. Some people think that you can tell if a person is retarded by looking at them. If you think that way, you don't give people the benefit of the doubt. You judge a person by how they look or how they talk or what the tests show, but you can never really tell what is inside the person. (pp. 50–51)

Certainly there is much merit to what this person thought. While the field may continue trying to reach agreement on what mental retardation is, we must not forget what mentally retarded people are. The above statement by Ed Murphy should be kept in mind. It may help us understand as much as do more formal definitions and concepts.

CONCLUSION

Determining the criteria for mental retardation is an important task. The role of a definition is to clearly present these criteria. At this time, the AAMD offers the most widely used definition. It includes the requirement that a person have both a reduced level of mental functioning as well as a deficit in adaptive behavior.

Ironically, the two criteria have undergone historical reversals in regard to their significance. Originally, before the development of intelligence tests, adaptive or social behavior deficits most clearly delineated the retarded from the nonretarded. When psychometric tests emerged, a more objective, quantifiable method of identifying retardation and its different degrees (including mild and borderline) became possible. The test scores also became seen as "true" measures of intelligence which in turn was generally perceived as a unitary concept.

In the past twenty years, the significance of adaptive behavior has resurfaced. It has gained particular importance as a criterion because of the role it plays in the designation or non-designation of some low socio-economic status minority individuals as being mentally retarded. Thus the definition of mental retardation has become not only a psychological/educational issue but a social/political issue. Much of the activity of defining mental retardation, regardless of the position one takes, will revolve around this issue for many years to come.

STUDY QUESTIONS

1. What variables have been considered in defining mental retardation? Which are predominantly used today?
2. What personal or social philosophies have influenced the definers of mental retardation?
3. How is the term "significantly subaverage general intellectual functioning" operationally defined by the AAMD?
4. Why is "adaptive behavior" difficult to define and measure? Who are its major proponents as part of the definition of mental retardation? Who opposed it?
5. What influenced the development of intelligence tests? What is their primary purpose?
6. In what major way did the 1959/1961 AAMD definition of mental retardation differ from the current AAMD definition?
7. Discuss the various criticisms of the AAMD definitions related to the use of intelligence tests and the IQ criteria.
8. What values influenced Mercer and Dunn in their conceptualization of who is retarded and who is not?
9. Contrast Bijou's concepts of mental retardation with Kolstoe's.
10. What is the general state of the public's understanding of mental retardation?

2

Classification and Prevalence

PART I: CLASSIFICATION

I.   The purpose of classification
II. Classification according to IQ level
    A.   The mildly retarded
    B.   The moderately retarded
    C.   The severely and profoundly retarded
III. Medical classification
IV. Some concluding remarks on classification

PART II: PREVALENCE

I.   The purpose of determining prevalence
II.   Defining prevalence
III. Problems in determining prevalence
IV.   Statistical expectations of prevalence
V.   Actual prevalence: 1% or 3%
VI.   Prevalence in the public schools
VII. Prevalence according to severity level
VIII. Variations in prevalence
    A.   Type of community
    B.   Age range
    C.   Gender
    D.   Socioeconomic and ethnic status
IX.   Some concluding remarks on prevalence
X.   Study questions

THE PURPOSE OF CLASSIFICATION

It would be difficult to find a group of people, animals, plants, objects, or nearly anything else that isn't subject to at least one type of classification. Basically, when we classify something we place it in a group with other "items" so that in some particular way it has something in common with others in the same class or group. Chapter 1 discussed a very general classification system: differentiation of the mentally retarded and the nonretarded. In this chapter we will discuss different classes of mentally retarded people.

CLASSIFICATION ACCORDING TO IQ LEVEL

The most common classification system used with the mentally retarded is classification by level of IQ. Traditionally special educators and psychologists have classified mentally retarded persons into three or four groups according to where they fell within a range of IQs. One system, often referred to as the *special education system,* allows mentally retarded persons to be classified as *educable* mentally retarded (EMR), *trainable* mentally retarded (TMR) or *profoundly* mentally retarded (PMR). The ranges of IQs for each of these three groups are about 50 to 70 (or 75) for the EMR group, 25 to 50 for the TMR group, and below 25 for the PMR group. (You should note that often the term "handicapped" is substituted for "retarded," thus rendering EMH, TMH, and PMH groups.)

Originally the terms preceding the words "mentally retarded" were used to describe the educational prognosis of the individual. To some degree the educable child was assumed to be capable of learning some traditional academic subjects such as reading, writing, and arithmetic. The trainable child was not supposed to be capable of such activity but could be taught daily living skills such as self-feeding, using the toilet, and dressing. The profoundly retarded (who has also been referred to as the "custodial" retarded) was assumed to have very little potential and capable of not learning very much at all.

The American Association on Mental Deficiency provided another classification by IQ system (Heber, 1959, 1961; Grossman, 1973, 1977, 1983). In its latest manual on the classification of mentally retarded persons (Grossman, 1983), the Association outlined the following IQ ranges for its classification system:

Mild mental retardation:	50–55 to approximately 70
Moderate mental retardation:	35–40 to 50–55

Severe mental retardation: 20–25 to 35–40
Profound mental retardation: Below 20–25

It can be noted that specific upper and lower IQ scores have been avoided in favor of bands of scores for each level of retardation. The AAMD suggested that when an individual fell between two levels, the actual classification of that person should be based more on clinical judgment and less on the specific score. This judgment would have to be made in light of all available information, particularly that relating to the degree of adaptive behavior demonstrated. Prior to the 1973 definition (Grossman), the AAMD classification system (Heber, 1961) included the borderline mentally retarded group whose IQs fell between about 70 and 85 points.

Over the years, a variety of classification systems based on IQ have been developed (Gelof, 1963). For our purposes, however, the special educators' system and AAMD system and their respective levels of retardation will be used most often throughout this text.

Each level of retardation has certain characteristics that are common among many of its members. Additionally, each level seems to be affected by certain issues or problems. The particular levels, their members, and their unique aspects are discussed below.

The Mildly Retarded

This group of individuals includes those functioning between about 50 to 55 and 70 IQ points or sometimes higher. Generally they are capable of daily self-care and academic skills up to about the fourth or fifth grade level. They can develop acceptable social skills and, as adults, often participate in competitive, nonsheltered employment. Their most obvious manifestation of retardation appears during their school years when they fall behind their chronological-age peers in traditional school subjects. This discrepancy increases with increasing age. It is their academic limitations that most often cause them to be classified as mentally retarded. Most have no recognizable physical etiology and are referred to as "cultural-familial" mentally retarded or retarded due to psychosocial disadvantage. A smaller portion of the mildly retarded (10% to 20%) have identifiable organic pathologies and may "appear" to be retarded.

The inclusion of many minority individuals within the classification of mild, cultural-familial mental retardation has been questioned since the late 1960s and early 1970s by the courts, through legislation, and by a number of professionals (e.g., Dunn, 1968; Mercer, 1973). These challenges questioned the appropriateness of identifying and placing many minority students in EMR classes for several reasons. These included:

The intelligence tests used for placement and procedures for their administration were thought to be discriminatory.

Due process procedures, guaranteed by the U.S. Constitution, were not followed in the placement.

The placement was thought to be a form of racial segregation.

Parents were not involved in the placement process.

The special classes were not thought to be beneficial to many of the students.

Subsequent federal legislation, PL 94–142, passed in 1975, was intended to remediate these problems. This legislation, along with various court rulings, has modified the composite of the mild classification. MacMillan, Meyers, and Morrison (1980) clearly indicated this change when they suggested that "sociopolitical and legal forces" have changed the EMR population over the last twenty years. They detailed five stages of changes in this group:

1. Pre–World War II "special training classes" enrolled well-behaved slow-learning students with IQs into the 80's who fit into the mildly retarded and borderline categories. These classes were not necessarily designed to serve a clinically defined deficit group.
2. Post World War II saw the development of special classes and programs promoted by the National Association of Retarded Children and associated state organizations. The term *mentally retarded* was increasingly accepted for the slow learner.
3. The Kennedy administration ushered in an era where services were expanded to "all who needed them." Available funding invited schools to fill classes. A continuity of mildly retarded children with more seriously impaired children was achieved through common labeling. The EMR classification during this era (1959–1968) included children with IQs into the mid-80 range.
4. Civil rights concerns over labeling ethnic minority children as EMR (from approximately 1969 to 1973) resulted in a great reduction in the total number of children labeled for EMR services. In California, and elsewhere, the more able EMR students were decertified. Only children with IQs below 70 were candidates for EMR placement.
5. Since 1975 and the implementation of PL 94–142, the labeling of only clear-cut cases as EMR, and then only after meeting extensive procedural safeguards, seems to have reduced drastically the number of children labeled EMR (p. 112)

The net effect of this is that the group of individuals classified as EMR by the schools has varied over time. It is safe to assume that variations in EMR grouping still occur from school to school, district to district, and state to state. The outcome is that there is no "solid" group of

EMR individuals. Generally, however, we may expect fewer minority students to be placed within this classification.

As an alternative to classifying children as mildly retarded, some have suggested the more generic (and perhaps less offensive) term "mildly handicapped" be used. This group would include not only the mildly retarded but also those with other academic problems such as learning disabled and emotionally disturbed students. Proponents of this approach feel that little differences exist between the different categories in terms of academic needs and thus grouping them together would be educationally sound (Blackhurst, 1977; Neisworth & Greer, 1975; Schwartz & Oseroff, 1975; Smith & Neisworth, 1975). This noncategorical position contains merit particularly for young, elementary school age children. As the children grow toward adulthood, however, the general cognitive deficits of the mildly retarded may clearly distinguish them from their nonretarded peers. This would have implications for curriculum and other facets of educational programming. Koegel and Edgerton (1982) have recently noted the difficulties faced as adults by many minority individuals formerly classified as educable retarded. Their work suggests that special and unique needs continue to exist for these persons even beyond the school years.

The Moderately Retarded

Moderately retarded individuals score between about 35–40 and 50–55 IQ points on an intelligence test. They can usually develop communication skills, fairly good motor coordination, self-help skills, generally acceptable social skills, and basic vocational skills. Their academic abilities are somewhat limited, but with intense training they can achieve first or second grade level reading, writing, and arithmetic skills. Most academic learning for this group will focus on functional needs.

Many moderately retarded persons (as well as those who are severely or profoundly retarded) will have physiological etiologies as a source of their retardation. Unlike most of the mildly retarded, moderately retarded persons can usually be identified even by an untrained individual who observes their physical appearance and behavior. Most noticeable will be their speech, language, and social interactions. The moderately retarded are perhaps the most visible mentally retarded persons to the public.

Moderately, severely, and profoundly retarded persons are rather a "solid" population in terms of their acceptance as retarded. In other words, a person with an IQ below about 50 or 55 will generally not be the subject of social debate about the appropriateness of their categorization as mentally retarded.

The Severely and Profoundly Retarded

Individuals classified as severely and profoundly retarded have been the focus of much attention in the last several years. Severely retarded persons fall in the lower end of the trainable retarded group with IQs between 20–25 and 35–40. The profoundly retarded comprise the lowest group having IQs below 20–25 points. Until PL 94–142 required it, they were often not provided with public school education.

Many individuals considered severely retarded are able to acquire some functional daily living skills. Generally, however, in contrast to the moderately retarded, the severely retarded will probably not become even semi-independent insofar as living abilities. In other words, if they attain placement in group living homes, much support will still be required.

The abilities of profoundly retarded individuals may vary a great deal. Some people with measured IQs of 17 to 19 will seem to be eons above others from whom it is not possible to obtain a reliable IQ score. Some profoundly retarded people can learn to walk, communicate in a functional manner, and tend to their own bodily needs. In such a case there is little difference between a severely retarded person and a profoundly retarded person except for a few IQ points. Other profoundly retarded people are nonambulatory, multiply handicapped, and/or have little apparent awareness of their environment.

Switzky, Haywood and Rotatori (1982) pointed out some important differences between the severely retarded and the profoundly retarded. Most notable is the degree of severity of their conditions. For example, while the severely retarded may attain a mental age (MA) of about three to five years, the profoundly retarded person's MA will not exceed three years. Furthermore, the profoundly retarded will have a higher incidence of motor, sensory, and physical handicaps and will be more prone to an earlier death. Cleland (1979) reported that the profoundly retarded, when compared to the severely retarded, more often had delayed puberty, active seizures, enuresis, abnormal electroencephalograms, lack of socialization skills, and several other debilitating conditions.

Miller (1976, as cited by Switzky et al., 1982) suggested that the profoundly retarded could be divided into two groups: the "relative" profoundly retarded and the "absolute" profoundly retarded. The first group consisted of older, less impaired persons who generally had some ambulatory, communication, and self-help abilities. The "absolute" profoundly retarded included persons lacking all adaptive behaviors and who had extremely delicate medical conditions.

When we combine the severely and profoundly retarded, as is often done in textbooks and articles, we are making reference to individuals with a wide range of abilities, a very heterogeneous group. Such references to the "severely and profoundly" retarded should be made carefully and full descriptions of the type of individual we are discussing should be made clear (Robinson, 1980; Taylor, 1980).

In recent years, the generic term "severely handicapped" has emerged to encompass the severely retarded, the profoundly retarded, and other persons with seriously impeding disabilities. Several definitions of "severely handicapped" have been suggested (Abt Associates, 1974; Justen, 1976; U.S. Department of Health, Education & Welfare, 1975; Sontag, Smith & Sailor, 1977; Baker, 1979; Sailor & Haring, 1977). Most of the definitions tend to avoid tying the severely handicapped to a particular, more traditional disability such as mental retardation. Instead, the definitions consider the functional behavior of the individual. Sometimes associated behaviors are also included such as self-mutilation and stereotyped behavior.

At times there has not been a clear understanding about the distinction between the severely handicapped and the severely or profoundly retarded. Consider the definition offered by Baker (1979) for the severely handicapped:

> The severely handicapped individual is one whose ability to provide for his or her own basic life-sustaining and safety needs is so limited, relative to the proficiency expected on the basis of chronological age, that it could pose a serious threat to his or her survival (p. 60).

If we accept this definition, we may conclude that the severely mentally retarded, the profoundly mentally retarded, and perhaps a portion of the moderately retarded, as well as others, could be included under the rubric of "severely handicapped." However, we should not make the mistake of saying that the severely handicapped is a group synonymous with the severely (and/or profoundly) retarded. The severely handicapped, as a group, may be comprised of various disability categories; for example, deaf, blind, and autistic.

MEDICAL CLASSIFICATION

Classification according to medical condition is primarily of interest to physicians and those involved in research on the effects of physiological factors resulting in mental retardation. Some of the earliest systems used to classify retarded persons were based on etiological diagnoses or physical characteristics (Scheerenberger, 1983). By the beginning of the twentieth century, D. M. Bourneville's pathological forms of mental retardation were widely used in both Europe and the United States. The eight major categories included:

1. Hycrocephalic idiocy
2. Microcephalic idiocy
3. Idiocy from arrested development of the convolutions
4. Idiocy from congenital malformation of the brain
5. Idiocy from hypertrophied or tuberous sclerosis
6. Idiocy from atrophied sclerosis
   a. Sclerosis of one hemisphere, or of two hemispheres
   b. Sclerosis of one lobe of the brain
   c. Sclerosis of isolated convolutions
   d. Mortified sclerosis of the brain
7. Idiocy from meningitis or from chronic meningo-encephalitis
8. Idiocy from pachydermical cachexia or myxoedamatous idiocy combined with absence of the thyroid gland. (Scheerenberger, 1983, p. 66)

A more contemporary medical classification system is used today by the AAMD. Grossman (1983) presented ten medical classes which may be associated with, or be the cause of, a person's retarded development. The classes were written to generally correspond with classes presented in the *International classification of diseases* (World Health Organization, 1978) and the *Diagnostic and statistical manual of mental disorders* (American Psychiatric Association, 1980). The classes include mental retardation due to:

Infection and intoxications
Trauma or physical agent
Metabolism or nutrition disorders
Gross brain disease (postnatal)
Unknown prenatal influence
Chromosomal anomalies
Other conditions originating in the perinatal period
Following psychiatric disorder
Environmental influences
Other conditions

A more general etiological classification system has been described by various writers over the years using different terminology. Basically, this system divides mentally retarded persons into two groups: those who are mentally retarded because of some *pathological* cause; for example, who have their normal development insulted prenatally, perinatally, or postnatally; and those who, although their development is normal, simply do not attain average mental development. The source of their retarded development is *nonpathological*.

The former group has certain characteristics in common. First of all, the cause of their retardation is physiological and can often be identified through medical diagnoses. Second, most of these individuals will fall into the moderate, severe, or profound range of retardation, although some may be mildly retarded. Third, they often "look" retarded; that is, they tend to fit the popular image of mental retardation. Fourth, they tend to have various concomitant physical disabilities. Individuals comprising this group have been referred to as having *pathological, extrinsic, physiological, exogenous,* or *organic* mental retardation.

The second group includes individuals for whom there is no readily identifiable source of their retardation. These individuals are referred to as being *non-pathological, intrinsic, subcultural, garden-variety, endogenous, psychosocially, cultural-familial,* or *familial* mentally retarded persons. Generally, they fall into the mild class of mental retardation. While there is no physiological identifiable cause of this group's retarded mental development, different people have speculated that it is either a result of their polygenetically inherited ability, the influence of their environment, or an interaction of the two.

SOME CONCLUDING REMARKS ON CLASSIFICATION

The classification by IQ systems (mild, moderate, severe, or profound; educable, trainable, or profound) serves four basic functions. First, it provides a communication system among professionals. Generally speaking, two people talking about "moderate retardation" would have some idea of the level of people each was talking about. Second, the system is of use in research since it allows the researcher to make statements about a relatively specific group and allows the consumer of research to make inferences about research for a specific group.

The third function of the classification system is that it serves an administrative purpose. Students are classified and placed in certain groups so that they can be taught and so they can generate funds to pay for the teaching and related services. The fourth function of the system allows special appeals to be made to certain organizations or agencies on behalf of specific groups of children. For example, legislative bodies or charitable organizations might be more likely to provide funds for the severely or profoundly retarded than for the mildly or moderately retarded.

Given these important functions, the classification by IQ system seems viable. However, it is important to look at the weaknesses of the system. The greatest weakness is that the system has limited educational utility. We cannot and should not develop individual educational plans based on a person's level of classification. Hobbs (1975) points out that we grossly oversimplify the situation when we place children into such classes or categories. He suggests two major changes in classification systems. The first is that profiles be developed for each student which fully describes his or her status within individual ecological systems. As opposed to saying a child is "educable" and placing him into a class for the rest of his school career, the profile would be developed, would dictate the child's needs, and would be subject to continued evaluation and analysis. Hobbs suggests that the computer age we live in makes this possible.

The second suggestion by Hobbs is that we develop a system of funding based on *services needed* by students rather than on a particular classification that child may fall into. Such an approach would allow a more specific expenditure of funds and would not require the constraints of traditional categorical placement.

Some of the functions of the current classification system will continue; for example, general communication. Others may be improved, such as those related to education and funding. Historically, terminology related to the mentally retarded has changed but the general system has remained. It probably will for quite a while. The basis of what Hobbs has suggested may emerge although it probably will take some time for it to be perfected. The development of individual educational plans as required by PL 94–142 is a step in this direction.

PART II: PREVALENCE

THE PURPOSE OF DETERMINING PREVALENCE

The most important reason for determining the prevalence of mental retardation is to know how many such people will be in need of special services. How many should we plan to serve in the public schools? How many before and after the school years? How many at each level of retardation? We may also need to determine if any major fluctuations in the population are occurring across settings. Are there more or less mentally retarded persons in one state than another? In one town than another? In one school district than another? In order to answer these and similar questions, we study prevalence.

DEFINING PREVALENCE

For our purpose, prevalence of mental retardation means the number of mentally retarded persons existing at a given point in time. Sometimes the term "prevalence" is confused or used synonymously with "incidence." To do so in the study of mental retardation would be a mistake.

According to Marozas, May, and Lehman (1980) *incidence* refers to the number of *new* cases emerging over a period of time, whereas *prevalence* is the *current* number of cases at a given time. Tarjan, Wright, Eyman, and Keeran (1973) point out that the incidence of mental retardation will always be higher than the prevalence because the concept of mental retardation allows some individuals, particularly at the mild level, to be considered mentally retarded at one point in life (e.g, the school years) but not at another (e.g., as adults).

Our primary concern is with prevalence since this figure will determine degree of need.

PROBLEMS IN DETERMINING PREVALENCE

Problems in determining the prevalence of mental retardation result from variations in the definition and criteria used to determine who is considered to be mentally retarded (Farber, 1968; Luckey & Neman, 1976). If we consider the lower levels of mental retardation (moderate, severe, and profound), the determination can generally be straightforward. There is little doubt at the sub-50 IQ level as to whom should be included. On the other hand, when we attempt to count the mildly retarded, there is considerable debate over whom we should include. Since there are different concepts of mental retardation, we can expect different numbers of people to be counted. Another problem in determining prevalence is that various methods have been used to count or estimate the number of retarded persons, and some variation in the findings might be attributable to these different procedures.

When we consider these two problems together, it can be seen how difficult it is to get a "true" picture of prevalence. As an indication of this, Heber (1970) summarized twenty-eight prevalence studies and found that reported levels of mental retardation ranged from .16% to 23% of the various populations.

STATISTICAL EXPECTATIONS OF PREVALENCE

Given a population of individuals with various levels of intelligence (IQs), normal distribution theory predicts the relationship of different numbers of people to the mean of the distribution curve. Examine Figure 2–1. This curve represents a theoretically expected normal distribution. The height of the curve represents the number of people. Along the bottom is the mean which is right in the center. Going out from the mean in either direction are the standard deviations. As we get further and further away from the mean, moving either way, there are fewer and fewer people. As Figure 2–1 indicates between + 1 and − 1 standard deviations, we will have a total of 68.26% of the population. If the IQ test we were using had a mean of 100 and a standard deviation of 16 points, then 68.26% of the population would be expected to score between 84 and 116 IQ points. If we go out to a + 2 and − 2 standard deviation, 95.44% of the population could be expected to score within this range. That would leave 4.56% of the population to score either above + 2 standard deviations (132 +) or below − 2 standard deviations. If we split this figure in half (4.56 ÷ 2), we could estimate that about 2.28% of the population would score below − 2 S.D. from the mean. Thus, based on a normal distribution of IQs with a mean of 100 and a standard deviation of 16, we would expect about 2.28% of the population to be mentally retarded if we only considered the measured intelligence criterion and did not include the adaptive behavior criterion. Actually, a commonly presented prevalence figure for mental retardation is about 3% of the population.

Dingman and Tarjan (1960) challenged the normal distribution theory by pointing out that actually there were more mentally retarded individuals at the sub-50 IQ level than would be expected according to the normal distribution curve. This, they said, was because of the many cases of mental retardation due to pathological conditions. These conditions are not accounted for by normal distribution theory. Figure 2–2 was proposed by Dingman and Tarjan. In this figure, toward the left side of the curve, another superimposed curve is presented. Dingman and Tarjan suggested that this smaller curve represented a distribution of mentally retarded persons with pathological etiologies. This group violates the as-

FIGURE 2–1   Normal Distribution of the Population

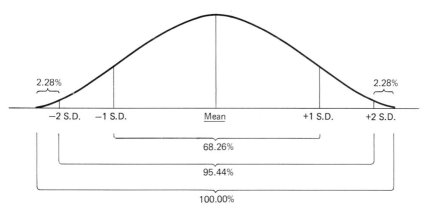

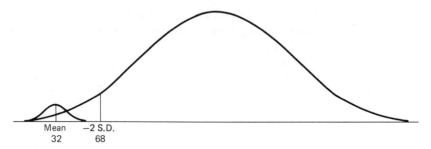

Mean   −2 S.D.
32   68

FIGURE 2–2   Adjusted Distribution Accounting for Pathological Etiologies of Mental Retardation

Adapted from H. Dingman, and G. Tarjan, "Mental retardation and the normal distribution curve," *American Journal of Mental Deficiency*, 1960, *64*, 991–994. Reprinted by permission.

sumptions of normal distribution theory and inflates the number of mentally retarded persons.

ACTUAL PREVALENCE: 1% OR 3%

Traditionally, 3% has been the prevalence figure that was most often quoted. In other words, it was estimated that three out of every one hundred people would be mentally retarded. This was based on a number of early studies (see Farber, 1968, for a review) that suggested this prevalence figure. Generally these studies used some IQ cutoff (e.g., 70–75) score as a criterion for determining whether or not people were mentally retarded and did not consider adaptive behavior performance.

With the adoption of adaptive behavior as an additional criteria, some have suggested that a 3% figure is unrealistic and that if we take adaptive behavior into consideration, the actual prevalence of mental retardation is closer to 1% of the population (Baroff, 1982; Tarjan, Wright, Eyman & Keeran, 1973; Mercer, 1973).

Tarjan et al. (1973) explained that the 3% figure may be appropriate for considering the total number of people who will probably *ever* be considered mentally retarded during their lives. This does not, however, mean that at any one time 3% will be mentally retarded. This figure, they said, will be closer to 1%. This may seem a little strange, but it is quite possible under the "here and now" concept proposed by the AAMD definition (Grossman, 1983).

Tarjan et al. (1973) said that in order to accept the 3% prevalence figure, four conditions would have to exist: "(a) the diagnosis of mental retardation is always based on an IQ below 70; (b) mental retardation is identified in infancy; (c) the diagnosis does not change; and (d) the mortality of individuals is similar to that of the general population." In reality, none of these conditions are met. Table 2–1 presents the distribution of mental retardation under the 3% and 1% prevalence figures based on a theoretical city of 100,000 people. Tarjan et al. pointed out that Mercer's (1973) study in Riverside, California, tended to confirm their numbers.

As can be seen in Table 2–1, the big differences under the 1% model and the 3% model occurs at the 50+ IQ level (mild) before and after the school years. The 1% figure shows a drastically reduced number of mildly retarded persons both before and after formal schooling. This accounts for the major difference between the two sets of numbers.

It is reasonably safe to assume that the overall prevalence of mental retardation is no more than 1%. Based on a 1982 population of approximately 230 million in the United States (The World Almanac and Book of Facts, 1983), this would mean that there were about 2,300,000 mentally retarded people in the country at that time. Increases in the population would result in a proportional increase in the number of persons identified as mentally retarded at a given time.

PREVALENCE IN THE PUBLIC SCHOOLS

The prevalence of mental retardation in the schools is higher than in the general population. Mentally retarded children in the public schools com-

TABLE 2–1 Estimated Prevalence of Mental Retardation in a Prototype Community of 100,000

	IQ	AGES				
		0–5	6–19	20–24	25+	TOTAL
Prevalence = 3%	0–19	12	24	8	56	100
	20–49	48	96	32	224	400
	50+	300	600	200	1400	2500
	Total	360	720	240	1690	3000
Prevalence = 1%	0–19	8	18	4	20	50
	20–49	36	70	20	74	200
	50+	25	600	25	100	750
	Total	69	688	49	194	1000

From G. Tarjan, S. Wright, R. Eyman, and C. Keeran, "Natural history of mental retardation: some aspects of epidemiology," *American Journal of Mental Deficiency*, 1973, 77, 369–379. Reprinted by permission.

prise about 25% of all exceptional children in the schools. During the 1977–78 school year, 3.8 million exceptional students were being served. Of these, 944,909 were classified as mentally retarded (U.S. Department of Health, Education and Welfare 1979). This number represented 1.84% of the total school population. In the following year the percentage decreased to 1.63% (Patrick & Reschly, 1982).

Because all levels of retardation are identified during the school years, including the mildly retarded, it should be expected that some increase in the 1% prevalence figure would occur. Additionally, most school systems, while they include adaptive behavior in their definition of mental retardation, tend to rely more on IQ score to identify their retarded students (Huberty, Koller & Ten Brink, 1980; Patrick & Reschly, 1982). Based on a psychometric criterion, then, we might expect schools to have prevalence figures closer to 3% than 1%. The fact is, however, that many states are restricting the identification of educable mentally retarded children. This in turn has reduced the overall prevalence of identified retarded school-age students to the 1.63% (or lower) figure stated above. This prevalence varies greatly from state to state as can be seen in Table 2–2.

TABLE 2–2   Percent of School-aged Children Classified as Mentally Retarded in Different States During 1978–79

0–1%	1%–1.5%	1.5%–2%	2%–2.5%	2.5%–3%	>3%
Alaska	Arizona	Florida	Missouri	Georgia	Alabama
California	Connecticut	Idaho	Nebraska	Kentucky	Arkansas
Colorado	Delaware	Illinois	Ohio	Mississippi	N. Carolina
D. C.	Maryland	Indiana	Oklahoma	Tennessee	S. Carolina
Hawaii	Michigan	Iowa		W. Virginia	
Nevada	Montana	Kansas			
New	New Jersey	Louisiana			
Hamphire	New	Maine			
Oregon	Mexico	Massachusetts			
Rhode Island	New York	Minnesota			
S. Dakota	N. Dakota	Pennsylvania			
Texas	Washington	Virginia			
Utah	Wisconsin				
Vermont					
Wyoming					

From J. L. Patrick and D. J. Reschly, "Relationship of state educational criteria and demographic variables to school-system prevalence of mental retardation," *American Journal of Mental Deficiency*, 1982, 86, 351–360. Reprinted by permission.

PREVALENCE ACCORDING TO SEVERITY LEVEL

Although the prevalence of mild retardation may be shifting downward, the prevalence of moderate, severe, and profound mental retardation remains more or less stable. Even though genetic counseling, prenatal identification, and therapeutic abortion may reduce some instances of more critical forms of mental retardation, it will probably be several years before these procedures will make a noticeable impact on the overall prevalence of mental retardation.

A large number of studies have been conducted in Europe and the United States to determine the prevalence of more severe levels of retardation in children. Often these investigations have considered moderate, severe, and profound levels of retardation in combination. Abramowicz and Richardson (1975) reviewed twenty-seven such prevalence studies that were conducted between 1925 and 1970. Defining "severe" mental retardation as retardation with IQ below 50, these authors reported that the prevalence rate for this group, at 0–20 years, appeared to be between 3 and 5 per 1,000, with the average being about 4 per 1,000 or .4%. This is slightly higher than estimates for the total population in this IQ range; but this is because many of these individuals die as they grow into adulthood; therefore, a greater prevalence would be found during the pre-adult years (Farber, 1968; Tarjan, et al., 1973).

Nine of the studies reviewed by Abramowicz and Richardson (1975) analyzed the prevalence of moderate retardation vis à vis severe/profound retardation. The criterion for differentiation varied. In five studies, the cutoff IQ was 20, in three it was 25, and in one it was 31. Those above these marks were considered moderate or trainable, those below were severe or profound. Despite the lack of uniformity, the data provided useful information. The average prevalence of the moderately retarded children in these nine studies was 2.14 per 1,000 or .21%. This is consistent with earlier estimates (Dingman & Tarjan, 1960; Robinson & Robinson, 1976). The average prevalence of severely or profoundly retarded children was .78 per 1,000 or about .08%.

VARIATIONS IN PREVALENCE

It would be difficult to generalize to any great degree the overall prevalence to a particular setting since various factors will affect specific prevalence figures. These factors include the *type of community,* the *age range* of a particular group of people, the *gender* of the people, and the *socioeconomic and ethnic status* of the people.

Type of Community

Rural versus urban setting has been considered as a factor in terms of the prevalence of mental retardation with a proportionately greater number of cases occurring in rural areas (Farber, 1968). The majority of individuals in these studies have been mildly retarded. As Table 2–2 indicates, many states with large rural populations tend to have relatively large percentages of their public school students identified as mentally retarded. Farber (1968) suggested that migratory practices may have some bearing on the prevalence finding in these rural areas. He cited studies that suggested more intelligent persons are more apt to leave rural settings than are less intelligent individuals. This could at least explain to some degree the relative difference in prevalence figures.

In their study in Pima County, Arizona, Reschley and Jipson (1976) found that the location of residence made a difference in the prevalence of retardation among Mexican-Americans but not Anglo-Americans. According to their criterion (IQ ≤69), there were significantly more mentally retarded Mexican-Americans living in rural areas than in urban areas.

Living in a rural or urban setting doesn't seem to affect the prevalence of moderately, severely, and profoundly retarded groups so much as it does the mildly retarded. Abramowicz and Richardson (1975) found only one study that reported a disproportionate number of severely retarded children in rural over urban areas (Lewis, 1929). They suggested that Lewis' finding was probably due more to the visibility of severely retarded children in rural areas as compared to the urban areas. More recent studies have not found urban/rural differences among the more severely retarded.

Age Range

Age is another factor that has been shown to have some bearing on prevalence. The prevalence for people in certain age ranges will be different than the prevalence in other age ranges. Farber (1968) pointed out that "those periods in a person's life when he has most contact with the official agencies gauging his intellectual competence must also be those in which case-finding is most accurate" (pp. 69–70). Usually this will be during the school age years.

We know that most mildly retarded persons are identified during the school-age years (Tarjan et al., 1973). Farber reviewed two studies that demonstrated that the prevalence of mentally retarded persons increases up to about the age of fourteen or fifteen (Farber, 1959; Levinson, 1962). He suggested that this was due to increasingly obvious discrepancies between mildly retarded individuals and nonretarded persons as the academic competencies became more abstract. Lemkau and Imre (1969) found that the age "peak" was a bit higher, occurring between fifteen and nineteen years of age. Within this range they reported a prevalence of 9.6%. This seems a little high; but their overall prevalence for children between six and nineteen was 7.4%, which is itself quite high. In contrast to these studies, Reschly and Jipson (1976) found no significant differences in prevalences among students in first, third, fifth, seventh and ninth grades.

The prevalence of moderately, severely, and profoundly retarded individuals tends to be reduced during adulthood due to many early deaths (Tarjan et al., 1973). Cleland (1979) reported that the average age of death for the profoundly retarded was about thirty-eight. Moderately and severely retarded persons will live somewhat longer. This fact, coupled with the fact that more individuals in these groups are "reported" or "found" as they get older, tends to make the maximum time for identification (and thus prevalence determination) probably between about five and fourteen years. However, it should be noted that these children are usually seriously handicapped from birth and, if they survive the first few years, will be a consistent part of this group until their death. Unlike the mildly retarded individual, there is not much probability that they will ever be considered nonretarded.

Gender

As with every other disability, a person's sex influences the probability of being mentally retarded. There may be as many as 30% more males considered mentally retarded than females. In one study reviewed by Farber (1968), the number of males surpassing females was related to IQ level, with proportionally more males at the higher levels than at the lower levels (Kirk & Weiner, 1959).

Several reasons might account for prevalence differences due to gender. One possibility is that different cultural expectations might make boys more obvious when they are mentally delayed. Another is that boys have a higher probability of being affected by some sex-linked genetic influence. The former may be more likely for at least higher level individuals. Reschly and Jipson's (1976) finding of no difference in sex based on IQ across different cultural groups tends to make one think that it is more societal expectations than intellectual differences that separate the males from the females in this area.

In their review of prevalence studies on children with IQs below 50, Abramowicz and Richardson (1975) also found consistent sex differences in prevalence figures. Ten of the studies they reviewed investigated sex differences and all ten found higher prevalences among boys. On the average, 4.01 boys per 1,000 (boys) were moderately, severely, or profoundly retarded whereas only 3.01 girls per 1,000 (girls) were so classified.

Socioeconomic and Ethnic Status

A final factor that may be considered to affect prevalence is ethnicity and socioeconomic status. Again, we must separate traditional practices from current and emerging practices. As we have noted, there has been a historical tendency for more mildly retarded children to come from poor, minority families. Usually it is difficult to separate the two factors as they influence prevalence (Patrick & Reschly, 1982). Although some minorities have been erroneously identified as mentally retarded, others so identified continue to have difficulties during the adult years which leads one to suspect the original diagnosis was more correct than incorrect (Koegel & Edgerton, 1982). Regardless, there is an obvious trend in some places to reduce the number of minorities in classes for the mildly retarded.

Of paramount influence will be the criterion used to judge mental retardation and the concept of retardation formally acknowledged in a state or locality. In comparing Mexican-American, Anglo, Black, and Papago Indian children on WISC IQ scores, Reschly and Jipson (1976) found significant differences in prevalence based on a Full-Scale IQ score of 69 or less. Using this criterion, prevalence rates included 14.2% of the Papago Indian children, 8.1% of the Blacks, 6.7% of the Mexican-Americans, and 1.6% of the Anglos. However, when assessing prevalence differences based on *Performance* IQ of 69 or less, they found 4.7% of the Blacks below this criterion, 4.2% of the Papagos, 2.2% of the Mexican-Americans, and 1.2% of the Anglos. This clearly demonstrates how different criterion may affect prevalence rates.

Socioeconomic conditions tend not to be related to the prevalence of more severe retardation as much as they do to the mildly retarded. Lewis (1929) found 30.1% of the severely retarded persons in his survey living in superior or good homes and 30.7% living in poor or very poor homes. On the other hand, only 11.3% of the mildly retarded lived in superior to good homes while 61.7% lived in poor to very poor homes. A similar finding was reported by Birch, Richardson, Baird, Horobin, and Illsley (1970).

SOME CONCLUDING REMARKS ON PREVALENCE

Like classification systems, prevalence is important for the administration of special education programs. In order to be able to provide services to a group of people, it is necessary to know about how many people will need the services. This is essentially why prevalence studies are done. If the population of a given area is known, one should be able to estimate those who would be mentally retarded.

Of course there are limits to this proposition because there are, as we saw, a number of factors that influence prevalence. This is often a problem for administrators. The type of information that is contained in this chapter might be considered a knowledge foundation. If someone needs to know the number of mentally retarded people that exist in a particular community, this information will give them an *idea* of the number they might be looking for but may not predict the actual figure.

STUDY QUESTIONS

1. State the levels of retardation based on IQ. What terms are used for similar levels according to the special educators' system and the AAMD system?
2. What differences might exist in the class of "mildly" retarded people today and those in the same class during the 1950s, 1960s, and 1970s?
3. What are the advantages and disadvantages of categorical vs. noncategorical classification of the mildly retarded (or the mildly handicapped)?
4. Why do most people typically picture a moderately retarded person when asked to describe a mentally retarded individual?
5. What distinctions can be made between the severely and the profoundly retarded? Between the "relative" profoundly retarded and the "absolute" profoundly retarded?
6. Discuss the major functions and limitations of the classification by IQ system.
7. Why is knowledge of the prevalence of mental retardation important?
8. Why is it difficult to determine the prevalence of mental retardation?
9. What effect does *pathological* retardation have on the expected normal distribution of measured intelligence?
10. What trends are becoming evident in the prevalence of school-aged mentally retarded persons in the different states? What is causing these trends?
11. Why can the prevalence of the moderately, severely, and profoundly retarded be considered more stable than the prevalence of the mildly retarded?
12. Discuss how gender, community, socioeconomic and ethnic status can affect the prevalence of mental retardation.

3

Identification Procedures

Overview: The purpose and complexity of assessment and identification

PART I: IDENTIFICATION OF THE MILDLY RETARDED IN THE PUBLIC SCHOOLS

PART II: IDENTIFICATION OF THE MODERATELY, SEVERELY, AND PROFOUNDLY RETARDED

OVERVIEW: THE PURPOSE AND COMPLEXITY OF
ASSESSMENT AND IDENTIFICATION

There are several reasons why an individual might be assessed or evaluated. One would be to determine what the person knows or does not know. Another might be to see what one has learned or needs to learn. A third might be to find out if a particular teaching technique has made a difference in acquired knowledge or skills. A fourth would be to decide if a person should be classified in a particular way such as mentally retarded. It is this last reason that is the major focus of the present chapter.

Providing services to mentally retarded individuals requires that some process be available to accurately identify them. The process is not a simple one. In most public school systems, it requires a great deal of time and considerable involvement by professional personnel. While moderately, severely, and profoundly retarded persons may be easily identified, the identification of many mildly retarded persons may be quite difficult. The difficulty arises because of two potential dangers:

1. Identifying a person as retarded who *should not* be identified as retarded; and,
2. Not identifying a person as retarded who *should* be identified as retarded.

Either type of error may have serious consequences. In order to avoid such mistakes, identification procedures today require more involvement than ever before. Guidelines must be followed carefully, tests must be given fairly, and results must be interpreted judiciously. No one test or one individual can make the decision to classify a person as mentally retarded. Unlike earlier procedures, multidisciplinary teams using various sources of information ultimately make the final determination. This approach is generally thought to be safer, resulting in more accurate placements (Pfeiffer, 1982).

In this chapter, we will examine the procedures used to identify a person as mentally retarded. In preface to this, the reader should realize two facts. First, for all the objectivity toward which we strive, subjective influences cannot be avoided. We are humans dealing with a human problem and mistakes can be made. A major goal is to reduce the number of these mistakes. Second, the identification of mentally retarded persons, especially the mildly retarded, is not only a psychological and educational issue, it is also a social and legal one. We should become aware of the significance of this added dimension of the assessment process.

Before a person is formally identified as being mentally retarded, there is generally some suspicion that he or she may be retarded. Depending on the possible degree of retardation, this suspicion or idea may occur at different points in the person's life and be held by different key individuals. With more severely retarded individuals (IQ≤50), who are usually organically impaired, the parent or physician may be the first to suspect a problem. This will often occur shortly after birth or during the first few years of life. Some mildly retarded children may also be informally identified by their parents or physicians, especially if these children are organically involved. However, the majority of mildly retarded children, the cultural-familial retarded, will first become suspect during their early school years. Generally one of the child's elementary school teachers will recognize the potential problem. This recognition will often be based on academic difficulties. Sometimes these will be accompanied by social behavior deficits.

Regardless of who suspects the child to be retarded or when it is suspected, a formal diagnosis will ultimately validate or reject the condition of mental retardation. The procedures and implications for formally identifying the different levels of retardation at the different times vary and must be considered separately. Identification of the mildly retarded within the public school system presents the more complex issue. Thus it will be discussed first in some detail. Following this discussion, we will consider the identification of moderately, severely, and profoundly retarded persons.

PART I: IDENTIFICATION OF THE MILDLY RETARDED IN THE PUBLIC SCHOOLS

THE PROCESS OF IDENTIFICATION

Three steps are necessary in order for a child to become formally classified as educable or mildly retarded within the public school system: a referral, an evaluation, and an identification and placement. With this last step, there will be a formal conference to determine the most appropriate placement for the child and to plan an individual educational program (IEP). The child will not be classified as mentally retarded without each of these steps being completed.

The Referral

The student is usually referred for evaluation by a teacher who recognizes he or she is having some difficulty. The teacher may not know for sure what the source of the problem is, but might simply realize the child is not keeping pace with the other children academically or socially.

Usually there is a certain person within the school to whom the teacher will send the referral. This may be the guidance counselor, assistant principal, principal, or some other designated person. A standard form will be filled out by the teacher and sent to this person who will forward it to the central school board office for processing. The pupil services section of the central administration will then usually schedule the child for formal evaluation.

It must be realized that the decision by the teacher to refer the child for formal evaluation (and hence the possible identification) is very subjective. A teacher often has no set criteria for deciding whether or not to refer the child. Some teachers may, for one reason or another, be reluctant to make a referral or feel that he or she can adequately serve the child. In such cases, the process may stop here or at least be delayed. In other cases, a teacher may refer a child who could be adequately handled in the regular classroom. Such an event might occur if the teacher had a relatively low tolerance for children with learning problems of any sort. As we can see, a slight bias in one direction or the other may portend difficulty.

The Evaluation

Following a referral by the teacher, and after permission is received from the child's parents, an evaluation of the child will be made. Here we reach another subjective decision point. In the large majority of cases, the child will be formally evaluated. However, in some instances this may not occur. Algozzine, Christenson, and Ysseldyke (1982) found that 92% of all referred cases were evaluated. If a psychologist or psychometrist does not test the child, the child cannot be identified as mentally retarded.

A primary instrument used during the evaluation will be the intelligence test. However, this global measure (i.e., the IQ) cannot be the sole source of information. Alley and Foster (1978) noted that the regulations governing PL 94–142 clearly call for multiple sources of information to be available for the ultimate decision-making process. These additional evaluative techniques must include:

A provision for the assessment of educational needs

Tests that reflect specific abilities rather than any impaired sensory, manual, or speaking skills (except when these are the areas the test is supposed to test)

A multidisciplinary or team approach that includes at least one individual knowledgeable about the suspected deficit area

An assessment of areas that may be related to the suspected disability. When appropriate, this may include health, vision, hearing, social and emotional status, general intelligence, academic performance, communicative status, and motor abilities

In addition to these guidelines, in order to avoid potential biases, each test must:

Be administered in the child's native language or another appropriate mode of communication if feasible

Have been validated for its specific use

Be administered by a competent evaluator

Clearly, the Federal law and regulations require that a fair and non-discriminatory assessment procedure be followed.

Planning and Placement

The third phase of the classification process involves the interpretation of the data collected, planning an appropriate educational program in the least restrictive environment, and placing the child in that program. Correct interpretation of the data should result in correct identification and placement. The more relevant data available and the more professional thought given to the particular case, the more likely a correct decision will be made. Turnbull, Strickland, and Brantley (1978) noted that the following individuals *must* be involved in the planning conference:

The student's teacher (regular and/or special)

A person responsible for providing and/or supervising special education programs

The student's parent(s)

The student, if appropriate, and

The person(s) who conducted the evaluation or someone knowledgeable about the interpretation of the tests' results

Additional persons may also be involved if their presence will facilitate the planning conference. They may include health personnel, social workers, therapists, vocational rehabilitation specialists, or physical education specialists (Turnbull et al., 1978).

The involvement of these various professionals is usually thought to result in more accurate placement decisions. Pfeiffer (1982) found that in mock situations, teams of professionals were able to make more accurate placement decisions than they were able to as individuals. He wrote:

A cooperative work group brings to bear on a complex task differing values as well as unique professional perspectives. (p. 69)

In their collective effort, these individuals are to decide the most valid categorization of the student but, perhaps more important, the most appropriate educational placement and individual education plan. In so doing, they will examine all the available information. The significance of this information may be perceived differently by different individuals. Knoff (1983) found that many psychologists and special educators felt that observation of the student in the classroom would provide the most useful information. Unfortunately, sometimes more subtle factors may influence placement decisions such as individual professional biases, the geographical proximity of services, or the vested interests of certain individuals or agencies (Holland, 1980). Needless to say, such influences should be avoided.

Undoubtedly, formal test results will have an important influence on the identification and placement of students. In the following section we will examine the instruments used to help the school system decide if a child should be classified as mildly retarded.

INSTRUMENTS USED TO IDENTIFY AND PLAN

From our earlier reading, we know that the AAMD presents two major criteria for a child to be classified as mentally retarded: "significantly subaverage general intellectual functioning" as measured by an intelligence test and a concomitant deficit in adaptive behavior (Grossman, 1983). Additionally, as just discussed, other information will be necessary for planning individualized educational programs. Given this information, it would be beneficial for us to examine in more detail the nature of formal assessment instruments and procedures. Since intelligence tests have historically been the mainstay in the identification process, they will be examined first. Adaptive behavior scales will also be reviewed. While they tend to have taken a back seat to intelligence tests (Huberty et al., 1980; Patrick & Reschly, 1982), especially in the identification of the mildly retarded, some of the concerns expressed about intelligence tests and the trend toward broader assessment approaches warrant their inclusion in this section.

Intelligence Tests

Intelligence quotients are derived by asking someone to demonstrate a sample of their knowlege, skills, or abilities under a standard set of conditions. The procedure for administering and interpreting an intelligence test is quite clinical and requires a great deal of training and expertise (Cegelka, 1978). Unless a person is trained to administer a specific intelligence test, he or she should not do so.

There are many intelligence tests and they include many different test items or, in other words, allow for several different behaviors to be sampled. Salvia and Ysseldyke (1978) listed thirteen kinds of behaviors that are most often measured on tests of intelligence. These include the following:

Discrimination: A number of items are presented and the subject selects the one that differs from the rest.

Generalization: An item is presented and the subject is asked which of several other items goes with it.

Motor behavior: The subject is asked to copy a design, trace a path through a maze, or perform some other eye-hand coordination task. Memory is sometimes required.

General information: The subject is requested to answer factual questions.

Vocabulary: The subject must name pictures or point to the correct picture named by the examiner.

Induction: From a series of examples, the student is asked to induce a general principle.

Comprehension: The student is asked questions about a specific situation, either factual questions or judgmental questions.

Sequencing: A series of items with a progressive relationship is presented, and the subject must select an item which continues the sequence.

Detail recognition: The subject has to provide detail as in the drawing of a picture of a man.

Analogies: Given one relationship; for example, A is to B, the subject must complete a second relationship that has the same properties as the first; for example, as C is to _____ .

Abstract reasoning: The subject is required to determine the answer to some problem, such as in a particular situation or an arithmetic problem.

Memory: The subject is presented with an auditory or visual stimulus and asked to replicate it.

Pattern completion: The subject is asked to select an item which correctly completes a pattern that has been started.

Not all intelligence tests will measure all of these skills but many do measure most in one way or another.

In determining a school-age child's IQ, two tests are most commonly used: the Stanford-Binet Intelligence Scale (Terman & Merrill, 1973) and Wechsler Intelligence Scale for Children–Revised (or simply the WISC-R, Wechsler, 1974).

Totally, the Stanford-Binet contains 142 items distributed across age ranges. A variety of different items are found at each level. The examiner starts testing the child on items after a basal level is determined and continues testing until the subject reaches a ceiling (misses six items). Based on the individual's performance, two scores are determined: a mental age (MA) and a deviation intelligence quotient (IQ). The mean IQ is 100 with a standard deviation of 16 points. The MA is equal to the chronological age of a "normal" individual who has an IQ of 100; that is, one who passes the items within his or her age level.

The WISC-R is divided into two parts: the verbal scales and the performance scales. The verbal subtests include *information, comprehension, arithmetic, vocabulary, similarities,* and *digit span.* The performance subtests include *picture completion, picture arrangement, block design, object assembly, coding,* and *mazes.* Unlike the Stanford-Binet, the WISC-R divides similar items into the separate subtests listed above. Within each subtest, the procedure for administering the WISC-R is similar to the procedure for the Binet. The examiner starts at a basal level and continues until a ceiling level is reached. Throughout the test, standard administration procedures are rigorously adhered to by the examiner.

Three IQ scores are yielded by the WISC-R: a verbal IQ, a performance IQ, and a full-scale IQ. Each has a mean of 100 and a standard deviation of 15 points. Additionally, examiners may look at performance on each of the subtests to determine abilities on specific types of tasks.

Intelligence, as defined and tested by intelligence tests, is relative. A person's score is reported in relation to others' scores. Such tests are called norm-referenced tests. Thus one of the outcomes is the ability to compare the individual to others in terms of his or her measured intelligence. In describing this relationship, we may conclude whether the individual is at about the same level as others, is "below" others, or is "above" others. We can also state the degree of this deviation. Based on the IQ the person earns, we can state the relation of the person to others in terms of standard deviations. If a person is within a plus or minus one standard deviation from the mean, we say the person is "normal." Greater differences from the mean may indicate the person is "different." If the direction is far enough below the mean, it may indicate that the person is mentally retarded.

Adaptive Behavior Scales

In recent years there has been a significant increase in the development of adaptive behavior scales. There are three reasons for this: (1) the inclusion of "deficits in adaptive behavior" as a part of the AAMD definition of mental retardation; (2) the increased number of programs for the training of severely and profoundly retarded persons; and (3) the utility of the scales for evaluating training effects (Meyers, Nihira & Zetlin, 1979). Meyers et al. estimated that over 100 adaptive behavior scales have been developed.

Adaptive behavior scales are generally different from intelligence tests. The major differences include their purpose, the types of behaviors they evaluate, and their administration. Adaptive behavior scales were developed to measure "the effectiveness of an individual in coping with the natural and social demands of his or her environment" (Nihira, Foster, Shellhaas & Leland, 1974, p. 5). The purpose of these scales is not to measure an individual's intellectual or mental ability but, more straight-forwardly, to describe the individual's day-to-day behavioral repertoire. Unlike intelligence scales, adaptive behavior scales are intended to provide a picture of what someone actually does in his or her environment.

One use of adaptive behavior measurement may be to distinguish between school (psychometric, clinical) retardation and retardation within the social system of an individual. Serving this function, adaptive behavior scales will be of primary interest to those attempting to eliminate the designation of the "six-hour retarded child." The Adaptive Behavior Inventory for Children, which is a part of the System of Multicultural Pluralistic Assessment (Mercer & Lewis, 1978), was designed explicitly for this reason.

Another, perhaps more common use of adaptive behavior scales is to provide useful information for planning instructional programs for mentally retarded individuals, particularly for those in the moderate to profound range of retardation. They therefore serve a dual function: they may describe a person's current behavioral status (Gully & Hosch, 1979) and, at the same time, suggest important areas of learning for an individual (Windmiller, 1977).

With such a large number of scales available and with only a loosely defined concept, a variety of items may be assessed on any one or several adaptive behavior scales. Figure 3–1 duplicates two pages of items from the AAMD Adaptive Behavior Scale (Nihira et al., 1974), one of the most commonly used scales. The examples demonstrate behaviors ranging from self-help skills ("never has toilet accidents") to destructive behaviors ("cries and screams"). Meyers et al. (1979) identified seven behavior domains common to most adaptive behavior scales. These include the following:

> Self-help skills: feeding, dressing, toilet training, and grooming.
>
> Physical development: perceptual motor development, fine and gross motor coordination, ambulation, and the development of auditory and visual abilities.
>
> Communication skills: primarily the social use of expressive and receptive language.
>
> Cognitive functioning: primarily the development of reading and writing skills and number, time, and money concepts.
>
> Domestic and occupational activities: the productive use of time, vocational and avocational activities, and home chores.
>
> Self-direction and responsibility: voluntary involvement in purposeful activities, caring for personal belongings, and completing assigned tasks.
>
> Socialization: the degree of interaction and cooperation with others.

In addition to such areas, several scales include behaviors generally considered to be maladaptive or inappropriate. These would include stereotyped behavior, self-stimulation, inappropriate contact with others, verbal and physical aggression, and destructive behavior. Part II of the AAMD Adaptive Behavior Scale is completely devoted to the measurement of maladaptive behaviors (Nihira et al., 1974).

The items on most adaptive behavior scales would prove to be "too easy" for many children classified as educable mentally retarded. Some may therefore conclude that these scales can not adequately diagnose this level. Conversely others would suggest that some of these children should not be classified as mentally retarded. One adaptive behavior scale was developed, however, that might reflect impaired functioning in some potential mildly retarded individuals. It is the Social and Prevocational Information Battery (SPIB) (Halpern, Raffield, Irvin & Link, 1975). This test was designed to measure functional, individual skills often considered to be important for mildly and moderately retarded adolescents and adults. It includes measures of job searching skills, job related behavior, banking, budgeting, purchasing, home management, health care, hygiene and grooming, and functional signs. It has been reported to be valid and reliable for measuring these behaviors of individuals classified as mildly or educable mentally retarded (Irvin and Halpern 1977). While most cultural-familial mildly retarded persons could be expected to do fairly well on a scale such as the AAMD ABS, when tested using the SPIB, they may not fare as well because the skills measured are of a higher level.

The procedure for judging a person's level of adaptive behavior is quite different from judging a person's intelligence. Scales used to evaluate adaptive behavior do not call for clinical rigor in their administration. Their main purpose is to learn broadly what someone can or cannot do. There are two main techniques used to ascertain this information. One is for someone who knows the individual to be rated to fill out the scale's checklist. A second is for another person, who perhaps does not know the individual, to interview someone who does know the person. Generally it is assumed that the person being rated does not have the ability to report on his or her own behavioral abilities. One study, however, found that in some instances mildly retarded persons were more accurate at reporting their own behavior than were their group living home counselors (Millham, Atkinson, & Nathan, 1980).

For the most part, adaptive behavior scales, unlike intelligence tests, do not actually require behavior to be demonstrated at the time the evaluation is conducted. Instead, recalling what the person has done or is able to do is used in the rating. However, there are at least a couple of exceptions to this. The Balthazar Scales of Adaptive Behavior I (Balthazar, 1971) has an actual test of dressing and undressing. The Social and

PART ONE

I. INDEPENDENT FUNCTIONING

A. Eating

[1] Use of Table Utensils (Circle only ONE)

Uses knife and fork correctly and neatly	6
Uses table knife for cutting or spreading	5
Feeds self with spoon and fork - neatly	4
Feeds self with spoon and fork - considerable spilling	3
Feeds self with spoon - neatly	2
Feeds self with spoon - considerable spilling	1
Feeds self with fingers or must be fed	0

[2] Eating in Public (Circle only ONE)

Orders complete meals in restaurants	3
Orders simple meals like hamburgers or hot dogs	2
Orders soft drinks at soda fountain or canteen	1
Does not order at public eating places	0

[3] Drinking (Circle only ONE)

Drinks without spilling, holding glass in one hand	3
Drinks from cup or glass unassisted - neatly	2
Drinks from cup or glass unassisted considerable spilling	1
Does not drink from cup or glass unassisted	0

[4] Table Manners (Check ALL statements which apply)

Swallows food without chewing	___
Chews food with mouth open	___
Drops food on table or floor	___
Uses napkin incorrectly or not at all	___
Talks with mouth full	___
Takes food off others' plates	___
Eats too fast or too slow	___
Plays in food with fingers	___
None of the above ___	
Does not apply, e.g., because he or she is bedfast, and/or has liquid food only. (If checked, enter "0" in the circle to the right.)	___

8-number checked =

A. Eating ——————— ADD 1-4

B. Toilet Use

[5] Toilet Training (Circle only ONE)

Never has toilet accidents	4
Never has toilet accidents during the day	3
Occasionally has toilet accidents during the day	2
Frequently has toilet accidents during the day	1
Is not toilet trained at all	0

[6] Self-Care at Toilet
(Check ALL statements which apply)

Lowers pants at the toilet without help	___
Sits on toilet seat without help	___
Uses toilet tissue appropriately	___
Flushes toilet after use	___
Puts on clothes without help	___
Washes hands without help	___
None of the above ___	

B. Toilet Use ——————— ADD 5-6

C. Cleanliness

[7] Washing Hands and Face
(Check ALL statements which apply)

Washes hands with soap	___
Washes face with soap	___
Washes hands and face with water	___
Dries hands and face	___
None of the above ___	

[8] Bathing (Circle only ONE)

Prepares and completes bathing unaided	6
Washes and dries self completely without prompting or helping	5
Washes and dries self reasonably well with prompting	4
Washes and dries self with help	3
Attempts to soap and wash self	2
Cooperates when being washed and dried by others	1
Makes no attempt to wash or dry self	0

[9] Personal Hygiene
(Check ALL statements which apply)

Has strong underarm odor	___
Does not change underwear regularly by self	___
Skin is often dirty if not assisted	___
Does not keep nails clean by self	___
None of the above ___	
Does not apply, e.g., because he or she is completely dependent on others. (If checked, enter "0" in the circle to the right.)	___

4-number checked =

[10] Tooth Brushing (Circle only ONE)

Applies toothpaste and brushes teeth with up and down motion	5
Applies toothpaste and brushes teeth	4
Brushes teeth without help, but cannot apply toothpaste	3
Brushes teeth with supervision	2
Cooperates in having teeth brushed	1
Makes no attempt to brush teeth	0

FIGURE 3–1   Sample Pages from the AAMD Adaptive Behavior Scale

From K. Nihira, R. Foster, M. Shellhaas, and H. Leland, *"AAMD adaptive behavior scale."* (Washington, D. C.: American Association on Mental Deficiency, 1974). Reprinted by permission.

PART TWO

I. VIOLENT AND DESTRUCTIVE BEHAVIOR

	Occasionally	Frequently
[1] Threatens or Does Physical Violence		
Uses threatening gestures	1	2
Indirectly causes injury to others	1	2
Spits on others	1	2
Pushes, scratches or pinches others	1	2
Pulls others' hair, ears, etc.	1	2
Bites others	1	2
Kicks, strikes or slaps others	1	2
Throws objects at others	1	2
Chokes others	1	2
Uses objects as weapons against others	1	2
Hurts animals	1	2
Other (specify: _____)	1	2
——None of the above Total		

[2] Damages Personal Property	Occasionally	Frequently
Rips, tears or chews own clothing	1	2
Soils own property	1	2
Tears up own magazines, books, or other possessions	1	2
Other (specify: _____)	1	2
——None of the above Total		

[3] Damages Others' Property		
Rips, tears, or chews others' clothing	1	2
Soils others' property	1	2
Tears up others' magazines, books, or personal possessions	1	2
Other (specify: _____)	1	2
——None of the above Total		

[4] Damages Public Property		
Tears up magazines, books or other public property	1	2
Is overly rough with furniture (kicks, mutilates, knocks it down)	1	2
Breaks windows	1	2
Stuffs toilet with paper, towels or other solid objects that cause an overflow	1	2
Attempts to set fires	1	2
Other (specify: _____)	1	2
——None of the above Total		

[5] Has Violent Temper, or Temper Tantrums	Occasionally	Frequently
Cries and screams	1	2
Stamps feet while banging objects or slamming doors, etc.	1	2
Stamps feet, screaming and yelling	1	2
Throws self on floor, screaming and yelling	1	2
Other (specify _____)	1	2
——None of the above Total		

I. VIOLENT AND DESTRUCTIVE BEHAVIOR ——— ADD 1-5 [ ]

II. ANTISOCIAL BEHAVIOR

[6] Teases or Gossips About Others	Occasionally	Frequently
Gossips about others	1	2
Tells untrue or exaggerated stories about others	1	2
Teases others	1	2
Picks on others	1	2
Makes fun of others	1	2
Other (specify: _____)	1	2
——None of the above Total		

[7] Bosses and Manipulates Others		
Tries to tell others what to do	1	2
Demands services from others	1	2
Pushes others around	1	2
Causes fights among other people	1	2
Manipulates others to get them in trouble	1	2
Other (specify _____)	1	2
——None of the above Total		

[8] Disrupts Others' Activities		
Is always in the way	1	2
Interferes with others' activities, e.g., by blocking passage, upsetting wheelchairs, etc	1	2
Upsets others' work	1	2
Knocks around articles that others are working with, e.g., puzzles, card games, etc.	1	2
Snatches things out of others' hands.	1	2
Other (specify _____)	1	2
——None of the above Total		

FIGURE 3–1 Continued

Prevocational Information Battery mentioned above requires responses to correct choices.

Scores derived from adaptive behavior scales differ from scale to scale. Some scales, such as the Vineland Social Maturity Scale, yield a single score; i.e., the Social Age (which may be converted to a Social Quotient). Most scales, however, are divided into subscales or domains and provide scores within each of these areas. The scores are derived from the reported performance on each item within the subscale or domain. These scores may then be used to compare the individual to the performance of other persons in the standardization sample of the particular adaptive behavior scale.

ISSUES RELATED TO IDENTIFICATION AND PLACEMENT

In recent years, two controversial issues have been associated with the identification of children as educable or mildly mentally retarded. One is the overrepresentation of minorities within this category and the other is the effect of labels on the population. While the interrelation of the two can clearly be inferred, they are separated here for the purpose of discussion.

The Identification and Placement of Minority Students

The disproportionate overrepresentation of minorities in special classes for the educable mentally retarded has been a major issue and cause for concern for many years. After much discussion among professionals, the federal courts and Congress faced the issue and attempted to resolve it. The heavy thrust of the attack was on the use of intelligence tests (on which minority groups as a whole tend to score lower) as a major or sole criterion for classifying minority individuals as educable mentally retarded.

That minorities have historically been overly represented in EMR classes cannot be denied (Farber, 1968). Mercer (1973), in her study in Riverside, California, found that there were 49% fewer whites in special classes than would be expected proportionally. She also found that there were four times more Mexican-Americans and three times more blacks than would be expected if normal population proportions held true. The U.S. Department of Health, Education and Welfare Office of Civil Rights (1979) reported that in the 1978–79 school year, blacks comprised 17% of the public school population but accounted for 41% of all EMR placements. More recently, the Education Advocates Coalition (1980) reported that "Black children are misclassified and inappropriately placed in classes for the 'educable mentally retarded' at a rate of over three times that of white children. Other minorities are frequently misclassified as well" (p. 4).

Given this fact, we must ask why. One possible conclusion is that there are more minorities who are mentally retarded. By psychometric definition, this appears to be true. In fact, much research has been conducted to find out why minorities, especially low socioeconomic black individuals, score low on intelligence tests. But there may be another answer that lies within the intelligence tests and their administration. This is the contention of those who criticize the use of the tests with minorities (e.g., Mercer, 1973, 1975; Williams, 1970; Tolliver, 1975; Gonzalez, 1974). The three major criticisms presented by these writers and others are as follows.

Types of items. In order to answer some of the questions on intelligence tests, certain experiences are necessary. These questions and their answers may have value in the dominant culture but not in other cultures or subcultures. Thus, many minority children have not had the experiences necessary to answer the questions. Many times they provide answers considered to be wrong or incomplete and this lowers their score.

Language differences. In a testing situation, if the tester and testee are not communicating clearly, questions and/or answers might not be understood clearly. This may be a result of incomplete learning of the English language as with Mexican-American children, the use of dialect by black children, or simply limited vocabulary development. In some cases, if the problem were more clearly presented or the question better understood, more points might be earned.

Reaction to the testing situation. It is generally assumed that maximum performance is being given by the student in a testing situation. This may not always be the case. Critics have suggested that minority children may not provide their utmost effort because they do not see the significance of the test. Instead, it might be more important for them to rush through it in order to terminate the situation as soon as possible. It has also been suggested that the testing situation may arouse tensions and suspicion in the minority child.

In addition to these problems, intelligence tests have been criticized for their lack of utility. McClelland (1973) pointed out that one's IQ had very little to do with vocational success. Citing various studies, he noted that intelligence tests and other measures of aptitude were generally not related to how well a person could function as an adult. He also stated that more often such tests are used to screen certain applicants (e.g., minorities) who could probably do the job just as well as one who scored higher on the test.

Several cases have been brought into federal courts which have challenged the use of intelligence tests with minorities. Under different federal laws, the plaintiffs (those challenging the use of the tests) have charged that the defendants (usually the school officials who require the use of intelligence tests resulting in classifying the child as mildly retarded) have violated their civil rights. The federal laws often cited have included Title VI of the Civil Rights Act of 1964, the Fourteenth Amendment to the Constitution, the Education of the Handicapped Act (PL 93–112) and/or the Education for All Handicapped Children Act (PL 94–

142). These laws in combination prohibit any form of discrimination based on race, color, or national origin; and require due process in the identification, labeling, and placement of children in special classes. Three recent cases are discussed below.

Larry P. v. Riles, No. C–71–2270 RFP (W. D. Cal., October 11, 1979). In this federal case, the use of intelligence tests for determining whether or not a child should be classified as mildly retarded was challenged on the basis of being discriminatory against blacks. Federal District Court Judge Robert Peckham made his decision in October, 1979, ruling that the tests were indeed discriminatory. He said that such a test could not be used and required that a moratorium on the use of intelligence tests in California for the purpose of identifying EMR children be continued. The moratorium was initiated in 1974.

Not only did Judge Peckham say that the tests were discriminatory, but that those who used them should have known better. He said that the tests "are racially and culturally biased, have a discriminatory impact on black children, and have not been validated for the purpose of (consigning) black children into educationally dead-end, isolated, and stigmatizing classes" (Opton, 1979).

Judge Peckham did not feel that the discrimination was accidental although he also did not feel that the intent was necessarily to hurt black children. But he concluded that, based on the evidence, "there was less than a one in a million chance that the overenrollment of blacks and the underenrollment of whites in California EMR classes would have resulted from a color-blind placement system. This held true even if an unwarranted assumption was made that the incidence of mild retardation was 15% higher for blacks" (Education Advocates Coalition, 1980).

Mattie T. v. Holladay, No. DC–75–31–S (N.D. Miss., July 28, 1977). In Mississippi, an almost identical case occurred. The data provided to Federal District Judge Orma R. Smith showed that black children were being placed in EMR special classes at a rate of three to one over white children. On the other hand, it was pointed out that white children were placed in resource classes for the learning disabled twice as often as were black children.

According to expert witnesses, the racial disparities were occurring at three levels: teacher referral of students for EMR classes, IQ testing, and program placement. This was similar to Mercer's (1973) findings in California.

A court-approved consent decree was entered in February, 1979. It required "a significant reduction in the disparities by 1982, establishes a means of targeting state monitoring and technical assistance on the districts with the worst disparities, and sets up a process for development of new placement procedures" (Education Advocates Coalition, 1980).

Judge Smith realized that the children who had been classified as EMR would need help upon being decertified and reentering the regular classroom. It was ordered that "a program of tutoring and intensive academic assistance to bring the person up to a level of academic achievement which should allow the person to receive a high school diploma" be followed.

Parents in Action on Special Education (PASE) v. Hannon, No. 74–C–3586 (E.D. Ill., 1974). This suit was filed on behalf of minority students against the Chicago School Board. As in the *Larry P.* and *Mattie T.* cases, it was charged that the use of intelligence tests were discriminatory. However, in contrast to the rulings by Judges Peckham and Smith, Federal District Judge John Grady ruled that the tests were *not* culturally unfair because the school system used other criteria that prevented racial bias in the placement procedure. The ruling was appealed to the Seventh U.S. Circuit Court of Appeals.

Following Judge Grady's ruling, the Chicago School Board voted, in spite of the court's decision, to eliminate the use of intelligence tests in the procedure for placing students in EMR classes. The Board noted that more than 80% of the students in Chicago's EMR classes were black. "Such a condition," they said, "suggests potential bias in testing, assessment, and placement policies or their implementation" (Education Daily, 1981). The Board therefore established a task force to determine how to phase out the use of intelligence tests and return children to regular classrooms.

Is there any defense for the use of intelligence tests to classify minority children as educable mentally retarded? Some feel that we may actually be doing more harm than good in the elimination of the tests. There are at least two realms in which judgments of the use of intelligence tests may be based: the social system and the educational system. From a social or societal perspective, few in our society today would argue that racial segregation or discrimination is appropriate. However, educationally speaking, some defend the use of intelligence tests.

Sattler (1974) pointed out that several studies have demonstrated the validity of intelligence tests for describing current functioning and predicting academic functioning of minority children as well as of others. Indeed, he says, the tests do point out differences in groups of children. However, Sattler wrote that: "Because the tests may reveal inequality of opportunities available to various groups, they may also provide the stimulus for social interventions to facilitate the maximum development of each individual's potentialities" (p. 43).

A second point is that because the tests are objective, they may actually reduce bias rather than increase it. Other methods of identification may be more subjective and result in more biased assessment procedures. Educational opportunities and curriculum might be based more on ancestry, prejudice, and caprice and less on aptitude. In short, the consequence of not testing might be to increase bias and discrimination.

Finally, it might be argued that to judge individuals within their own environment or subculture as Jane Mercer has suggested does not reduce the value of intelligence tests. Because a person is capable of functioning in one specific environment does not indicate that they may do as well in other environments. An objectively measured level of intelligence, on the other hand, is a more universal measure of aptitude (Clausen, 1972). Since the assessment provides an index of standing in the total culture, it allows greater knowledge of the individual's potential in environments other than his or her immediate situation.

The Effects of Labeling

Labeling children has resulted in much discussion, debate, and research. The position taken by many is that when we place a label on someone, such as "mentally retarded," we stigmatize that person. It has been suggested that we may affect an individual to such a degree that he or she may never recover. Another concern is what the label does to the interaction between the labeled person and others. It may, for example, cause a teacher to treat a child as though he or she cannot learn. In other words, it might reduce expectations.

In an extensive review of the literature by MacMillan, Jones, and Aloia (1974), many issues were presented with regard to the real and hypothesized effects of labeling on mildly retarded children. Based on their review, MacMillan and his colleagues concluded that the evidence of the effects of labeling was not sufficient to allow any firm conclusions to be drawn regarding their adverse effects. The main reason for this is that any effect of the label may interact with other variables to such a degree that it is difficult to separate the impact of the label from the other variables such as academic or social behavior. For example, suppose a child has been labeled mildly retarded and it was found that the teacher was providing the child with material that was less difficult than that being provided to the other children. We might also find that the other children did not play as often with the labeled child as they did with others. Can we conclude that the teacher's behavior and that of the children was a result of the child being labeled? It may be that the child's *behavior* and *ability* caused the reactions. In fact, these reactions may have occurred whether the child had been labeled or not.

If we consider the effect of the label on how the child thinks or feels about himself, the same type of confounding situation occurs. We may say labels reduce an individual's self-concept. But is it the label or is it how others treat him or her? Is it the label, or is it the number of failures the child has experienced because of an inability to cope successfully? It would be difficult to conclude that if the child had not been labeled, these problems would not occur.

A number of studies have been reported since the review by MacMillan et al. (1974) that have attempted to isolate the effects of labels on various groups' reactions. Most of these studies have used bogus case reports or films in which the subject was or was not labeled. The participants who read about or viewed the subjects were divided into groups, some being told the child was labeled retarded, others being given no label. In some of the studies, other variables were also introduced such as attributes of the child. The differences in the subjects' attitudes or opinions about the child were then recorded and analyzed in light of the information provided to them.

In summarizing several of these studies, three tentative conclusions can be drawn. First, if a child is labeled as mentally retarded, most people are probably going to feel that the child's capacity to learn is below normal and that he or she should be placed in a special class (Gillung & Rucker, 1977). This seems to hold true even though the labeled child may be described with some positive attribute (Taylor, Smiley & Ziegler, 1983).

A second point, however, is that other kinds of information can also affect such an opinion. Knowing the nature of a child's behavior, for example, changed some stereotyped views of educable retarded children in a study by Foster and Keech (1977). Additionally, Palmer (1980, 1983) found that a low IQ or other deficit information (e.g., academic ability) was as likely to result in a special class placement suggestion as was the EMR label.

It is perhaps unfortunate that many other kinds of information reduce ratings or opinions of students' ability to the same degree as do labels. Aloia (1975) found that physical unattractiveness had this effect and Aloia, Maxwell, and Aloia (1981) found ethnicity also had such an effect. Smith and Greenberg (1975) found lower social class status increased expectations that a child would be classified as mildly retarded. Based on findings like these, then, we cannot conclude that labels alone affect people's expectations of others.

A third conclusion that can be drawn from recent research, and maybe a bit on the positive side, is that labels sometimes serve to increase tolerance, acceptability, or understanding of the inappropriate or nonnormal behavior of the individuals who are labeled. Seitz and Geske (1978) found this, as did Severance and Gasstrom (1977). Using children as judges, acceptability was increased when a poor academic performer was labeled as mentally retarded (Budoff & Siperstein, 1978; Foley, 1979). Also with children, when the behavior remained the same, the label made no difference although described attributes did affect the ratings (Freeman & Algozzine, 1980; Young, Algozzine, and Schmid, 1979).

While we can conclude that other types of information besides the EMR label may affect one's opinion of a child, we should not assume that labels are benign artifacts of the process. While they are necessary for professional communication, their use must be considered a serious matter. This is but another reason why we must be extremely cautious when classifying a child as educable mentally retarded.

CONCLUSIONS

At one time, the process for identifying a child as mildly or educable retarded within the public schools was quite simple. If a teacher felt the child was failing because of mental retardation, the child was tested and, if the IQ was appropriately low, placement in an EMR class followed.

Because society today is more concerned about individual rights and potential infringement upon those rights, we now use more caution. More information about the student and more professional time is entered into the decision-making process. Additionally, the decision is seen as a beginning because individual educational planning must follow.

With such caution, we might expect fewer students to be placed in EMR classes, particularly minority students. Certain areas in the country have already seen this trend (MacMillan et al., 1980). When intelligence tests are banned, or strict adaptive behavior criteria are applied, we can expect to see a reduction in the EMR population (Childs, 1982). While proponents of a social-system perspective of mental retardation would applaud this, many educators would question the value of its net effect on some children's welfare as it may preclude necessary special educational services.

In the end, errors of one type or another cannot be avoided. However, we can do much to lessen their probability. One approach is to increase the information being used. To some degree adaptive behavior scales may be helpful but may not be enough to solve the problem. Concerned professionals must realize the complexity of the dilemma and work to solve it. We should hope that not too many children suffer along the way.

PART II: IDENTIFICATION OF THE MODERATELY, SEVERELY, AND PROFOUNDLY RETARDED

Unlike determining who is mildly retarded and who is not, determination of who is moderately, severely, or profoundly retarded is not a controversial issue. Their deviation from the norm in both measured intelligence and adaptive behavior is generally so noticeable that regardless of their home or community environment, they clearly stand out as being mentally retarded. By the time these individuals reach the age to begin school, in all probability they will already have been diagnosed as mentally retarded. Many will have been in private preschool programs while others will have been placed in public or community residential facilities.

Diagnosis of developmentally lower functioning children will primarily be concerned with the *degree* of retardation more than the *presence* of retardation. For the purpose of program planning, professionals will want to know the approximate functioning level of the child. Typically, parents will want to know the prognosis. "What will he be like when he grows up?" Of course, so many variables will affect the answer to this question that it is often difficult to answer except in the most general terms.

There are several ways that a child of this level can be diagnosed. Intelligence tests and adaptive behavior scales are used in the diagnosis of more severely retarded individuals just as with mildly retarded persons. Other methods are also used. However, note that these formal measures often merely confirm what parents or professionals have already suspected.

PARENT OBSERVATIONS

Most parents know their children quite well. Either from reading or from observing other children, they know what infants, toddlers, and preschoolers are supposed to do. When they do not observe these actions in their own children, or when they observe them at a later time than usual, they often become suspicious. This is how many retarded children are first "identified."

There are many things that parents may notice. Batshaw and Perret (1981) have highlighted some of these clues to developmental delay. They include such behavioral deficits as showing little regard for the environment, sitting in one position for a long time without complaining, weak sucking, high-pitched crying, and not responding to parents' attention. Physical characteristics sometimes include weak muscle tone, delays of two or more months in holding up the head, rolling over, sitting up, standing, or walking. The normal time for development for these and other behaviors are presented in Table 3–1 (Batshaw and Perret, 1981). Parents might notice the lag of development in several of these areas.

MEDICAL DIAGNOSIS

While mental retardation is not an illness or disease, various physiological problems sometimes do result in retarded mental development. A medi-

TABLE 3–1 Development in the First Years of Life

MONTH	GROSS MOTOR	FINE MOTOR	SOCIAL-ADAPTIVE	LANGUAGE
1	Partial head control Primitive reflexes predominate	Clenched fists	Fixates objects and follows 90°	Alerts to sound
2	Good head control Lifts chin in prone		Follows 180° Smiles responsively	
3	Lifts chest off bed Hands held open Primitive reflexes less prominent	Hands held open Reaches toward objects Pulls at clothing	Follows 360° Recognizes mother	Coos
4	Swimming movements	Hands come to midline	Shakes rattle Anticipates food Belly laugh	
5	Rolls prone to supine			Orients toward sound "Razzes"
6	Anterior propping response	Transfers objects Holds bottle Palmar grasp	Looks after lost toy Peek-a-boo Mirror play	Babbles
7	Bounces when standing Sits without support	Feeds self cookie		Imitates noise Responds to name
8	Lateral propping responses	Rings bell Radial raking grasp		Nonspecific "Mama" Understands "no"

Age	Gross Motor	Fine Motor	Adaptive/Social	Language
9	Crawls		Mouths objects	
10	Stands with support	Plays with bell Claps	Waves "bye-bye" Pat-a-cake	
11	Cruises around objects	Finger grasp		Follows gesture command
12	Makes first steps	Throws objects	Aids in dressing	2–3 specific words
15		Marks with pencils	Indicates when wet Spoon feeds Builds tower with blocks Gives kisses Imitates chores	Low jargon Follows 1-step commands
18	Runs stiffly Handedness is determined Jumps	Scribbles	Places formboard Turns pages Parallel play Takes off clothes Does puzzles	High jargon Body parts Follows 2-step commands Points to one picture
24	Walks up and down steps	Imitates vertical lines Draws circle with pencil	Puts on and takes off shoes Plays with children	Uses "I" Four body parts Points to pictures Can form three-word sentences

From Batshaw, M. L., and Perret, Y. M. Children with handicaps: A medical primer. Baltimore: Paul H. Brookes Publishing Co., © 1981. (Table 11.1, pp. 140–141, used with permission.)

cal diagnosis cannot say absolutely that a child will be retarded to a certain degree, but it can predict that some delay will occur.

There are several different processes that may be involved in a medical diagnosis of mental retardation. However, these are omitted here because they are discussed in the next chapter.

DIAGNOSTIC INSTRUMENTS

Developmental Screening

Most children develop according to the same sequence. The characteristics that are listed in Table 3–1 are generally observable. However, more formal screening methods are available and these will be conducted by physicians in cases where the parents suspect a problem. Frankenburg (1977) recommended that all children be screened at three, six, nine, twelve, eighteen, twenty-four, and thirty-six months. This is important as an earlier identification can result in earlier intervention.

A commonly used screening device for infants is the Denver Developmental Screening Test (Frankenburg & Dodd, 1969). This instrument is administered by asking the parent about the child's performance on various behaviors. The items are divided into gross motor, fine motor, language, and personal-social domains. Since the device is norm-referenced, it can detect if a child is at, below, or about where he or she should be in comparison to like-aged children. It is useful for children between two weeks and six years of age.

Infant Development Scales

Infant development scales or infant intelligence tests are similar to regular intelligence tests in their design and use. The only difference is that they contain items appropriate for younger children (i.e. motor and perceptual motor items) instead of those used with older individuals (i.e. verbal items). They are considered to be downward extensions of regular intelligence tests and have standardized methods for administration and scoring. They are also norm-referenced so that it is possible to determine a child's relative standing in the population. The tests typically yield age-equivalent scores, social quotients, developmental quotients, or intelligence quotients (Simeonsson, 1977).

There are several tests of this nature. The Bayley Scales of Infant Development (Bayley, 1969) are probably the most widely used. The Bayley, which contains mental and motor subscales, is useful for assessment during the first two and a half years of life. Other tests of this nature include the Gesell (Gesell & Amatrude, 1952) and the Cattell (1960).

While these scales do not have academic predictive ability as do tests such as the Stanford-Binet and the WISC-R, they do show a child's standing in relation to other children at the same age level. If a child is to be moderately, severely, or profoundly retarded, these scales will predict this (Hatcher, 1976). However, they are heavily loaded with nonverbal items and thus tend not to correlate with later academic performance or intelligence test scores.

Tests of Cognitive Processes

Like regular intelligence tests, the infant developmental scales do not tell us how a person arrived at a score, simply that the item was passed or failed. The score yielded is a quantification of relative standing. We know the product but we do not know the process. Tests of cognitive processes are designed to show how a child achieves a product. These tests are based on Piaget's theory of qualitative cognitive development. The examiner determines the child's level of cognitive development by analyzing how well the child performs on different items requiring different processes, not simply on whether or not a certain item is passed.

These scales are ordinal in nature in that they are arranged in the order in which cognitive development normally occurs. The development is not expected to occur at the same time for every individual but is expected to occur in the same order. Kahn (1976) has shown that the order is followed with the severely and profoundly retarded and therefore can be used with this population.

The most commonly used scales of cognitive process development are the Ordinal Scales of Psychological Development (Uzgiris & Hunt, 1975) and the Albert Einstein Scale of Sensory-Motor Intelligence (Corman & Escalona, 1969). These measures not only allow for the identification of deficits but also help in the development of instructional training programs.

Intelligence Tests and Adaptive Behavior Scales

The intelligence tests and adaptive behavior scales described earlier in this chapter are also used with the moderately, severely, and profoundly retarded. (Intelligence tests might not be useful with some very low-level profoundly retarded persons.) When they are used with lower functioning individuals, administration and scoring procedures are the same as described earlier. Adaptive behavior scales can be used for classifying lower-functioning retarded students but they can also assist in program development. In this role, they serve a very useful function.

CONCLUSIONS

There are several ways by which the presence of moderate, severe, or profound retardation can be confirmed. The most useful way will also provide direction for intervention and program development. The early identification via medical methods can play this dual role in some cases as can the Piagetian assessment procedures and the adaptive behavior measures.

STUDY QUESTIONS

1. Why are mildly retarded persons more difficult to identify than lower level retarded persons?
2. Who are the first to recognize that a child may be mildly retarded? Moderately, severely, or profoundly retarded? When does this recognition occur?
3. What provisions are required by law to reduce test biases? What is the significance of the multidisciplinary team approach?
4. What individuals must be involved in the planning process? What others *may* be involved?
5. What does an intelligence test do?
6. Discuss the major differences between adaptive behavior scales and intelligence tests including purpose, types of items, and administration.
7. Why have critics of intelligence tests suggested that minority children do poorly on those tests? How have others defended their use?
8. To what degree can we conclude that labels affect the acceptance of educable mentally retarded students?
9. In what ways are most moderately, severely, and profoundly retarded children identified? Describe the types of instruments used.

Physiological Causes of Mental Retardation

THE RELATIONSHIP OF MENTAL RETARDATION
AND PHYSIOLOGICAL CAUSES

A relatively small number of people who demonstrate retarded functioning do so because of a *physiological* disorder. In other words, at some point during the complex process of becoming a person, some incident occurred that resulted in abnormal development and functioning. Physiological etiologies will be more common among the moderately, severely, and profoundly retarded and less so with the mildly retarded. This chapter addresses several of these causes.

CHROMOSOMAL AND GENETIC FUNCTIONING

The cell is the basic unit of life. In a multicellular organism such as man, there will be many different kinds of cells which will perform a variety of jobs. For example, muscle cells, nerve cells, blood cells, and so on all contribute in a special way to make the body work. In normal humans, each cell contains 46 chromosomes within its nucleus. The chromosomes are matched in 23 pairs. The first 22 pairs of the chromosomes (44) are called autosomes; the twenty-third pair are the sex chromosomes. The sex chromosomes determine whether a person is female (XX) or male (XY). The autosomes determine other features of the person.

The chromosomes of the cell appear during mitosis, the process of cell division. At this time, the chromatin in the nucleus forms into the strands of chromosomes. It is at this time that the 46 chromosomes can be clearly identified. After the chromosomes develop from the chromatin (prophase), they line up in the center of the cell (metaphase) and then begin to divide (anaphase). Generally each of the daughter cells formed from the miotic division gets a complete set of 46 chromosomes. These then elongate (telephase) and return to a chromatin state (interphase) until the next cell division (Simpson & Beck, 1965).

The process of mitosis affects all cells. Another process, meiosis, occurs only in the sex cells, i.e. the male sperm and the female ovum. Meiosis involves two cell divisions resulting in four daughter cells from one parent cell. Each of the daughter cells contains only 23 chromosomes instead of 46. During fertilization, the two gametes (the sex cells) combine and result in a fertilized egg containing 46 chromosomes, that is, 23 plus 23.

Each of the 46 chromosomes in the body's cells contain a series of chemicals called *genes*. There are hundreds of genes on each chromosome. The genes determine certain features (e.g. eye color, bone structure, etc.) They also synthesize certain proteins which allow the body to function. Cells in the pancreas, for example, produce insulin which enables the body to use glucose. Sometimes *single-gene mutations* occur. This happens when one chemical is substituted for another in the gene's structure. When this occurs, the cell and subsequent cell generations may not function properly. Associated physical characteristics and metabolic functions will be abnormal. The mutation will become a part of the genetic structure and can be passed on from parent to child.

Genes contained on one chromosome are paired with the genes on the other chromosome that completes the pair. If two genes on a pair contain the same information-producing characteristic, they are called *homozygous*. If they are different in terms of the trait they produce, they are called *heterozygous*. Homozygous gene pairs will always produce the trait that both recessive genes are mandating. Heterozygous pairs will produce only one trait, the one called for by the *dominant* gene.

When fertilization occurs, each parent contributes 23 chromosomes. Each chromosome will contain genes to be matched with the genes on the respective chromosomes from the other parent. Remember that within each parent, meiosis has left the gametes with only half (23) of the normal complement of chromosomes. Which gamete, containing which chromosomes with which genes, that a parent delivers is pure chance (50–50). But what is actually delivered will have a definite bearing on the trait that is manifested. Traits or characteristics may be inherited through autosomal recessive genes, autosomal dominant genes, and X-linked (sex-linked) genes. Many normal traits will be inherited in one of these ways. Sometimes, however, syndromes of mental retardation will result from genetically inherited disorders.

SYNDROMES DUE TO AUTOSOMAL RECESSIVE GENE DISORDERS

Manifestations of autosomal recessive genes can only occur if *both* parents contribute a recessive gene. Look at Figure 4–1A. Here you see two people, both "carriers" of an autosomal recessive gene—*a*. What will this mean for their child? There are three possibilities, each with a different probability. At the point of fertilization each parent may contribute either the *a* gene or the *n* (normal) gene. If they both contribute the *a* gene, the child will inherit and manifest the characteristic *(aa)*. There is a 25% chance that this will happen. If one parent contributes the *a* gene and another contributes the *n* gene, regardless of who contributes which, the child will become like both parents: a carrier. This means that he or she will have the capability to pass the gene on to his or her own child but will not manifest it. There is a 50% chance that this will happen. If both parents contribute the *n* gene, the child will neither manifest the characteristic nor be a carrier. There is a 25% chance that this will happen.

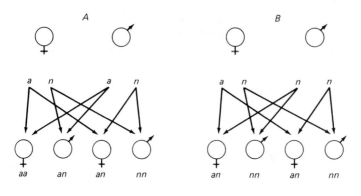

a = recessive gene with characteristic
n = normal gene with some other characteristic
aa = affected, characteristic manifested
an = carrier, characteristic not manifested
nn = normal

FIGURE 4–1 Possibilities of Recessive Gene Transmission

Look now at the B side of Figure 4–1. In this situation one parent is a carrier *(an)* while the other is not *(nn)*. As you can see, none of the offspring will manifest the characteristic but there is a 50% chance that a child will be a carrier.

Genes serve to provide the body with different kinds of enzymes. Enzymes are proteins that act as biochemical catalysts to metabolize nutrients that the body needs to function. When a basic molecule such as sugar enters the body, it passes through a series of steps with each step being controlled by an enzyme. These steps are referred to together as a metabolic pathway. At each step, the product is altered to serve a special need.

The enzymes are normally produced according to the direction of the specific amino acid code found on the strands of DNA, the genetic material of the chromosomes. Sometimes mutations occur on single genes. That is, the DNA provides an incorrect amino acid and thus an improper enzyme structure. Two results occur. First the enzyme will be deficient and will fail to serve its function on the metabolic pathway. Second, the mutation becomes a part of the genetic code and may be passed on to children. Many children develop genetic disorders because of mutations that occurred at some time in their ancestry.

When an enzyme deficiency occurs, certain molecules cannot be further metabolized so they build up in the body. This may affect different bodily tissues including the brain. Additionally, other products, which are metabolized in the pathway at a later time, will be deficient. Thus there will be high levels of certain metabolic products and low levels of other products. The results may range from having no effect to causing profoundly retarded functioning. Disorders due to enzyme dysfunctions are sometimes called inborn errors of metabolism.

One of the positive aspects about such an etiology is that the particular enzyme-related disorder can sometimes be identified and dietary restrictions and supplements can be used to prevent the impact of the inherited disease. This type of procedure can prevent the occurrence of mental retardation or reduce the potential level of severity.

Phenylketonuria

One of the most commonly known enzyme-deficient diseases resulting in mental retardation is phenylketonuria or PKU. Children born with PKU are deficient in the enzyme phenylalanine hydrozylase. This enzyme normally converts phenylalanine to tyrosine. Since this conversion cannot occur, the phenylalanine builds up in the body's fluids and tissues when the newborn begins to ingest milk. Progressively the increase in phenylalanine will lead to brain damage and severe mental retardation.

Children with PKU appear normal at birth but if the disorder is not treated through dietary intervention, at three to four months they begin to show progressive deterioration; and at two or three years mental retardation is usually quite apparent. Phenylketonurics tend to have normal physical development but may not learn to walk or talk. Often they are blonder than their siblings, frequently have autistic-like behavior, are hyperirritable, and have convulsions (Carpenter, 1975a). Fortunately PKU can be discovered at birth through blood screening tests and can be successfully treated through dietary intervention (Guthrie, 1972).

In addition to PKU, there are several other syndromes due to autosomal recessive gene defects that result in mental retardation. Carter (1975) and Batshaw and Perret (1981) provide analyses and descriptions of many of them. A number are listed in Table 4–1.

SYNDROMES DUE TO AUTOSOMAL DOMINANT GENE DISORDERS

Unlike autosomal recessive genes which require two recessive genes to be matched, a characteristic can be caused to occur if just one parent delivers an autosomal dominant gene. A recessive gene can be carried without being manifested but if a person has a dominant gene, the manifestation will usually be present. In Figure 4–2A one parent is normal *(nn)* while the second has the dominant gene characteristic *(An* or *nA)*. Statistically, half of the children can be expected to receive the dominant gene from the affected parent and have an *An* composite whereas half the time they

TABLE 4–1   Mental Retardation Syndromes Due to Autosomal Recessive and Dominant Genes

SYNDROME	ETIOLOGY	DESCRIPTION
Galactosemia	Autosomal recessive	Liver disease and an enlarged liver, along with jaundice, occurs in the newborn period. Cataracts, convulsions, diarrhea, and vomiting also occur. Mental retardation will occur but a galactose- and lactose-free diet will prevent the mental retardation.
Hurler's syndrome	Autosomal recessive	At some time between shortly after birth and about six years, the characteristics of this syndrome begin to appear. Besides mental retardation, the person's physical features will also be affected. This will include contracture of the limbs, hump back, short neck, heavy eyebrows, saddle nose, enlarged stomach, and widely spaced peg teeth, among other features. No treatment is widely effective.
Maple syrup urine disease	Autosomal recessive	The urine of these children smells like maple syrup—thus the name. Often they die during the first week after birth. If they do not, they will be mentally retarded. They may alternate between being rigid and flacid and will have convulsions. The involved amino acids can be eliminated from the diet. This will save the lives of many children; but mental retardation may still occur.
Tay Sachs disease	Autosomal recessive	A toxic product is not metabolized and thus leads to brain damage and death. The mutation originally occurred in eastern Poland in the early 1800s. At about six months, the child loses the ability to sit and babble; soon the child becomes blind, deaf, convulsive, and severely retarded. The children usually die by age 5. In some cases, kidney transplant has been an effective treatment.
Hypothyroidism (Cretinism)	Autosomal recessive	These children are large for their age, are floppy, have a hoarse cry and, untreated, become mentally retarded. The treatment consists of the administration of the thyroid hormone. If this treatment is prompt, prognosis is good and the child will not be mentally retarded. Cretinism was one of the earliest distinguished syndromes of mental retardation.

TABLE 4–1 *Continued*

SYNDROME	ETIOLOGY	DESCRIPTION
Apert syndrome	Autosomal dominant	Children with this disorder have a high and steep forehead. Their nose and ears are large and their face is depressed toward the central portion. Their fingers and toes are webbed; and they may be hydrocephalic. Mental retardation can occur, but sometimes these children have average or above-average intelligence.
Huntington's chorea	Autosomal dominant	This disorder may appear any time in life but often does not do so until the person is between 40 and 60 years old. Chorea means that uncontrolled movements occur. In this case tremors, drooling, and difficulty in swallowing occur. Sometimes mental deterioration occurs, but sometimes it does not.
Neurofibromatosis	Autosomal dominant	This disorder, also called Von Rechlinghansen's disease, is characterized by café au lait (coffee with cream), yellowish, brown patches of skin. Tumors may also form on the skin and on other body parts. If tumors develop in the central nervous system, mental retardation may result, but this is not always the case.
Tuberous sclerosis	Autosomal dominant	The symptoms of this syndrome are similar to those in neurofibromatosis. Tumors are found throughout most of the body's tissue. The tumors on the face often form a butterfly-shaped pattern across the nose and onto the cheeks. Tumors sometimes form on the retina and cause blindness to occur. Mental retardation is a frequent result.

would receive the *n* gene from the affected parent (and, of course, an *n* gene from the normal parent) and therefore would not be affected.

In a case where two parents both manifest the dominant gene characteristic (see Figure 4–2B), one out of four times a child might expect to receive the dominant gene from both parents. Sometimes this "double dose" is fatal. Half the time, the children would manifest the characteristic *(An)* while a fourth of the time they would receive the nondominant gene from both parents and would be normal.

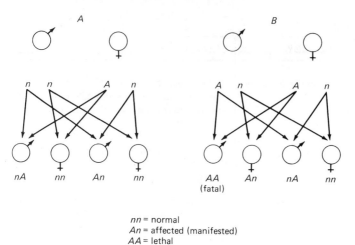

nn = normal
An = affected (manifested)
AA = lethal

FIGURE 4–2 Possibilities of Dominant Gene Transmission

Since only one parent must be affected in order to transmit a dominant gene disorder, it would seem that the incidence of autosomal dominant disorders would be higher than that of autosomal recessive disorders (in which both parents must be at least carriers). This, in fact, is not true about mental retardation syndromes due to dominant gene defects. Why not? It is because in order to reproduce a child, people have to reach a certain age and have the opportunity for sexual relations. Many mentally retarded people who have dominant gene defects meet neither of these requirements; therefore dominant gene defects are more difficult to transmit to a new generation. (Keep in mind that recessive disorders are usually passed on by parents who are carriers but who do not manifest the mental retardation themselves.)

A legitimate question is, how does any retardation due to dominant gene inheritance occur at all? There are three reasons. Sometimes, even though the person has the genotype, the phenotype (the manifestation) is not completely expressed. This is called *reduced penetrance*. The individual carries the dominant gene but for various reasons the expression of the disorder does not occur.

Another reason is that there is sometimes *variability in the expression*. That is, sometimes the disorder is not as severe as in other cases. Neurofibromatosis is an example (see Table 4–1). In some cases the characteristics are only slightly expressed. In other cases, severe mental retardation occurs. Still, even in the slighter manifestations, the person is carrying a dominant gene and if children are ever born, there is a 50% chance that they will inherit the dominant gene. The phenotype they express may be much more severe than that of their parent and may include mental retardation.

Finally, different autosomal dominant syndromes will have their deleterious effects expressed at different ages. Huntington's chorea (see Table 4–1), for example, often has an age of onset during the adult years. This allows an individual time to procreate. Because of this reason, and those above, dominant gene defects continue to occur. Comparatively speaking, however, they result in fewer cases of mental retardation than do autosomal defects. The bulk of dominant gene defects have more bearing on physical development than on mental development. Table 4–1 contains some of the syndromes due to dominant genes that sometimes result in mental retardation.

SYNDROMES DUE TO X-LINKED GENE DISORDERS

The previously described recessive and dominant gene defects are all tied to the first 22 chromosomal pairs, the autosomes. Genetic characteristics derived from the 23rd pair of chromosomes are called X-linked (or sex-linked) characteristics. The controlling genes are on the female (X) chromosome.

Females have two X chromosomes (XX) within each of their cells. When a man and woman contribute their gametes during fertilization, the woman (XX) must always contribute a female chromosome while the man, who has an X and a Y chromosome (XY) can contribute either the X or the Y chromosome. Thus the man determines the sex of the child.

The X chromosome carries various controlling genes besides those related to the sex of the child. The Y, however, is generally considered to be barren of genes except for its ability to control maleness. Therefore, whatever X-linked characteristic a boy gets, it will be inherited from the mother.

There are various characteristics which result from genes inherited from the mother on the X chromosome but most are innocuous. Some, however, are more serious. Hemophilia, Duchenne muscular dystrophy, and Lesch-Nyhan syndrome are examples. While the first two are life-threatening and often result in early death, the latter is a syndrome characterized by severe to profound mental retardation.

Lesch-Nyhan Syndrome

Lesch-Nyhan syndrome generally has no symptoms manifested at birth. Shortly thereafter, however, within about the first two years, uncontrolled movements and spasticity appear as neurological and physical growth deteriorates. The cause of the disorder is an enzyme deficiency in the metabolism of purine. One of the symptoms of the syndrome is a strong tendency toward self-mutilation with the affected boys often doing severe damage to their lips, hands, and fingers through biting.

SYNDROMES DUE TO CHROMOSOMAL ANOMALIES

In the previous sections, syndromes were presented that resulted from problems associated with specific genes. As mentioned earlier, genes are minute chemical arrangements comprising complete chromosome strands. Sometimes entire strands of chromosomes, one or more of the 46, will in some way be defective. This, of course, will have a direct bearing on the functioning of all of the genes of the involved chromosome(s). Figure 4–3A is a normal karyotype of the human male and Figure 4–3B is a normal karyotype of the human female. Karyotyping is a process which takes a cell from the body in order to study the size and shapes of the chromosomes. Karyotypes of some syndromes will show that chromosomal anomalies exist. These anomalies will have different forms and will involve either the autosomes or the sex chromosomes. Sometimes extra chromo-

FIGURE4–3 A   Normal Male Karyotype

From C. H. Carter, (Ed.), *Handbook of mental retardation syndromes*, 3rd Ed., 1975. Courtesy of Charles C Thomas, Publisher, Springfield, Illinois.

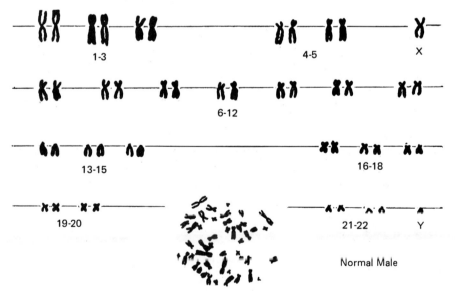

somes are present while others may be missing. Sometimes different chromosomes will be inappropriately joined together.

During both mitosis (normal cell division) and meiosis (division of the sex cells), problems can occur in the normal separation and arrangement of chromosomes. *Nondisjunction* can result in daughter cells forming with uneven numbers of chromosomes. This happens during anaphase when one of the chromosomes does not divide. Thus one new daughter cell gets an extra chromosome (trisomic), while the other daughter cell will lack a chromosome (monosomic). This can happen during mitosis or meiosis, but it most often occurs in meiosis during the first division (Batshaw & Perret, 1981). Down's syndrome results when the two number 21 chromosomes end up in one daughter cell while the other has no number 21 chromosome. The first daughter cell then has a total of 24 chromosomes while the latter cell has only 22. The gamete with 22 chromosomes cannot survive. However, the one with 24 can; and if it is fertilized by a sperm cell, with the normal 23 chromosomes, a zygote with 47 chromosomes will occur. The extra chromosome will be attached to pair number 21. Thus trisomy 21, or Down's syndrome, occurs. As the embryo develops into a fetus, every body cell will contain the trisomy 21 arrangement. This affects both mental development and physical characteristics. Figure 4–4 is a karyotype of a Down's syndrome person's cellular structure.

FIGURE 4–3 B Normal Female Karyotype

From C. H. Carter, (Ed.), *Handbook of mental retardation syndromes*, 3rd Ed., 1975. Courtesy of Charles C Thomas, Publisher, Springfield, Illinois.

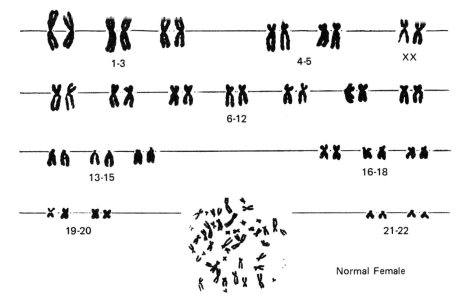

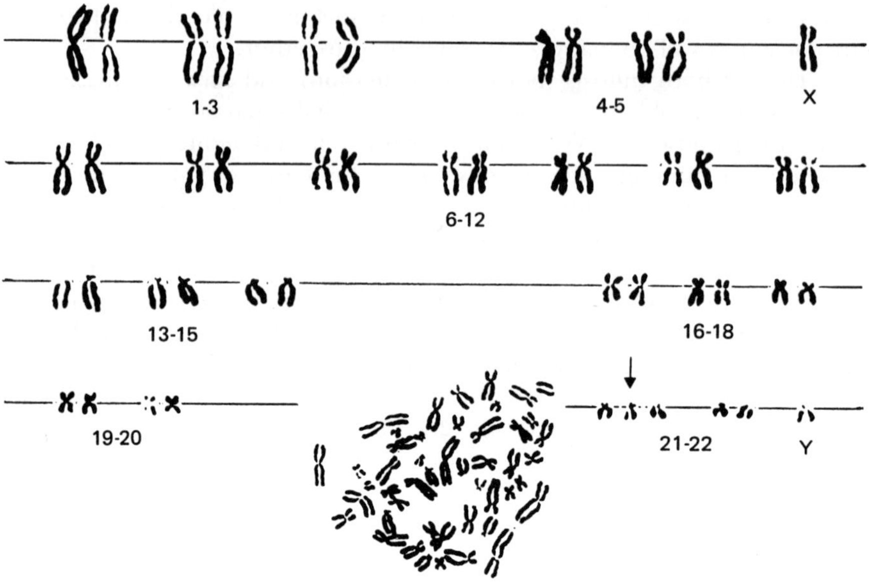

FIGURE 4–4 Down's Syndrome Karyotype
(arrow indicates extra number 21 chromosome)

From C. H. Carter, (Ed.), *Handbook of mental retardation syndromes,* 3rd Ed., 1975. Courtesy of Charles C Thomas, Publisher, Springfield, Illinois.

Down's Syndrome

Down's syndrome is the most prevalent syndrome resulting from chromosomal disorders. It was first identified by Langdon Down in 1854 who included it in part of his classification system. It has traditionally been referred to as mongolism, and the individuals as mongoloids, because of the belief that those with the disorder looked like Mongolian people. We know now that this is not true but we still hear the terms mongoloid or mongolian idiot from time to time. LeJeune, Gautier, and Turpin (1963) reported the discovery that Down's syndrome individuals had an additional chromosome at pair number 21, that is, trisomy 21. Other chromosomal disorders have been reported since this time.

Probably because of their distinctive features (see Figure 4–5) and the relatively high incidence as compared to other physiological syndromes, people often picture a Down's syndrome individual when they hear the term mental retardation. While their physical features may vary, they often include "simian crease on the palms, short in-curving little fingers, short broad hands, hyperflexibility of the joints, upward slanting of the eyes, epicanthic folds, furrowed protruding tongue, flat broad face, wide space between first and second toes and (of course) mental retardation" (Connolly, 1975, p. 41).

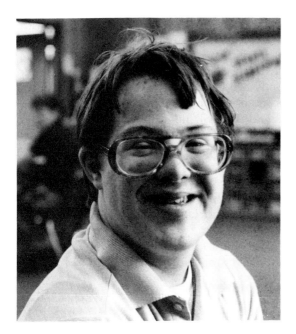

FIGURE 4–5 Down's Syndrome
Trisomy 21 (Down's syndrome)

Down's syndrome is usually caused by nondisjunction during meiosis. This accounts for about 90% to 95% of all cases (Abroms & Bennett, 1983). The remaining cases are due to *translocation* or *mosaicism*.

Translocation occurs when a fragment of chromosomal material breaks off from one chromosome and attaches itself to another one. If it attaches to pair number 21, the translocation form of Down's syndrome will occur. When translocation occurs, the resultant cell will divide through meiosis, and four gametes will develop. One will be normal, another will be "balanced." That is, it will contain all of the genetic material, but not in the appropriate arrangement. The two other gametes will be unbalanced and will result in zygotes that are trisomic or monosomic. If a person has a balanced translocation chromosome, he or she will be a carrier and may transmit the balanced chromosome to his or her offspring. This, of course, is extremely rare. Most cases of Down's syndrome occur *de novo*.

Mosaicism is another rare form of Down's syndrome. Nondisjunction and translocation as described previously occur *before* fertilization. Sometimes, however, after the egg and sperm unite to form the zygote, around the first or second cellular division, nondisjunction occurs. During mitosis, one of the chromosomes, usually number 21, does not divide appropriately and one cell ends up with 47 chromosomes (trisomy 21) while the other gets only 45. The one with 45 will die. But the one with 47 will continue to live and will produce generations of trisomy 21 cells. However, there are other cells in the cluster that are normal. They will remain unaffected and will proceed to produce normal cells. The ultimate outcome is a *mosaic,* a body composed of cells with different chromosomal structures. This mosaicism will produce a child that will be considered a Down's syndrome child but will not be "completely" Down's syndrome as is the case when the nondisjunction occurs before fertilization. Usually the physical abnormalities of these children are not as extensive as with "normal" Down's syndrome and the degree of retardation is less severe. Rynders, Spiker, and Horrabin (1978), based on their review of the literature, found trisomy 21 individuals to have a mean IQ of 45 with a range from 18 to 75. Down's syndrome resulting from translocation has a mean of 53 with a range from 28 to 85; and those resulting from mosaicism had a mean of 57 with a range from 14 to 100.

The incidence of Down's syndrome has usually been linked to maternal age, with older women (35 years or more) being considered greater risks. The reason attributed to this is that the woman's ova is believed to deteriorate as she grows older. Recent data, however, seems to indicate that in some cases, nondisjunction may occur within the sperm. Thus the age of the father may be a factor in at least some (20% to 25%) cases of nondisjunction. This seems to hold true for fathers over 55. Additionally, it seems that as older women become more aware of the risks related to childbirth, young women are producing a proportionally larger number of Down's syndrome infants (Abroms & Bennett, 1980; 1983).

Other Syndromes Related to Chromosomal Disorders

In addition to Down's syndrome, several other chromosomal problems may occur that will result in other syndromes of mental retardation. Trisomies may occur on one of the other chromosome pairs. Chromosome pairs 13, 14, and 15 (the D group) are susceptible as are pairs 16, 17, and 18 (the E group). D trisomy (13–15) results in very grossly deformed children. They will commonly have a cleft palate, seizures, eye defects, ear defects, extra fingers or toes, and severe retardation. E trisomy children have several distinct characteristics including low-set ears, an elfin facial appearance, abnormal fingerprints, excess body hair, heart defects, and a number of other maladies (Connolly, 1975).

The *cri-du-chat* (cat cry) syndrome results when the short arm of chromosome number 5 is deleted during meiosis. Besides being mentally retarded, these children have a broad bridged nose, a small receding chin, slightly slanted eyes, and a weak, cat-like cry during infancy. In addition, they can have heart defects, growth retardation, and microcephaly (Batshaw & Perret, 1981).

NEURAL TUBE DEFECTS

Two major neural tube defect syndromes can occur: *anencephaly* and *spina bifida*. Often *hydrocephalus* accompanies spina bifida. The reason these defects occur is because the cells do not migrate far enough during embryogenesis for the bodily structures to be completed.

It is during the fourth week following conception that the neural tube develops from the neural plate to form the basis of the central nervous system. Usually on the twenty-eighth day, the edges of the neural plate meet and close together to form the neural tube. The cells in this structure then continue to differentiate, ultimately becoming the brain, the spinal cord, and the spinal membranes. Later the skull and the spinal column will form to provide protection for these delicate tissues.

In anencephaly, the neural tube does not close at all and the brain does not form. In spina bifida a portion of the neural tube does not close and there is an incomplete formation of the spinal column. The opening allows the cord and peripheral nerves to slip out of the spinal column. Nerves below the meningomyelocele (the part of the spine that is disrupted) do not function. If the fetus survives, the child may be without the use of body parts below this lesion; that is, will probably not have bowel and bladder control or be able to walk. In many cases children with spina bifida will be physically disabled but will not be mentally retarded.

Neural tube defects can have quite serious implications. Newborns with anencephaly usually die shortly after birth. Besides paralysis below the lesion, children with spina bifida sometimes develop hydrocephaly. This occurs because circulation of the cerebrospinal fluid does not drain properly. This fluid builds up in the skull, places pressure on the brain, and the skull enlarges in order to accommodate the surplus amount of fluid. Surgery can repair the spinal opening and a shunt can be placed within the skull and under the skin in order to allow the fluid to drain into another part of the body. These procedures, however, will not always prevent serious consequences.

PROBLEMS DURING PRENATAL DEVELOPMENT

Throughout the nine months of pregnancy, the embryo or fetus is susceptible to various factors which may affect the process of normal development. Some of these factors, or *teratogens*, may affect ultimate mental development as well as physical development.

There are several different types of teratogens. The most common are *infections, chemicals or drugs,* and *radiation. Malnutrition* may also affect normal fetal development.

Infections

The placenta will serve to screen out many harmful substances. Others, however, will pass through. These may affect the mother in only a very mild way but the fetus may suffer more severe consequences. *Rubella* (German measles), *cytomegalovirus, herpes, syphilis,* and *toxoplasmosis* are examples of viruses that may infect the fetus.

With most infections, the first eight weeks of life seem to be the most critical insofar as consequences to the fetus are concerned. At this time the infection will cause serious damage to the developing central nervous system. Inflammation will occur and will destroy certain tissues, often cortical tissue. If the fetus survives the remaining period of gestation, it will often be born with brain damage and will be mentally retarded. Additional physiological problems may also occur. These might include blindness, deafness, congenital heart lesions, jaundice, hepatitis, and seizures.

The degree to which the infection causes problems is related to the location and extent of damage it does to the brain. In some cases the damage may be very localized and produce only a minor mental or physical handicap. In other cases it may be widespread, causing severe to profound retardation along with other physical defects. The damage is also related to when the infection occurs.

Rubella is probably the best known infection resulting in mental retardation. In the mid-1960s, a rubella epidemic resulted in many children being born deaf, blind, microcephalic, cerebral palsied, with heart defects and/or mental retardation. The rubella vaccine, which was developed after the epidemic, is the most common method of prevention.

A similar viral infection, cytomegalic inclusion body disease or cytomegaloviral (CMV) is now believed to be more common than previously thought. It is thought that about 80% of all adults have been infected by CMV (Carter, 1975). If the infection occurs during early pregnancy, it will be passed on through the placenta to the fetus. The infection, which has symptoms similar to mononucleosis or the flu, affects the lining of the brain. Abnormalities including hydrocephaly, microcephaly, intercranial hemorrhaging, generalized brain damage, and seizures may result. In addition, blindness and deafness may occur.

Herpesvirus (herpes simplex and herpes zoster) has been implicated in some cases as causing brain damage and mental retardation following infection by the mother. The greatest danger, however, occurs at the time of birth. If the mother's infection is active at this time, the child will become infected when passing through the cervix and vagina. Since the baby has no immunity, the infection generalizes and covers the entire body of the newborn, causing encephalitis and brain damage. If a mother has an active case of herpes when she is about to deliver, the physician will often perform a caesarean section in order to avoid contact between the child and the location of the infection.

Congenital syphilis is an infection which is transmitted as a venereal disease. The manifestation of the disorder in infants will vary. However, the general result, as with other infections, is an inflammation of the cortical tissue. The children often have rashes and skin disorders, poorly developed teeth, heart defects, and hydrocephaly. In milder cases, children may have close to normal levels of intelligence or be only mildly retarded. In more severe cases, profound retardation may occur, facial features and extremities may be absent or grossly defected, and large ulcerations may occur throughout the body.

Toxoplasmosis is considered to be the most damaging of all prenatal infections (Carter, 1975). About 75% of the infants of all affected mothers will show some degree of abnormality. These may be present at birth or appear shortly thereafter and may include cerebral calcifications, hydrocephalus, microcephalus, seizures, spasticity, rashes, jaundice, and an enlarged liver, spleen, and lymph glands. Mental retardation occurs most often and may become more severe as the child grows older.

Besides those mentioned above, other sources of infections may have damaging effects on the developing fetus. These include mumps, Asian flu, chickenpox, infectuous mononucleosis, and other viral infections.

Chemicals and Drugs

Like infections, various drugs and chemicals ingested by the mother can result in serious consequences to the fetus. A variety of drugs can affect the structure and functioning of cells. This can result in either abnormal body growth and development (as with thalidomide) or serious brain damage (as with alcohol). In addition to thalidomide and alcohol, drugs which may serve as teratogens include anticonvulsant drugs and anticancer drugs (Batshaw & Perret, 1981).

Anticonvulsant drugs, such as Dilantin and phenabarbital, may result in facial and limb malformations and heart lesions. Additionally, microcephaly and mild mental retardation may occur. The drugs are used to control seizures. Because of these problems, however, physicians will often discontinue the use of anticonvulsant drugs during the first trimester of pregnancy if the seizures are infrequent. If the seizures are too severe, the medication may be continued at a smaller dosage.

Taken in sufficiently large quantities (although the precise amount is not clear), alcohol can have serious damaging effects on the embryo or fetus. The alcohol breaks down into a toxic substance which affects the normal growth of embryonic tissue. Most of the children are moderately retarded, have droopy eyelids, heart defects, and are small in size. If pregnant women drink alcohol, physicians advise moderation.

While there is a lack of strong empirical evidence, other drugs such as LSD and heroin may also have adverse effects on the fetus. Children of heroin addicts often experience severe withdrawal symptoms at birth.

This may result in brain damage or even death. Fetal abnormalities have not been found to result from smoking tobacco. However, relatively low birth weight may result particularly if the woman is a heavy smoker (i.e. two packs a day); and this may place the infant in physical risk.

Anticancer drugs or chemotherapeutic agents may have an effect on the embryo similar to the effect they have on cells within the malignant tumor. The purpose of these drugs is to reduce the speed of cell division of the cancer. The embryo also is developing through rapid cellular division. The anticancer drug can cross the placenta and affect the growth of the embryo. Abortion is often suggested if the woman must receive chemotherapy during the first trimester.

The effects of various drugs and chemicals on the embryo and fetus are not well known. Only since the early 1960s, when the effects of thalidomide became apparent, have medical scientists started to investigate these problems. Laboratory animals have been used in many experiments in order to try to determine what potential adverse results might occur.

Radiation

Radiation was first seen to have deleterious effects on human development following the bombing of Hiroshima and Nagasaki during World War II. Today physicians show a great deal of concern about exposing pregnant women to even brief amounts of X-ray. While it is not clear how much radiation may be harmful to the developing fetus, complete avoidance is usually recommended to pregnant women. Infants whose mothers have been exposed to X-rays often show damaged or destroyed brain tissue, changes in nerve cells, and tumors on the brain.

Besides the effect of radiation on a developing embryo, many authorities express concern about preconception exposure to high doses of radiation or X-ray. Their fear is that the effects on the sex glands (the testes or the ovaries) may result in genetic or chromosomal problems in the sperm or ovum. This may result in genetic mutations or chromosomal anomalies similar to those that have been discussed previously.

Malnutrition

The effect of maternal malnutrition on the developing fetus is not entirely clear. Some contend that malnutrition of the mother can have harmful effects. Others contend that the effects are negligible. The particular time of interest is during the last trimester of fetal development. At this time the brain is growing at a very fast pace. It would seem that important nutrients, especially protein, would be necessary in order for proper cellular development. Carter (1975) maintained that "the incidence of congenital abnormalities, low birth weight infants, and prematures is significantly higher in mothers with malnutrition and hypoprotei-nemia. Children of these mothers often have pre- and postnatal failure to thrive. The brains have a decreased weight and number of neurones in the cortex. A decrease in the average intelligence in these children has been shown in large studies" (p. 223).

Others disagree with the effect of maternal malnutrition on mental development. Some of this disagreement is based on the Dutch famine of 1944–45. At this time, because of World War II, many people in Holland suffered from famine. It was a period of time that lasted for about six months. Hundreds of peope died. People, including pregnant women, were placed on dietary rations that allowed them only about one-half of their dietary nutritional needs. In a study of the children who were born shortly after the famine, Smith (1947) found that the infants were small for their age but otherwise healthy. In a later analysis, however, Stein, Susser, Saengar, and Marella (1975) found a marked increase in the mortality of infants (up to 90 days) that were in their third trimester of development during the famine. Deaths during days 7 to 29 occurred at a rate of about 24/1,000. Deaths during days 30 to 89 occurred at about the same rate. The remarkable finding of the Stein et al. study however was that individuals who were born during the famine and lived, twenty years later were found to be functioning in the range of normal mental development. The prevalence of mental retardation among this group was no higher than within the normal population.

PROBLEMS THAT OCCUR AT BIRTH

Besides the various difficulties that can occur prenatally, there are other difficulties that can occur at the time of birth and shortly afterwards. These can generally be related to the health of the mother during both pregnancy and delivery.

Chronic Illness

In some situations the mother may be suffering from an ongoing disease and this may affect the health of her baby. The nature of this effect may bear on the child's later mental development. A primary disease of concern is diabetes. In some cases, but not all, children of diabetic mothers will be premature. This has serious implications and will warrant close attention by the obstetrician. These mothers may also be prone to toxemia. This means they will tend to have high blood pressure, edema (retention of fluid in body tissues), and other biochemical disturbances. In its worst state, toxemia can result in the mother having seizures. If this occurs before birth, it can impede the supply of oxygen to the child. Some children of diabetic mothers can experience severe neurological delays and may ultimately develop lower than average IQs though they will not always become classified as mentally retarded.

Besides diabetes, mothers with chronic illnesses such as thyroid disease, hypertension, heart problems, or respiratory disorders can also produce children who will evidence growth retardation and perhaps mental retardation.

Acute Illness

At the time of birth, or shortly before, if the mother develops some illness, this may adversely affect the child. Such illnesses may include bacterial or viral infections. If the mother develops such an infection, it may be passed on to the child through the placenta prior to birth, or at the time of birth, through contact with the vagina. The problem is that the child has not lived long enough to build up any immunities. Therefore, even relatively harmless infections can be dangerous.

One of the most dangerous is streptococcal sepsis. Sepsis is another word for blood poisoning. This particular infection spreads quickly throughout the child's blood. Fortunately, like most bacterial infections, it can be controlled with antibiotics. However, if this is not done, the infection can spread to the brain and cause meningitis to occur. When this occurs, if the child lives, he or she will have severe brain damage.

Viral infections such as herpes are different. There is no treatment for this type of condition and if contracted by the child, death will often occur. In the case of herpes, as mentioned earlier, the physician will perform a caesarean section in order to prevent the child from coming into contact with the disease during delivery.

Placenta Previa

Sometimes during the final months of pregnancy, the location of the placenta will become a problem. Normally, the placenta is attached to an upper part of the uterine wall. In placenta previa, the placenta attaches itself just above the cervical opening. This causes a problem to occur at the time of delivery. The child will place pressure on the placenta causing it to tear and bleed. This, of course, could result in the child not getting an adequate supply of blood. A great deal of blood loss could also place the mother in jeopardy (Batshaw & Perret, 1981). Without blood, the child will suffer extreme brain damage if not death. The physician will usually advise the mother to stay off her feet as much as possible and ultimately a caesarean section will be performed if the placenta overlays the cervix to a great extent.

Kernicterus

Many newborns develop jaundice, a yellowish coloring of the skin and eyes. This is not an uncommon occurrence. It develops because the particular liver enzyme has not adequately developed to metabolize bilirubin. Bilirubin is a by-product of old, broken-down red blood cells. Usually, within a week or so, the child will develop the enzyme adequately and normal coloration will occur. If not, the child will be placed under flourescent lights and this will speed up the enzyme process.

In some situations, however, Rh incompatibility exists between the mother and child. This means that a minor aspect of the child's blood differs from that of the mother. If the mother is Rh − and the child is Rh + and the newborn is the first child, there will be no problems. However, if he or she is a later child, there may be problems.

When the mother (Rh −) had her first child (Rh +), some of the child's blood cells got into the mother's blood system. In response, her blood system developed antibodies to counteract to destroy the incompatible blood cells. During subsequent pregnancies with Rh + children, the antibodies the mother developed after the first child would cross through the placenta and kill the red blood cells of the fetus. This would result in severe anemia and a massive buildup of bilirubin in the child's system. In the past, this would kill most fetuses while still in utero. Those that did not die suffered brain damage. They were mentally retarded, had cerebral palsy, upward-gaze paralysis, discoloration of the teeth, and high-frequency hearing loss. This syndrome was called kernicterus.

During the 1950s and 1960s, treatment consisted of blood transfusions given in utero and then continued after the child was born in order to reduce the bilirubin. Today a drug, RhoGAM, is given to the Rh mother following the first delivery. RhoGAM works to block the formation of antibodies in the mother's blood system. Subsequent children will develop without risk.

PROBLEMS AFTER BIRTH

Most physiological sources of mental retardation have their origin prior to conception, during embryogenesis, fetal development, or around the time of birth. There are, however, events during life which may leave a person, child or adult, functioning at some level of retardation.

Any occurrence that results in sufficiently severe damage to the brain can cause it to cease functioning or at least reduce its functional ability. We typically do not think of such things but they happen from time to time. For example, a person may nearly drown and receive no oxygen for a short period of time. In this case, the brain may cease its electrochemical operations. Functionally, the person would be mentally retarded. Several postnatal causes of mental retardation have been documented (Carter, 1975). Among these are child abuse, cerebral hemorrhaging (stroke), congenital heart disease, heat stroke, decompression illness, blast injuries, electric shock, asphyxia, and poisonous gases.

PREVENTING MENTAL RETARDATION DUE TO PHYSIOLOGICAL ETIOLOGIES

There are several ways to combat the causes of some of the syndromes that have been discussed. These techniques are not used in isolation but are used together in many ways to prevent the occurrence of mental retardation (Sells & Bennett, 1977).

Carrier Detection

Certain disorders transmitted through autosomal recessive genes or X-linked genes can be identified through blood screening techniques. For certain populations with certain diseases such as Ashkenazic Jews (a sect of Jews with Eastern European origin) with Tay Sachs, in which the probability that a recessive gene defect may be present is relatively high, this procedure is particularly useful (Kabeck, Becker & Ruth, 1974). It allows the clinicians to examine cells for the existence or lack of a certain enzyme. If this key enzyme is missing in the prospective parents, they will at least know the chance exists that they may have a defective child. In other cases, they may be relieved to learn that they are not carrying the disease. This approach would not work for the general population because the incidence of a given disorder is extremely low. In contrast, with Tay Sachs, about one in thirty Ashkenazic Jews is a carrier.

Not all enzyme deficiencies can be as easily detected as in Tay Sachs. Thoene, Higgins, Krieger, Schmickel, and Weiss (1981), using a variety of screening techniques, were able to identify seven metabolic disorders due to an enzyme deficiency. Again, the problem is that carriers are so rare that any general screening procedure would have to serve massive numbers of people in order to be effective. Because of this, genetic screening will most often be used by those who have already had one child with a disorder or who know the condition exists in their family.

Prenatal Monitoring

The most common form of prenatal monitoring is *amniocentesis*. This process draws some of the amniotic fluid surrounding the fetus for cellular examination. Amniocentesis can be used to detect three different types of problems: those indicated by the chromosomal structure (this would include nondisjunction, translocation, and sex chromosomes); those indicated through enzyme deficiencies; and neural tube defects such as spina bifida. Typically, three groups of parents seek chromosomal analysis through amniocentesis: women who are over thirty-five, couples in which one parent is a balanced carrier of translocation, and parents who have already had one Down's syndrome child (Milunsky, 1976).

Besides amniocentesis, fetal monitoring may also be done through *fetoscopy* and *senography*. Fetoscopy allows the physician to insert a small tube through the mother's abdominal wall and, by using a fibro-optic light source, examine parts of the fetus. This will sometimes allow the determination of physical characteristics that may indicate whether or not a problem exists. For example, the physician may see an extra toe which would indicate a certain syndrome exists. Senography uses ultrasound waves to outline the fetus. Structures are identified through different densities. The "visualization" of a deformity such as spina bifida or microcephaly is then possible (Batshaw & Perret, 1981).

Through amniocentesis and the other techniques, over one hundred inherited disorders can be identified (Sells & Bennett, 1977). Unfortunately, work on in-utero treatment has only started in recent years. Therefore, when the disorder is identified, therapeutic abortion is the only alternative parents may have to prevent the occurrence of the disability.

Newborn Screening

Many children born with inborn errors of metabolism can be identified through newborn screening tests. In some cases such as PKU and galactosemia, mental retardation can be prevented through dietary alteration. The PKU test is conducted with newborns before they leave the hospital. The analysis of the blood sample takes about two weeks and if a positive finding results, intervention can proceed immediately. The dietary intervention can prevent the child from becoming mentally retarded if started soon enough.

Generally the diet is only continued until the child is about six years old (Carpenter, 1975). This is because most of the brain's growth has been completed by this age; and there is little chance that damage will occur because of too much phenylalanine. Sometimes, however, physicians suggest the diet be continued indefinitely. This often presents a problem with children who are eager to eat a variety of foods.

The detection of hypothyroidism through birth screening has become possible in the last few years. The process measures the level of thyroxine using the same blood samples used with PKU (Dussault, Coulumbe, Laberge, Letarte, Guyda & Khoury, 1975). Effective thyroid hormone replacement therapy is readily available. The only problem is the diagnostic signs sometime develop slowly during the first six months and unless follow-up screening is done, they will be missed. States are being encouraged to use a two-stage approach: early screening followed by testing during later infant examinations.

Other Preventative Measures

With different problem sources, different methods of prevention can be used. Some intrauterine bacterial infections can be fought through preconceptual vaccinations; for example, rubella. Research is underway for preventing other infections such as cytomegaloviral infections. For some disorders, the only current source of prevention is avoidance. Women with herpes virus at the time of delivery, for example, can have a caesarean-section birth. Radiation, specifically X-ray, is another deleterious source to be avoided. Also of critical significance is alcohol and other nonprescribed drugs which must be avoided. While some disorders such as those due to specific gene defects or chromosomal anomalies cannot be prevented (only aborted), these just mentioned *can* be avoided.

CONCLUSION

During the last couple of decades we have learned a great deal about why some people become mentally retarded. As can be seen, there are many possible reasons. Medical science will never give us a world without mentally retarded persons because of various reasons. For example, genetic mutations will always occur. We can see, however, that many problems can be avoided.

Professionals in the field of mental retardation serve various functions. Providing direct educational and training programs is one of the most important. Another, though, is educating the community about some of the causes of retarded mental functioning. A professional in this field must possess knowledge in various areas including etiology. Such knowledge can be useful when dealing with others concerned with retardation and perhaps with some who are less concerned. While one could not expect expertise on physiology to emerge from an introductory text of this nature, it is hoped that to some degree the material will prove beneficial.

One final note: Students encountering such material as presented in this chapter often express concern over their own plans to become parents. It is certainly not the intention of this book to restrict anyone from the joys of parenting. Two facts should be realized. First, some causes of mental retardation cannot be avoided such as those due to genetic or chromosomal disorders. But, their occurrence is *extremely* rare. The odds are very strong in a couple's favor for having a normal, healthy child. Second, many potential causes of mental retardation are clearly avoidable while still others are probably avoidable with good general health practices and prenatal care. Everyone can do a great deal to help themselves in this latter area and thus avoid many concerns that might otherwise develop.

STUDY QUESTIONS

1. What must happen if a child is to inherit an autosomal recessive gene disorder?
2. Name and describe one syndrome of mental retardation due to an autosomal recessive gene defect.
3. What is the probability that a child whose parent has a dominant gene defect will inherit the disability?
4. Why is Down's syndrome referred to as "trisomy 21"? When does trisomy 21 usually occur?
5. Why do neural tube defects occur?
6. List four prenatal teratogens that may adversely affect normal fetal development.
7. When do most viruses inflict the greatest damage to the developing fetus?
8. What types of problems may occur or be present at birth that may affect the child adversely?
9. Why is screening or carrier detection difficult in the general population? Why is it more possible in smaller, more defined populations such as Ashkenazic Jews?
10. What is amniocentesis most commonly used to detect?

5

Environmental and Social Variables Related to Mental Retardation

OVERVIEW: CORRELATES VERSUS CAUSES OF MENTAL RETARDATION

Not all persons identified as mentally retarded will have a physiological cause such as those described in Chapter 4. A number of them, in fact the majority, will have no known etiology. The purpose of this chapter is to explore some of the possible reasons these persons develop retarded mental functioning.

It is important to stress that the variables discussed cannot be considered "causes" in a strict sense. A more appropriate term for them would be "correlates" since they often occur with the condition but not in a one-to-one fashion. In contrast, when a person has Down's syndrome, he or she will invariably be found to have a trisomy 21 chromosomal pattern. We can conclude, then, that the chromosomal distribution *causes* the retarded level of development and the corresponding physical features of Down's syndrome persons. With the present group, often referred to as the *cultural-familial* mentally retarded (CFMR), we have not been able to identify specific variables that always precede the condition. Instead, we have found only variables that correlate with it. Before discussing a number of these, we will review pertinent descriptive characteristics of the population.

THE CULTURAL-FAMILIAL MENTALLY RETARDED PERSON

The term "cultural-familial" implies two possible sources of these individuals' intellectual status. "Cultural" suggests an environmental basis while "familial" indicates a polygenetic origin. The term was used by Heber (1959) in the AAMD manual on terminology. Previous terms describing these individuals included "subcultural mental deficiency" (Lewis, 1933), "garden-variety mental deficiency" (Sarason, 1953), "endogenous mental deficiency" (Strauss & Lehtinen, 1947), and "familial mental deficiency" (Allen, 1958). Grossman (1977, 1983) referred to this group as being retarded due to "psychosocial disadvantage."

Several writers have provided pertinent descriptions of population and their environs (Girardeau, 1971; Heber, 1959; Heber & Dever, 1970; Jensen, 1970; and Zigler, 1967). Four key descriptors of these individuals are often suggested. First, they generally fall within the psychometric range of mild retardation. Second, there is no "demonstrable biological pathology." Third, they usually have a parent and a brother or sister who are also mildly retarded, and fourth, they grow up in low socioeconomic status homes. Often associated with this last element is minority group membership. However, members of all races will be found in this category.

As stated earlier, the classification of many minorities, particularly blacks, as CFMR has been challenged. The fact is that identification of them as mildly retarded, when it does occur, usually is done within the public school system. It is at this time in life, that is when abstract reasoning abilities are most important, that these individuals tend to have difficulty. During the preschool and postschool years, they will usually not be formally labeled as mentally retarded. Within their cultural parameters, many may indeed function in an acceptable manner.

As children and adults, most cultural-familial retarded persons live predominantly in poor rural areas or in urban ghettos. In one study (Garber & Heber, 1973), it was found that 33% of the EMR school population in Milwaukee came from a portion of the city that had 2% of the city's population. This portion of the city had the lowest median educational level, the lowest median family income, the highest population density per living unit, and the highest rate of dilapidated housing.

As stated above, these individuals are usually classified as mildly retarded. More important, however, is that this intellectual deficit tends to start out at an average level and then decline through the years. Heber, Dever, and Conry (1968), studying children in high-risk environments, found that children under three years were developmentally average. When they examined progressively older children from the same environmental situations, whose mothers had IQs below 80, they found almost a linear decrease in IQ (see Figure 5—1). This cumulative deficit in intelligence has become considered to be a characteristic of these individuals (Miller, 1970).

In addition to this overall decline, different mental characteristics have been found to vary in terms of their relative strength. Individuals within the CFMR population have been shown to be deficient in some areas yet relatively proficient in others. Jensen (1970) formulated a hypothesis of Level I and Level II mental abilities. Level I abilities are primarily associative in nature. An example would be recalling simple facts or information, that is, using short-term memory. Level II abilities are more cognitive such as solving a problem and would require more abstract abilities. Jensen suggested that CFMR individuals are deficient in Level II abilities but not necessarily in Level I abilities.

Parallel to the development of intelligence is the development of language. We might well expect that individuals with lower levels of measured intelligence would have deficient language patterns (Das, 1973). Bernstein (1961) suggested that the language of lower social class individuals is more restricted and descriptive rather than elaborative and analytical. Thus it would seem that the quality and quantity of verbalization is at a lower level in homes that produce CFMR individuals. It should be pointed out, however, that this position has been challenged. Labov (1969) and Cole and Brunner (1971) have taken the position that the language characteristics of lower social class individuals are *different* from the

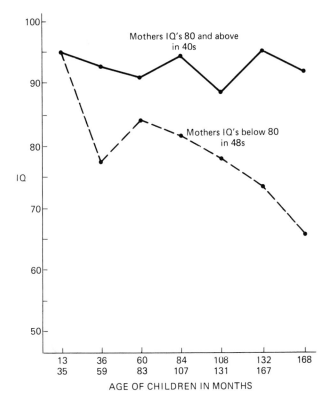

FIGURE 5–1   IQ Change in the Offspring of Disadvantaged Mothers as a Function of Maternal IQ

From Heber, R., Dever, R. B. and Conry, J. The influence of environmental and genetic variables on intellectual development In H .I. Prehm, L, A, Hamerlynck, & J. E. Crosson (Eds.), *Behavioral Research in Mental Retardation.* Eugene, Oregon: University of Oregon, 1968).

middle class, not *deficient*. Still, a distinguishing feature of the CFMR child is often the language he or she uses.

Various other characteristics have also been used to describe many individuals who are cultural-familial mentally retarded. These include being externally motivated, having low levels of self-esteem, lacking in personal control, and being impulsive (Miller, 1970). The applicability of these characteristics will certainly vary with each individual.

CORRELATES OF CULTURAL-FAMILIAL MENTAL RETARDATION

Two different views have been used to "explain" the occurrence of cultural-familial mental retardation. One view purports that a child inherits intellectual abilities from the parents and these abilities are more or less fixed. This is referred to as the "nature" position. The second view posits that the environment of the child affects his or her intellectual ability more than the genetic scheme transmitted by the parents. This is called the "nurture" position. The most commonly held position today is that the two sources interact in some fashion to affect the ultimate level of mature intelligence. The question is more one of degree than one of absolute influence.

Those who believe that intelligence is primarily an inherited trait propose a polygenetic model of inheritance. In contrast to a simple gene, Mendelian type of inheritance (such as is responsible for many of the metabolic disorders and resultant syndromes reviewed in the previous chapter), a polygenetic process of transmission assumes that intelligence is affected by many genes. Such a multiple source of influence is considered to be responsible for the normal distribution of intelligence (Jensen, 1969, 1970).

One of the main areas of research used to support the idea of genetic influence is the IQ correlations found to exist, in varying degrees, between relatives (Jensen, 1970; Vandenberg, 1971; Erlenmeyer-Kimling & Jarvik, 1963; Reed & Reed, 1965). What is shown in these studies is that close relatives (e.g., parent-child, siblings) have highly correlated IQs. As the degree of relatedness decreases, so does the similarity of the IQ. Unrelated persons, including foster parents and their adopted children, have low positive and sometimes even negatively correlated scores. Figure 5–2 displays these different relationships and their corresponding degrees of IQ correlation as reported by Erlenmeyer-Kimling & Jarvik (1963). As you can see in Figure 5–2, the highest correlation is found between monozygotic (one-egg) twins. This is exactly what would be expected because these individuals share an identical set of genes. As the degree of blood relation decreases, so does the range of correlations between IQ scores. From the geneticists' view, this would also be expected since closer relatives would have more genetic similarities. Vandenberg (1971) pointed out that there is nearly a perfect correspondence between median correlations and degree of relatedness.

Another type of evidence used to argue on behalf of genetic influence is the *lack* of change in intelligence following some form of environmental intervention. This was the basis of Jensen's (1969) controversial paper criticizing Head Start and compensatory education programs. Jensen contended that these programs failed to provide substantial gains in the low socioeconomic status (SES) children they served because the children did not inherit the necessary intelligence to learn adequately. Furthermore, Jensen felt that the environment could only serve as a "threshold" variable to influence the development of intelligence. According to this view, in an extremely deprived environment, the effect may serve to restrict the development of intelligence. However, most family environments, according to Jensen (1969), including most of those of low SES

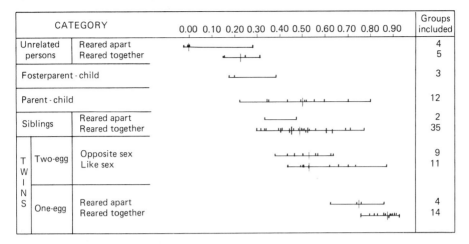

FIGURE 5–2 Correlation Coefficients for "Intelligence" Test Scores From 52 Studies

Correlation coefficients for "intelligence" test scores from 52 studies. Some studies reported data for more than one relationship category; some included more than one sample per category, giving a total of 99 groups. Over two-thirds of the correlation coefficients were derived from I.Q.'s, the remainder from special tests (for example, Primary Mental Abilities). Midparent-child correlation was used when available, otherwise mother-child correlation. Correlation coefficients obtained in each study are indicated by dark circles; medians are shown by vertical lines intersecting the horizontal lines which represent the ranges.

From L. Erlenmeyer-Kimling, and L. F. Jarvik, "Genetics and intelligence: A review," *Science*, December 13, 1963, *142*, 1477–1479. Copyright 1963 by the American Association for the Advancement of Science.

individuals, do not slip below this threshold level. Das (1973) agreed with Jensen on this point, saying that "the extent of sensory deprivation that produces these deleterious effects (in animal studies) can hardly be duplicated in human real-life situations" (p. 10).

The third type of evidence sometimes presented by those who defend genetic influences, is the demonstration of some behavior which can be considered to have a genetic basis. Zigler (1970) pointed out several studies of infants and young children that revealed various individual differences (such as crying) existed among the children prior to a time in their lives when they might have been influenced by the environment. Regarding these studies, he says that "they certainly indicate that individual differences potentially important for later social behavior are present at birth or shortly thereafter" (p. 88). Zigler does acknowledge, however, that the prenatal environment (as opposed to the genetic composition) may have an influence on the differentiation of these infant behaviors. He cites other studies as well purporting to indicate a more or less direct relation between "particular chromosomal properties and general behavioral status." Zigler notes that in regard to these studies, environmental influences have been considered to be a source of the behavioral variation "but a genetic interpretation appears just as plausible" (p. 89).

Probably the single most influential person in promoting the role of the environment as a major determinant of intelligence was J. McVickers Hunt. In his classic book, *Intelligence and Experience* (1961), Hunt challenged the predominant view of the day that intelligence was primarily "predetermined" and "fixed." He offered substantial theoretical and empirical support for the role played by the environment. His position was primarily based on the theories and research of Piaget and Hebb and was presented as an *interactionist* position. This position states that an individual's experience along with his or her genetic draw determines the development of intelligence. Hunt (1961) wrote:

> The encounters that the infant and the child have with the environment in the course of development collaborate with the human genotype in determining the development of those structures and those organizations of central processes within the child's brain that mediate his intelligent behavior. (p. 42)

Leading up to the publication of Hunt's book and subsequent to that time, many studies were conducted with both animals and humans that have shown the environment to be a significant contributor to intelligence. Various writers have reviewed and summarized many of these studies (Haywood & Tapp, 1966; Thomson & Grusec, 1970; Uzgiris, 1970; McCandless, 1964; Hunt & Kirk, 1971). One type of study cited most often is the "early intervention" study. These studies have reported interventions with young children who at the time of the intervention either were considered to be mentally retarded or were considered to be "high risk" children; that is, likely to later be considered retarded.

The idea of early intervention for high-risk children grew out of the concept of a "critical period" of development. Thompson and Grusec (1970) wrote that this concept suggests that at a particular early age, certain responses are learned which are more or less irreversible and that this early learning will have an impact on later functioning. A stronger position is that if the organism misses an opportunity for learning or developing during the critical period, the opportunity may be lost forever (Haywood & Tapp, 1966).

If one believes that the early environment influences intellectual development, then it should be possible to isolate some components of the environment that affect intellectual development. This involves an analysis of the learning process including the effect of specific environmental variables. In this area of research (variables affecting the development of CFMR individuals), there has been little specificity as to what these variables are. More often, researchers have presented the "environment" in a more global way (Girardeau, 1971). Therefore, the importance of some variables can only be inferred. Some of these are presented below.

Motivational Influences

One set of variables that may be relevant to the intellectual development of CFMR individuals are those of a motivational nature. Pavenstedt (1965) noted that low SES children are often taught by their parents to obey, conform, and work hard for teacher approval, but are not motivated for the purpose of knowledge acquisition. Taba (1964) reported that greater stress was placed on "getting by" rather than "getting ahead" in deprived homes. Similarly, Terrell, Durkin, and Wiesley (1959) reported that disadvantaged children showed a preference for concrete rewards. The attainment of more abstract types of reinforcement (e.g., the attainment of knowledge for knowledge's sake) did not seem to be as motivating. Furthermore, research has indicated that these children do not do well under situations of delayed gratification (Miller, 1970). We should note that normal school conditions do not provide concrete rewards, and the abstract reinforcement provided (i.e., grades) is often delayed.

Stimulational Influences

We can also look at environmental events that may stimulate perceptual and cognitive behavior. It is believed that a fairly consistent, uniform environment is necessary for the child to acquire many basic perceptual and cognitive processes. This seems to be lacking in the home of some cultural-familial retarded children. Klaus and Gray (1968), in a report on their project, wrote about the "temporal and spacial disorganization" found in many low SES homes. For example, no particular objects were located in one place consistently. They reported that "there is no undisturbed occasion for a toddler to explore an object thoroughly" (p. 7). They also found that most homes lacked a systematic scheduling of activities such as regular mealtimes and bedtimes. Such variation or discontinuity in the environment has been suggested by McCandless (1970) to have an adverse effect on cognitive behavior.

We may typically think of the deprived environment as being understimulating, but some have indicated that there is too much stimulation in some lower SES homes and that this is not beneficial for development. Pavenstedt (1965) noted that in many homes the television set was always on. The continual auditory stimulation may affect the infant's ability to discriminate auditorily and thus the auditory channel may become less well developed (Deutsch, 1964), or the child might learn to tune out the bombardment of sound.

The specific type of stimuli and stimulus conditions necessary for cognitive development is not known. The conditions that are found in many poverty-stricken homes are sometimes bleak and unstimulating. Many basic items found in middle-class homes such as mobiles, music boxes, storybooks, pictures, and games are not present in some low SES homes that generate many CFMR children. We cannot say that the presence of these items in middle-class homes or the absence of them in poor homes causes the typical level of intelligence and academic abilities attained by the respective groups. Again, we are left with essentially correlational data.

Language Influences

Language is generally considered to be an important component of intelligence if not the central aspect of it. In many poverty-stricken homes, language has been considered to be underdeveloped. A study by Hess and Shipman (1965) is one most often cited on this topic. Their findings indicated that a paucity of verbal communication existed in many low SES homes. The effect may be to restrict verbal development with the implication of restricting cognitive development. Both the quantity and quality of language is lower than that found in higher SES homes. Children interact less with adults (Keller, 1963) and their verbalizations are shorter in length (Deutsch, 1965). As might be expected, the development of expressive and receptive vocabulary and the complexity of sentence forms by disadvantaged children are all below the norms for the general population (Miller, 1970).

Nutritional and Health Influences

Certainly one of the most distinguishing characteristics of the low SES families that produce CFMR children is the level of nutritional intake. Simply stated, poor people have poor nutritional characteristics (Chan & Rueda, 1979; Das, 1973; Perkins, 1977). Perkins suggested that because of a lack of money and knowledge, these families tend to eat nutritionally insufficient foods. The prevalence of poor diets is at least four times as great for families with low SES status as for middle-class families (Perkins, 1977). Bakan (1970) wrote that "the most noxious of poverty's effects is malnutrition, and the most important cause of malnutrition is poverty." Even theorists who typically look more toward heredity than environmental variables as the source of CFMR acknowledge the role that malnutrition can play in reducing mental development (Das, 1973; Ginsburg & Laughlin, 1971).

While the significance of malnutrition of the mother during pregnancy has been debated by some, Perkins (1977) suggested that during the most rapid period of brain development (fifty days prenatal to forty days postnatal), severe malnutrition may stifle the rate of cellular division and thus reduce the ultimate number of cells in the brain. The effect of poor nutritional intake by older children, if not associated directly with brain growth and cognitive development, is certainly associated with poor health and a variety of diseases.

There are obviously more health problems within low SES homes as compared to the general population. MacDonald (1965) pointed out that the occurrence of health problems in disadvantaged homes is four times the number found in homes with higher income levels. Scrimshaw (1968) noted that in poorer developing countries, children between the ages of one and four have a mortality rate that is twenty to forty times greater than the rate in North America and Europe. Some of the diseases include meningitis, measles, encephalitis, diphtheria, whooping cough, scarlet fever, nephritis, and pneumonia (Perkins, 1977).

In order to fully experience and benefit from the environment, a healthy brain in a healthy body is essential. When considered in combination with prenatal and earlier postnatal nutritional deprivation, later poor nutrition and poor health could certainly be detrimental.

PREVENTING CULTURAL-FAMILIAL RETARDATION
THROUGH EARLY INTERVENTION

Covering a span of almost fifty years, various researchers have attempted to offset the effects of detrimental environmental conditions by intervening in the early lives of mentally retarded children or children who were apt to become mentally retarded. Three ideas promoted the practice of early intervention. These were the belief in the critical-period concept, the belief that intelligence is in a stage of plasticity during the early years, and the belief that cultural-familial mental retardation results in a gradual decline in intelligence, decreasing from an average to a below-average level (Caldwell, 1970).

The critical-period concept is based largely on animal studies but has been questioned as a narrow aspect of human cognitive development (Clarke & Clarke, 1976, 1977). Plasticity of intelligence has, of course, generally been accepted by environmentalists (Hunt, 1961) with major support for this concept provided by Bloom (1964). Through his analysis of several longitudinal studies on measured intellectual development, Bloom demonstrated that as a child grows older, more and more of his or her mature intelligence becomes obvious. The converse of this finding was that there was little or no correlation between a child's early measured intelligence and measured intelligence at maturity. It thus seemed logical that early intelligence was flexible, that is, it was not already determined. Early intervention was considered to be a way to influence intelligence before it reached a more fixed and depressed state at maturity. Additionally, evidence emerged (Heber et al, 1968) that high-risk children were actually *not* below average at birth but that intellectual deterioration occurred (see Figure 5—1). Some early intervention efforts were designed to prevent this occurrence.

There have been many attempts at early intervention and many reports of these attempts. In a sense, Head Start was such a project, but it was not meant specifically to prevent or ameliorate CFMR (Zigler & Cascione, 1978). Aside from this massive project, the separate individual programs that have been tried must certainly number in the hundreds. These programs have varied greatly in their philosophies, curricula, methods, durations, and outcomes. There have been several reviews of these studies that the interested reader would find most informative (Stedman, 1977; Tjossem, 1976; Horowitz & Paden, 1973; Kirk, 1970; Miller, 1970; Payne, Mercer & Epstein, 1974; Caldwell, 1970). A brief review of four prominent studies is presented below.

The earliest, most commonly cited study was conducted by Skeels and his coworkers at the Iowa Child Welfare Station (Skeels, 1966; Skeels & Dye, 1939). These researchers placed several retarded children below the age of three from a relatively depressive environment (an orphanage) into an institution for the mentally retarded and instructed some of the women in the institution in the proper care of the children. These women provided for the children's needs but, more importantly, provided them with a great deal of stimulation. Subsequent to the placement, the children were found to gain substantially on intelligence test scores while a control group of children who remained in the orphanage actually decreased in IQ points. Twenty-five years after the original placement, Skeels (1966) conducted a follow-up and found that the experimental group of individuals were all leading normal lives. None were considered to be mentally retarded. The control subjects, on the other hand, had only completed a median educational level of the third grade, four were institutionalized, and only two had married. This classic study was an important forerunner to more recent studies.

Bereiter and Engelmann (1966) reported a highly structured preschool program in which they attempted to improve the language functioning and cognitive development of 4½ year-old culturally deprived children. It was their belief that a well organized, systematic instructional environment was necessary for these children to show significant gains. In their instructional process they provided very distinct cues and consequences in the teaching of language and academic skills. Substantial gains were made by the children in the areas of language, arithmetic, and spelling. By the end of two years in the program (after the completion of kindergarten), the children were reading at a 1.5 grade level, doing arithmetic at a 2.6 grade level, and spelling at a 1.7 grade level.

Another study, the Early Training Project in Tennessee (Klaus & Gray, 1968) provided instruction to sixty-two disadvantaged children. There were four groups: a three-year experimental group, a two-year experimental group, a local control group, and a distal control group. For the experimental groups, two or three ten-week summer programs were provided along with a home-based instructional program during the rest of the year. The program was designed to develop specific skills but also healthy attitudes toward learning. Both experimental groups differed from control groups in word knowledge, word recognition, and reading, but not in arithmetic or spelling. What was more interesting, however, was that there was a "vertical diffusion" effect with the younger siblings of the experimental group. When compared to the siblings of the control subjects, the experimental group siblings had a mean IQ that was 13 points higher.

A study of particular interest was conducted by Heber and his colleagues (Garber & Heber, 1973; Heber & Dever, 1970; Heber & Garber, 1975) which has generally been referred to as the Milwaukee Project. This project was developed in an attempt to prevent a decline in the intelligence level of high risk, low socioeconomic black children (Garber & Heber, 1973). The developers of the project felt that most early intervention programs, which began just before the disadvantaged children began school, started too late. They felt a greater impact could occur if intervention was started earlier. They wanted to intervene before the children passed their "critical period" of development.

Over an eighteen-month period, Heber and his colleagues identified newborn infants born in a high risk area of Milwaukee. Forty mother-child pairs were ultimately included. As the children were born, they were assigned either to the experimental or the control group until there were twenty mother-child dyads in both groups.

In the infant stimulation program, project staff worked with the mothers and infants in the home until the child was three to six months of age. Between three and six months the infants began attending a special center. Until the child was twenty-four months old, one staff member was responsible for providing care and stimulation. At twenty-four months, the children were grouped three per teacher and began following a rigorous daily schedule that began at 8:45 A.M. and continued to 4:00 P.M. It included a breakfast, lunch, and snack; six structured learning periods; Sesame Street; self-directed free play; and a motor development period. The structured learning periods included language training, reading readiness, arithmetic, problem solving, reading, art, and music.

The researchers considered their model to be eclectic. They wanted to develop the children intellectually, socially, emotionally, and physically and prevent deficits in language, problem solving, and achievement motivation. The two main emphases of the program were language development and cognitive development.

The first important differences between the experimental and control groups were seen at eighteen months on the Gesell Scales, a measure of infant intellectual development. At this time the control group was about at the norm but was three to four months below the experimental group. At twenty-two months the experimental group was four and a half to six months ahead of the control group in all areas on the Gesell. In language development, between eighteen months and three years, the experimental group had relatively broad vocabulary and said more in conversation. The control group reached the same level of vocabulary development at two and a half years as the experimental group had achieved by one and a half years. On speech imitation, which started being assessed every six months beginning at three years of age, the experimental group had significantly less omissions, substitutions, and additions. At ages three, four, and five years, the experimental group had significantly better grammar, always scoring at least one year ahead of the control subjects. At fifty-four months, based on the Illinois Test of Psycholinguistic Abilities, the experimental children had a mean psycholinguistic age (PLA) of sixty-three months while the control children's mean PLA was forty-five months.

The mean IQ for the experimental children between twenty-four and sixty-six months was 123.4; for the control subjects, it was 94.8. At sixty-six months, the mean IQ for the experimental children was 125; for the control children, it was ninety-one.

After six years of operation, the project was ended in 1973. A follow-up of the children after they entered public schools was reported by Garber and Heber (1977). At seventy-two months, the experimental children had a mean IQ of 121 compared to eighty-seven for the control group. At eighty-six months, the means were 105 vs. 81; at ninety-six months, 106 vs. 84; and at 108 months, 109 vs. 81. While the mean IQ of the experimental group dropped somewhat, it remained 20 points greater than that of the control group. The two lowest experimental group children had IQs of 88—well above the EMR criterion. One-third of the control group had IQs below 75.

Of the many early intervention programs that have been conducted, the Milwaukee Project was certainly one of the most comprehensive. Yet this project and many others have been criticized. They have been criticized on experimental methodology, on results, and on theoretical grounds (Page, 1975; Brofenbrenner, 1976; Clarke & Clarke, 1976, 1977). Thus there has not been uniform acceptance of their results among professionals. Notwithstanding this and similar criticism, however,

Stedman (1977) examined forty longitudinal studies involving high-risk children and drew thirteen major conclusions from his analysis. These included the following:

1. The manner in which a child is reared and the environment into which he is born have a major impact on what he will become.
2. Factors such as race and sex do not appear to be related to the child's ability to profit from intervention programs.
3. The family's methods of establishing social roles leave little doubt that early family environment (parental language styles, attitudes toward achievement, parental involvement and concern for the child) has a significant impact on the child's development before he reaches his second birthday.
4. In situations where families are so disorganized that they cannot supply a supportive environment, an intensive external supportive environment may contribute to the child's development.
5. The effects of a stimulating or depriving environment appear to be most powerful in the early years of childhood when the most rapid growth and development take place. The primary focus of the child during these early years is the home. Therefore, home-based intervention programs or one-to-one teacher-child ratio stimulation activities appear to be the most appropriate and effective during this period.
6. There is evidence that the effects of early intervention programs for children are strengthened by the involvement of the child's parents.
7. It is only possible to describe the training conditions that handicap a child or lead to a child's success in general terms.
8. The socioeconomic status and entry level IQ of the child bear an uncertain relationship to the child's ability to profit from intervention. Design problems and the current state of the art in measurement render the effect of these factors difficult to determine.
9. Where access to children can be gained in early years, preferably during the language emergent years (one to two years of age) intervention programs will be more effective than those begun in later years.
10. A systematic, organized program can contribute significantly to a child's social and intellectual development between the ages of four and six years.
11. The effects of intervention programs appear to last only so long as the child remains in the intervention program. They appear to last longer in home training studies and to "wash out" sooner in school programs.
12. Follow-up studies of children in intervention programs usually show that initial gains are no longer measurable. This is partially attributable to the fact that we cannot determine at this point whether it is due to program failure, to problems of measurement, to inadequate criterion measures, or to the later interfering effects of competing environments, such as the home and school.
13. The quality and motivation of the staff are directly related to the success of the program and therefore are prime factors in determining the extent to which a program is exportable or replicable. (pp. 2—3)

It is clear that certain children can be considered at risk for becoming classified as cultural-familial mildly retarded. It is also apparent that many demographic factors can predict the problems these children will face. Ramey and his colleagues (Finkelstein & Ramey, 1980; Ramey & Brownlee, 1981; Ramey, Stedman, Borders-Patterson & Mengel, 1978) found that some of the information available on a child's birth certificate in many cases could predict that the child would have academic difficulty if not become classified as mentally retarded. It is unfortunate that such variables as the race of the child (black), the sex (male), and a low educational level of the mother foretold the difficulties for the child (Ramey et al., 1978).

CONCLUSION

Cultural-familial mental retardation is most obviously a baffling area. Many suggest it has a strong heredity basis. Others cite detrimental environmental effects as the source of the problem. Both groups concede that, at least to some extent, both genetics and environment must be involved, but the main question is to what degree. While the inferences are strong, there is no clear genetic structure that can be identified as being differentially responsible for intellectual development. It is the same with environmental factors. While certainly the typical poverty home environment seems to have many factors that correlate with depressed intelligence, nothing has been found to definitely cause such an effect.

Early intervention efforts may hold the greatest promise for preventing cultural-familial mental retardation or reducing its effect. Even though some notable researchers have questioned the efficacy of these efforts, there is enough evidence to warrant continued research if not full-scale program implementation. Current law (PL 94—142) requires public schools to provide services to handicapped children beginning at three years of age. This is clearly a positive direction. However, there are two major problems. One is that these children are often not identified as "handicapped" until they begin school, and they do not begin school until they are five or six years old. At this age, of course, they may not be as susceptible to early or preventative intervention as at an earlier time in their lives. A second problem is that the law, even if it is fully enacted for these children, may not be enough. At three years of age the children may already be beyond the potentially positive impact of early intervention. Furthermore, typical public school intervention may not include the element of home intervention and this appears to be an important aspect of successful projects.

Some researchers, such as Ramey and his colleagues, have begun providing important information on the identification of high-risk children. As their work and that of other professionals continue, society will have to decide whether serious efforts should be undertaken to try to prevent cultural-familial mental retardation.

STUDY QUESTIONS

1. Why is it not possible to say what causes cultural-familial retardation?
2. Name four descriptive characteristics of the cultural-familial mentally retarded population.
3. How does the measured intelligence of the cultural-familial mentally retarded vary over the years?
4. What is meant by "nature" and "nurture"?
5. Briefly discuss the evidence used to support the "nature" position.
6. What is meant by the "interactionist" position and how is it defended?
7. What type of studies are often used to defend the environmentalist position?
8. How might motivational, cognitive and perceptual, language, and nutritional and health factors influence the development of CFMR individuals?
9. Why has *early* intervention been considered a feasible approach to preventing CFMR?

Cognitive Development, Learning Processes, and Learning Products

OVERVIEW

In order to better understand mentally retarded people, researchers have studied their cognitive development, learning processes, and learning products or outcomes. Cognitive development implies a sequence or course of change that can be described in terms of mental age (MA) or developmental stages (such as Piaget's stages). Learning is a generic term that implies a change in an individual's responses or response potential (Scott, 1978). Learning processes are specific mechanisms that operate during the occurrence of learning, while learning products are the outcome of learning that allows us to function in our environment.

In this chapter, we will look at two indicators of cognitive development: mental age and various cognitive processes. In the area of learning, research on learning processes and products will be considered. Particular process abilities to be discussed include attention, memory, organizing information and using logic, operant learning, observational learning, and incidental learning. Additionally, learning products including language, reading, and arithmetic characteristics are reviewed in this chapter.

COGNITIVE DEVELOPMENT

A person's mental age theoretically describes his or her level of cognitive development. It does so in relation to other people; that is, it is a normative-referenced measure. If a person is of average intelligence (IQ = 100), his or her MA is assumed to equal his or her CA. The ratio formula for IQ is $\frac{MA}{CA} \times 100$. Therefore $MA = \frac{IQ \times CA}{100}$. A "normal" ten-year-old child's MA equals 10. A ten-year-old with a ratio IQ of 50 will have an MA of five years. If a person is of average intelligence, we can expect the MA to grow at the same rate as the CA, at least up to a point. While we know that retarded individuals will have MAs below their CA, it is also important to know how this MA develops.

Mental Age Development of Mentally Retarded Persons

Various studies have shown different kinds of changes of the MAs and IQs of mentally retarded people as their chronological ages increase. Some of the studies have shown decreases in IQ, others have shown increases, while still others have shown general stability of the IQ. One problem with many of these studies is that their samples have had limited age ranges.

In an effort to better understand this problem, Fisher and Zeaman (1970) investigated changes in MAs and IQs of over 1,000 mentally retarded people at different chronological ages. A semilongitudinal method of data collection was used (see Fisher & Zeaman [1970] for details). This allowed the researchers to look at MA and IQ changes that spanned from below five years of age to above 60 years of age. Figure 6–1 depicts what was found about MA development. This figure indicates that the MA growth at various levels of retardation is initially linear. The slopes of these linear portions of growth are all below that of normal growth. This means that the rate of MA growth is slower than that of normal persons. Additionally, the slopes decrease with lower levels of intelligence. In other words, the lower the level of intelligence, the lower the rate of MA growth. These findings were somewhat expected by Fisher and Zeaman (1970). However, the *length of time* of MA growth by the retarded subjects was *not* expected. It was found that maximum MA attainment came at 25 years for the severely retarded and as late as 35 years for the moderately,

FIGURE 6–1 Semilongitudinal Growth

Mean semilongitudinal MA growth functions for the five levels of retardation. Numbers on the curves refer to number of subjects measured.

From M. A. Fisher, and D. Zeaman, "Growth and decline of retardate intelligence," in N. R. Ellis (Ed.) *International review of research in mental retardation* (Vol. 4). New York: Academic Press, 1970. Reprinted by permission.

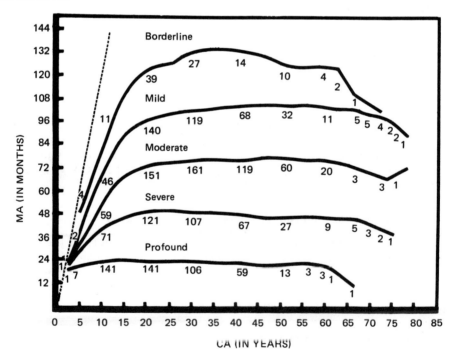

mildly, and borderline retarded groups. As Figure 6–1 also depicts, MA tended to drop off after 60 years of age. Fisher and Zeaman found no differences in MA development due to sex or etiology.

Figure 6–2 depicts Fisher and Zeaman's (1970) findings in terms of IQ scores. As can be seen, the IQs tend to *decrease* until about the age of twenty and then to *increase* or *stabilize* for a period of time at subsequent ages. This can be explained by the fact that the maximum CA denominator used to calculate IQs is usually sixteen or eighteen. This may also

FIGURE 6–2   Age Changes in IQ

Age changes in IQ for the five levels of retardation computed semilongitudinally.

From M. A. Fisher, and D. Zeaman, "Growth and decline of retardate intelligence," in N. R. Ellis (Ed.) *International review of research in mental retardation* (Vol. 4). New York: Academic Press, 1970. Reprinted by permission.

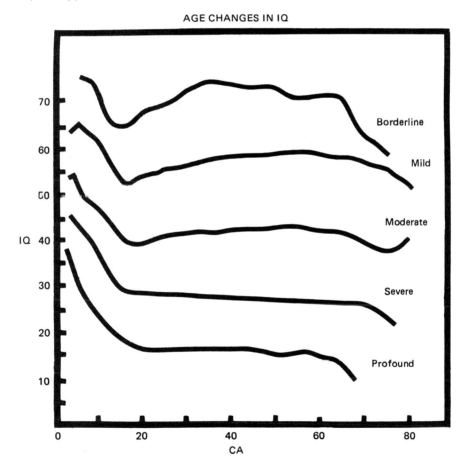

AGE CHANGES IN IQ

provide some explanation as to why previous studies of changes in IQs for retarded people had equivocal results; i.e., restricted age ranges were sampled.

Fisher and Zeaman's study has since been essentially replicated by Demaine and Silverstein (1978) with the same results. These studies offer two important implications. First, they provide a quantitative description of the mental development of retarded individuals representing several levels of intelligence. Second, this quantification describes a mental growth rate which does not stop at sixteen or eighteen as with normal persons (at least theoretically), but continues to develop well into the adult years. While the level of mental maturity attained does not reach normalcy, this pattern of growth indicates a relatively extensive period of cognitive development.

Qualitative vs. Quantitative Aspects of Mental Development

While mental age provides a useful quantitative description of cognitive functioning, some theorists have suggested that it does not provide a true picture of the *qualitative* aspects of cognition. They say that while a person with a measured level of retarded intelligence may have the same measured mental age as a younger child of average intelligence, the two would not demonstrate the same type of cognitive processing. There would be a difference in the quality of cognition.

This possibility is not difficult to understand. There are various ways by which one can achieve a certain mental age on an intelligence test. For example, a person might pass some items on the test while failing others. A different person might have just the opposite performance on some of the same items. Both may end up with the same mental age. Another possibility is that two people may use different strategies on the same item and be equally successful or unsuccessful.

The quantitative versus qualitative issue of mental development has generally been limited to mildly retarded individuals with cultural-familial etiologies. On one side of the issue are the developmental theorists (Zigler, 1967, 1969; Balla & Zigler, 1971; Humphreys & Parsons, 1979). Their position is that cultural-familial retardation simply represents the lower end of the continuum of the normal distribution of intelligence. Cultural-familial mildly retarded individuals, say the developmentalists, simply have a "naturally" lower level of intellectual ability. However, they maintain that although their IQs are lower, when matched with normal younger individuals of about the same level of mental development (generally meant to be mental age), CFMR persons operate in a cognitively similar fashion as do the normal individuals (Zigler, 1969). Figure 6–3 represents the developmentalist model suggested by Zigler (1969). The

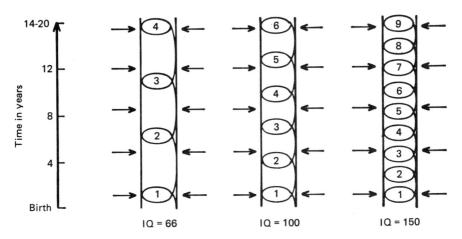

FIGURE 6–3 Developmental Model of Cognitive Growth

Developmental model of cognitive growth. The single vertical arrow represents the passage of time. The horizontal arrows represent environmental events impinging on the individual who is represented as a pair of vertical lines. The individual's cognitive development appears as an internal ascending spiral, in which the numbered loops represent successive stages of cognitive growth.

From E. Zigler, "Developmental versus difference theories of mental retardation and the problem of motivation," *American Journal of Mental Deficiency*, 1969, 73, 536–556. Reprinted by permission.

cultural-familial child is said to differ from the nonretarded child in only two ways cognitively: the rate of development is slower, and the final stage of development is lower than that achieved by normal individuals.

Various other theorists disagree with the developmental point of view (e.g., Das, 1972; Das, Kirby & Jarman, 1975; Ellis, 1969; Milgram, 1971). They suggest that the cognitive abilities of CFMR individuals and MA matched normal individuals are different. Their position is referred to as a "difference" position or in some cases a "defect" position. Basically, these theorists maintain that equal MA does not dictate equal cognitive processes.

Much research tends to support the difference position (Das, 1972; Das et al., 1975; Das & Cummins, 1978; Jarman, 1978; Stephens & McLaughlin, 1974). The Stephens and McLaughlin study serves as a good example because of its extensiveness. These researchers studied 75 mildly retarded and 75 nonretarded children with each group comprising three age levels. Twenty-nine Piagetian reasoning tasks were administered at different ages. When both CA and MA were controlled (matched), significant differences were found on twenty of the twenty-nine tasks. The differences were primarily in operational thought. The authors stated that "significant differences which are not accounted for by CA or MA do exist between the operational thought of nonretarded and retarded persons. These differences appear to involve the categorization, flexibility, and reversibility involved in tasks involving conservation and classification" (Stephens & McLaughlin, 1974, p. 126). This study and others seem to indicate that qualitative cognitive differences exist between the two groups.

For several reasons, however, firm conclusions cannot be drawn. One main problem is that MA may not be the right index to match when studying qualitative differences or similarities. Zigler (1969) suggests that MA is only a rough index of cognition. Thus a finer measure may be needed. Woodward (1979) agreed. She pointed out that "a mental age score is a hodgepodge of passes on a variety of items; even a narrow range of mental age scores in one group may comprise a number of different combinations of items that are passed, a variety that is not necessarily matched in the same way in the other group" (p. 174).

Another problem about accepting the qualitative difference hypothesis is that other subject variables not accounted for by mental age or cognitive development may affect performance. Zigler (1969) proposed that institutionalization, motivation, or "outerdirectedness" may have such a bearing. Additionally, it has been suggested that in some cases the etiology of the mentally retarded subjects used in some of the studies may not have been restricted to cultural-familial retardation. In other words, organically impaired individuals may have been included and confounded the results.

A study reported by Kamhi (1981) attempted to correct some of the flaws of earlier studies. In this study, all of the mentally retarded subjects "showed no history of organic etiology" (i.e., were cultural-familial). Additionally, they were narrowly matched on MA (± 3 months). Six Piagetian tasks were administered and performances were compared. The results contradicted many earlier findings. On one task, the mentally retarded children performed *better* than did the MA matched normal children. On the five other tasks, there were no significant differences. Kamhi suggested that "the similar performances of the retarded and non-retarded children on the six cognitive tasks clearly support the development theory of retardation; that is, that children matched for MA will demonstrate similar cognitive abilities" (p. 5).

Piaget's Theory of Cognitive Development and the Mentally Retarded

As Fisher and Zeaman (1970) showed us, the MA development of retarded persons is quite orderly. It should be of interest to us also to note the nature of Piagetian cognitive development regardless of its relationship to mental age. That is, given Piaget's well-known order of development, to what degree do mentally retarded persons of various levels follow this order and what cognitive stage is ultimately reached? Woodward (1963, 1979) has provided excellent and full reviews of this literature.

The early development of normal children (0–18 months) consists of the sensorimotor period. It might be expected that all mentally retarded persons, at different ages, would pass through this stage. For lower-level individuals, such as the severely and profoundly retarded, there may be no development beyond this stage. Wohlhueter and Sindberg (1975) studied object permanence in young, retarded children of various levels of intelligence. Tasks were given monthly for twelve to eighteen months, and the children's performances were observed. Children with major brain damage made little progress, remaining at a low level of sensorimotor development. Those who appeared to have less damage progressed more.

Woodward (1979) suggested that various factors could affect performance within the sensorimotor period although progressive sequential development seemed to be the rule. These factors might be expected to affect more severely retarded individuals. For example, seizures or the drug treatment used to control them may affect measured performance. Motivation may be another factor, particularly with institutionalized children. Another factor might be the lack of opportunity to interact with various aspects of the environment. These impediments could disallow the development of some processes or cause individuals to lose previously attained abilities. Silverstein, Pearson, Colbert, Cordeiro, Marwin, and Nakaji (1982) analyzed the development of severely and profoundly retarded persons over a five year period in the areas of object permanence and spatial relations. They found very slight gains in most of their subjects, primarily in spatial relations. While their gains were not particularly impressive, they were statistically significant. Silverstein and his colleagues suggested that more structured programs might have resulted in greater gains.

Piaget's preconceptual period, which normally occurs between one-and-a-half to four-and-a-half or five years, has not been extensively studied as it occurs in mentally retarded persons. Woodward (1962, 1972) and Woodward and Hunt (1972) analyzed the development of seriating, classifying, and handling spatial relations of moderately retarded children. They found that abilities in the preconceptual stage proceeded ordinally. Moderately retarded children between the ages of six and eleven years failed to reach an intuitive thought level, with the younger children remaining at a substantially lower preconceptual level and the older children advancing to a higher level. The frequency of intuitive thinking was found to increase in moderately retarded children when they advance beyond a CA of eleven years.

Research in the relatively higher levels of cognition, such as intuition and concrete operations, has generally focused on the developmental versus difference issue of MA discussed earlier. Some of the research, however, has also been concerned with the ontogeny of cognitive processes. Again the work of Stephens and her colleagues (Stephens, McLaughlin, Miller, & Glass, 1972; Stephens & McLaughlin, 1974) provides some of the most complete data on this topic, even though it dealt with only the mildly retarded. Development was found to occur sequentially from ages six to fourteen years, but not within the fourteen to eighteen year range. A two-year follow-up, however, showed gains in all groups including the oldest group. This indicates that like MA (Fisher & Zeaman, 1970), Piagetian cognitive development tends to continue occurring at least into the early years of adulthood for the mildly retarded.

LEARNING PROCESSES

A large number of studies have been conducted to determine what specific aspects of retarded persons' learning processes impede their ability to acquire knowledge and information in an adequate fashion. It is not enough to say that these individuals are simply not efficient learners because they are mentally retarded. Such logic can become quite circular. Instead we need to know more precisely how different mechanisms of learning operate. To this end various researchers have investigated some rather specific aspects of learning and have developed several theories which attempt to explain, at least in part, why mentally retarded individuals do not learn as well as do nonretarded persons.

Attention

One difficulty encountered by many retarded individuals is their inability to attend to the appropriate or necessary dimensions of a particular stimulus or object. Any given stimulus will have various dimensions such as shape, size, color, position, and weight. Normally a person learns which dimensions and which cues (square, red, large, etc.) within the dimensions hold the necessary information to select or act upon the stimulus. For example, we may select the correct key to open our front door by first attending to color, shape, and size, and then selecting the key that is gold in color, having a unique pattern, and longer than the others on one key ring. Researchers have found that mentally retarded individuals have a lower probability of attending to the correct dimensions and thus making the appropriate discrimination (Zeaman & House, 1963; Fisher & Zeaman, 1973; Zeaman and House, 1979). The lower the person's IQ and MA, the longer it will take to learn the appropriate attentional response and perform the discriminatory behavior. The greater the number of dimensions that must be attended to for the learning to occur, the longer the learning will take. Additionally, some mentally retarded learners may show preference for certain dimensions over others (Zeaman & House, 1979). If the preferred dimension is not the one necessary for them to perform correctly, their discrimination ability may be further hindered.

When we consider the attention/discrimination process and the almost continuous role it plays in our normal activities, we can see how a deficit in the area would hamper general learning. The discovery of this disability by researchers not only allows us to better understand the learning difficulty of retarded persons, it also helps us find more suitable instructional tactics.

Memory

Memory is demonstrated when a person acts in a specific fashion based on some form of stimulus or information that has been presented at an earlier point in time. Early research by Ellis (1963) proposed that mentally retarded individuals, specifically the mildly retarded, had a deficit in short-term memory, that is, recalling information that had just been presented. Ellis attributed this deficiency to an inadequate neurological structure that resulted in a quick attenuation of the "stimulus trace" mechanism. This meant that the impact of the stimulus did not remain physiologically in place long enough for the memory to function adequately. Later Ellis (1970) modified his theory and developed a multistore memory model. Under this scheme information was seen to pass through a number of memory stores including very short-term memory (VSTM, sometimes called iconic memory), primary memory (PM, sometimes referred to as an echoic buffer), secondary memory (SM), and tertiary memory (TM). In addition to these stores, two processes were included in the model: an attentional-perceptual process and a rehearsal process. The attentional-perceptual mechanism translates sensory impressions and selects stimulus material from VSTM and moves it to PM. Rehearsal does two things. It "recirculates" material through PM and keeps it from being forgotten and it moves information from PM to SM. Rehearsal may consist of the simple repetition of information such as saying a phone number over and over again or using a more complex strategy to organize and retain some bit of information.

Research on the use of different types of memory stores by mentally retarded persons has been conducted. Detterman (1979) and Mercer and Snell (1977) reviewed much of this research. From his review, Detterman tentatively concluded that mentally retarded individuals have relative deficits in all areas of memory. The greatest difference between retarded and nonretarded persons is probably in VSTM and the transfer from VSTM to PM. In PM, SM, and TM (sometimes the latter two are referred to together as long-term memory) the findings are mixed: some researchers have reported deficits, some have not. At present the safest conclusion is that retarded persons are most likely to have difficulty with immediate or short-term recall. If the material can pass through these stages, it may be retained for a period of time comparable to nonretarded persons.

One key to improving short-term memory and thus enhancing the amount of information stored in long-term memory, may be the use of rehearsal tactics. Detterman (1979) wrote:

> In general, rehearsal includes everything from relatively simple processes such as naming and repetition of items as they are presented to more complex operations like chunking and the formulation of retrieval plans. The major function of rehearsal seems to be to increase the probability of recalling information by maintaining it in PM for as long as possible, thereby moving it to SM; and by attempting to reduce the load the information places on the memory system. (p. 748)

There seems to be a general deficit in rehearsal ability by mentally retarded persons (Ellis, 1970). Given time to rehearse previously presented material, normal individuals benefit whereas many mentally retarded individuals do not. Similarly, various studies have been conducted on the use of mediational or elaboration strategies. In such studies, the procedures require the subjects to produce key words so as to associate the second item of paired-associates with the first. For example, if you are shown pictures of a dog and a house and are told to remember that they go together, you might say or think, "There's a *dog* in the *house*." Generally, mentally retarded subjects will not use such mediational or elaboration strategies to the same extent as do nonretarded persons. Subsequently, their recall is not as good as is that of average intelligence subjects. What is more interesting, however, is that some mentally retarded individuals can be taught to effectively use mediational strategies in some situations (Belmont & Butterfield, 1974; Brown, 1974). This finding has led to the belief that the problem is not so much in the ability to *use* a strategy but in *selecting* the correct strategy to use.

Organizing Information and Using Logic

The ability to take in a quantity of information, organize it, and then apply it to a problem or need in a logical fashion allows most of us to function adequately in our daily lives. Many mentally retarded people are at a disadvantage in this ability area, often not possessing the organizational and logical skills we use routinely. Spitz (1963, 1966, 1973, 1976, & 1979) has directed a considerable amount of thought, theory, and research toward understanding mentally retarded persons' functioning in this area. From his early research, Spitz (1963) concluded that because of cellular "sluggishness" in the cortex, mentally retarded persons are unable to organize input as well as do nonretarded persons. This could result in the short-term memory deficit discussed above. Equally problematic, it would impede the normal "chunking" of information (e.g. dog–house) used by most people to help store and retrieve information (Spitz, 1966). Spitz emphasized the necessity for a great deal of rehearsal in order to help mentally retarded persons retain information. Furthermore, in his later writing Spitz (1979) pointed out that some research indicated that if retarded persons were induced to organize or "chunk" material together, they could learn to do so and would benefit by recalling more material. Unfortunately, the ability to transfer this tactic to new situations was often found to be deficient making generalized problem-solving difficult.

In order to study the use of problem-solving strategies more directly, Spitz and his colleagues (e.g., Spitz & Borys, 1977; Byrnes & Spitz, 1977; Spitz & Winters, 1977) became interested in examining the logic used by mentally retarded individuals in playing games. Following an explanation of the rules of the games and several practice games to insure that the process was understood, the experimenters compared performances of retarded individuals and various groups of normal individuals. (The games were relatively simple ones such as tic-tac-toe and other activities generally requiring logic.) The primary finding in the studies was that the mentally retarded individuals operated at a level similar to children whose mental ages were one-and-a-half to three-and-a-half years below their own. In essence, for most of them, logic was not employed in attempting to solve the problems.

Operant Learning

Research in operant-learning investigates causal relations between environmental events and specific behaviors. Based on the work of Skinner (1938, 1953), operant researchers eschew traditional learning theories that attempt to explain behavior through intervening variables or hypothetical constructs. Instead, they focus on determining lawful relationships between environmental stimuli and the behavior of individuals. The particular behaviors studied and the stimuli that precede or follow them may vary but the purpose is the same: to demonstrate a particular environmental influence has modified the target behavior in some fashion.

The main source of behavioral control is the consequence of the behavior. Some observable consequence (an event or stimulus) follows a behavior and increases the probability that the behavior will occur again. This consequence is called a reinforcer. A positive reinforcer presents a stimulus or event that serves to increase the frequency of the behavior; a negative reinforcer removes a stimulus or event and also serves to increase the frequency of the behavior. Other environmental variables may also affect whether or not a behavior occurs. These may include discriminative stimuli that prompt the behavior or the schedule on which the reinforcer is delivered (Reynolds, 1975).

The application of the principles of operant learning (also termed applied behavior analysis and behavior modification) to mentally retarded individuals has provided us with a great deal of useful information. In this application, many effects have been documented between a variety of environmental manipulations and behavioral changes (Whitman & Sciback, 1979; Weisberg, 1971; Mercer & Snell, 1977). Most of these have been on the use of reinforcement.

Several different kinds of reinforcers have been found effective as can be illustrated by a few examples. Bailey and Meyerson (1969) used vibration effectively with a profoundly retarded boy. Remington, Foxen, and Hogg (1977) used rhymes and country music with multiply handicapped, profoundly retarded children. Piper and MacKinnon (1969) were able to show that food delivered through a stomach fistula could be used as a reinforcer. Other investigations have compared the effectiveness of different reinforcers. Rynders and Friedlander (1972) found the severely and profoundly retarded individuals preferred motion pictures to still slides. Blount (1970) found that retarded children preferred coins over bills; and Mithaug and Hanawalt (1978) found that severely retarded persons demonstrated preferences for various vocational tasks as opposed to other tasks.

Mentally retarded individuals respond to reinforcement just as do nonretarded persons. However, certain distinctions between retarded and most nonretarded persons are notable. Zigler (1966) stated that three factors would affect the potency of particular kinds of reinforcement for individuals. One is the developmental level of the individual. A second is the pairing of reinforcers with other stimuli which would allow the latter to become conditioned reinforcers. Finally, the degree to which the individual has been deprived of a reinforcer would affect its potency. It may be because some retarded individuals have been deprived of social reinforcement that they often tend to respond favorably to it. However, it may also be because of their history, as well as their developmental level, that some mentally retarded individuals will respond better to tangible reinforcers than to intangible, social reinforcement (Balla & Zigler, 1979).

Some theorists (e.g. Cromwell, 1963, 1967; Zigler, 1966) would predict that mentally retarded individuals would be more reinforced by immediate, tangible reinforcement than by delayed and/or intangible reinforcement. Generally this is considered to be true and there are many studies demonstrating the effectiveness of such reinforcement. Still there are many complexities. Individuals at a mild level of retardation may be reinforced socially or they may reject social contact. Moderately and severely retarded individuals usually tend to work for immediate, tangible reinforcement but are also often quite responsive to social reinforcement.

Some profoundly retarded individuals seem to show no preferences for any type of reinforcement while others respond well (Switzky et al., 1982).

Observational Learning

Observational learning, also referred to as imitation or modeling, is the ability to develop behaviors or skills through "an observer matching or being directly influenced by the behavior of a model" (Mercer & Algozzine, 1977, p. 345). This process warrants our attention because it possesses potential as a strong learning device (Bandura, 1971) and, as such, has generated a number of studies with mentally retarded individuals during the last few years (see Mercer & Snell, 1977, and Mercer & Algozzine, 1977, for reviews).

It is evident that normal children learn a great deal of their social skills and language by imitating those around them. This ability to imitate has often been misunderstood among the mentally retarded. For example, Belmont (1971) noted the history of clinically describing Down's syndrome individuals as being "outstanding in their mimicry." More recently, however, Silverstein, Aguilar, Jacobs, Levy, and Rubenstein (1979) found that these individuals were no more imitative than other retarded individuals of the same sex, IQ, and CA.

There are different things that can affect the retarded person's ability to learn through observation of another person (model). For example, we can consider the characteristics of the retarded individual who is supposed to imitate the model (e.g. IQ, MA), the task or behavior to be imitated (e.g. gross motor, fine motor, verbal behavior), and how the task is taught (e.g. with or without reinforcement).

From their reviews, Mercer and his colleagues (Mercer & Algozzine, 1977; Mercer & Snell, 1977) found that little systematic research had been conducted on the specific individual variables influencing the ability to imitate. It is safe to conclude that higher IQ individuals and higher MA individuals imitate more readily than lower-level individuals. Some ability to imitate has been reported among the severely and profoundly retarded, more among the moderately and mildly retarded.

The types of tasks taught through imitation have varied. Mercer and Algozzine (1977) noted that investigators have reported positive results with behaviors or skills as diverse as fine and gross motor movements, social skills, visual matching, and memory. Generally, the simpler the task, the more readily it can be learned by retarded persons (Yoder & Forehand, 1974). However, even more complex tasks are possible when systematic and structured techniques are used. A good example of this is the use of imitation and reinforcement in combination to teach verbal behaviors to severely and profoundly retarded persons (see Jones and Robson,

1979, for a review of the literature in this area). These techniques have been used to teach a range of skills from simple word production to the use of more complex grammatical statements (Baer & Guess, 1973; Garcia, Guess & Byrnes, 1973; Schroeder & Baer, 1972).

Incidental Learning

Incidental learning is learning something that is not intentionally meant to be learned. Often, mentally retarded people, particularly those with IQs below 50, do not do well on incidental learning tasks. One recent study, however, found that some moderately and severely retarded adults could benefit from observing what their peers were learning (Orelove, 1982).

According to Mercer and Snell (1977), much of the research in this area was spurred by the elicitation theory of Denny (1964, 1966; Denny & Adelman, 1955). This is essentially a behavioral theory that maintains that stimuli elicit behaviors and that various stimuli may compete in cueing the occurrence of different behaviors. Within the framework of this theory, retarded individuals are considered to have a short attention span, inhibition deficiency, and a deficiency in verbal control over motor responses (Mercer & Snell, 1977). One of the concomitant shortcomings is incidental learning ability.

Different types of incidental learning performance have been studied. Type I incidental learning presents some stimuli to the learner without any specific direction and then later asks the individual to recall some aspect of what was presented. Type II incidental learning presents the learner with directions to learn some relevant material of the stimuli presented, and then tests the individual on some irrelevant material that he or she was not instructed to learn. Type II can be intrinsic or extrinsic incidental learning. Intrinsic means that the irrelevant material is an integral part of the relevant material but not necessary to learning the material; for example, the color of the furniture to be remembered. Extrinsic material might be the people standing next to the furniture. Mercer and Snell (1977) concluded: ". . . it seems that now there is somewhat more evidence showing poorer incidental learning of Type I and some Type II intrinsic tasks in the mentally retarded when their learning is compared to that of normals who are MA or CA equal" (p. 174). The effect seems to be more apparent among the organically impaired than those in the cultural-familial classification.

Other incidental learning characteristics of retarded persons are also notable from the research. Difficulties increase as the task becomes more complex; incidental learning will be more successful at simpler task levels. Orientation or readiness activities tend to improve incidental learning. Hardman and Drew (1975) suggested the need to teach retarded individuals to be more aware of incidental environmental cues.

Implications of Learning Processes

The brief review of some learning processes and related theories that is presented should provide a little better understanding of retarded persons. With this knowledge, two conclusions may be drawn.

1. The learning processes of retarded persons may be at least partially responsible for their retarded functioning in certain, specific areas; and,
2. If we work around these learning deficiencies, we may be able to improve their functioning.

If we accept the second premise, certain strategies may be useful. For example:

Teach retarded students to focus on single distinct dimensions when initially teaching discriminations.

Show retarded learners how to use rehearsal strategies to improve memory and have them practice doing so when attempting to memorize.

Present information in relevant clusters; do not assume common associations will be obvious.

Seek and use appropriate reinforcement techniques realizing that each individual may require a different reinforcer.

Realize that observational and incidental learning tends to decrease with decreased IQs and structure the environment accordingly for effective learning.

By incorporating such tactics into the learning process, we may be able to improve functioning, if not the learning process per se. The interested reader is encouraged to review Mercer and Snell (1977) for a more extensive listing of teaching implications drawn from learning research.

LEARNING PRODUCTS

The material reviewed in this section describes the ability of retarded individuals to learn certain skills generally thought to be important for normal functioning. Key areas including language development, reading, and arithmetic, are addressed.

Language Development

Probably no other human characteristic parallels the development of intelligence as does language. The fact that intelligence tests rely greatly on both expressive and receptive language probably accounts for this to an extent. It should not be surprising, then, that mentally retarded individuals are also usually language-retarded individuals. Several aspects of their language are characteristically impaired, deficient, different, or delayed (Schiefelbusch & Lloyd, 1974; Sitko & Semmel, 1973).

One area of difficulty is often speech, the most common manifestation of language. Spradlin (1963) reported in his review that different studies found between 57% and 72% of institutionalized retarded persons had some type of speech defect. A similar percentage was found among noninstitutionalized retarded children. For the most part, these disorders were found in the moderately, severely, and profoundly retarded. Among mildly retarded children attending special classes, only about 8% to 26% had speech defects. In both groups of individuals, the most predominant defects were articulation and voice problems with stuttering accounting for a much smaller percentage.

Many early studies of mentally retarded individuals found them to be lacking in various aspects of language. Some commonly noted deficits included shortcomings in their vocabulary and vocabulary usage, sentence length, auditory discrimination, and grammatical structure. Various studies have shown general delays in language development with greater delays being associated with lower levels of intelligence (Sitko & Stemmel, 1973). While the delay in language is quite evident, the *order* of language development does not seem to vary from that of normal individuals (Lenneberg, 1967; Rosenberg, 1970). Lenneberg reported a study of the language of 61 Down's syndrome individuals over a three year period. The data analyzed included utterances, articulation, sentence repetition, vocabulary, and understanding directions. He concluded that the language development of these individuals occurred in the same order as in normal individuals. Rosenberg's (1970) review of the literature led him to a similar conclusion. Thus while language development is *slower* among retarded persons, it is generally *not different*. An important question may be *how* much slower?

Wiegel-Crump (1981) conducted a study with Down's syndrome children which provided data on this issue. The children's syntax usage was measured and compared to equal MA normal children's performance obtained from another study. Wiegel-Crump found a progressive increase in syntactic complexity from MA 2–0 to MA 6–11. However, equal MA comparisons (with data from normal subjects) revealed equal performances only at MAs 2–0 to 2–11. At this point, the Down's syndrome children were between the 50th and 60th percentile ranking of normal children. However, between MAs of 3–0 and 6–11 years, the Down's syndrome children attained mean scores between the 10th and 15th percentiles of the normal children. This finding suggested that at lower mental ages, language performances of Down's syndrome and normal children may be similar but at higher mental ages, it may not. It seems, then, that as mentally retarded children increase in age, their language development tends to slow down.

Woodward (1979) has pointed out that recently Piagetian research has moved toward studying the relationship of cognitive development and language. Two recent studies with Down's syndrome children investigated this relationship (Greenwald & Leonard, 1979; and Mahoney, Glover & Finger, 1981). A basic tenet according to Piaget's theory is that object permanence indicates the development of symbolic representation and is thus a prerequisite to language (Morehead & Morehead, 1974). Greenwald and Leonard investigated the relationship between early language tasks and children's sensorimotor development. Both Down's syndrome and normal children were included. The results indicated that both normal and retarded children at the lower level of sensorimotor development achieved scores below children at the higher sensorimotor level. Neither group of children (retarded or nonretarded) who performed at the lower sensorimotor stage showed much performance on more complex language tasks; only those at the higher level did, and the nonretarded children showed greater performance. The study by Mahoney, et al. (1981) addressed the same issue. Again, Down's syndrome children and normal children served as subjects of the study. The results indicated that although the Down's syndrome children and the normal children scored about the same on cognitive development scales, the normal children scored significantly higher on the receptive and expressive language scales.

From these studies, two tentative conclusions can be drawn: there seems to be a relationship between sensorimotor development and at least some aspect of language development; however, this relationship overall is not strong. Even though Mahoney et al. found their retarded subjects to be performing at a sensorimotor level similar to their normal subjects, they did not find the same level of language development. Thus while a certain level of sensorimotor development *may* be prerequisite to language development, it cannot alone account for it.

Language and the cultural-familial classification. The language of the cultural-familial child from a minority background presents a unique problem. At issue is whether or not the language is deficient or simply different. Dever (1972) noted that a number of researchers reported language deficiencies among this population. He contended, however, that the only deficit exhibited was knowledge of middle-class English and suggested that this might be taught as a second language. Labov (1970) demonstrated that black children follow a rule-abiding system of language. Even though it is different, it is as consistent as the middle-class standard system. Labov pointed out that the various formal procedures used to assess language are not valid for evaluating the linguistic competence of black children because they do not consider the child's dialect or culture.

Language and the profoundly retarded individual. Quite often profoundly retarded persons simply do not develop language skills at all. One of the main problems may not be their lack of potential, but the fact that they often live in nonstimulating environments. Traditionally, this has been the residential institution; but the individual's home as well may not provide the human, material, or verbal stimulation necessary to promote cognitive and linguistic development.

Phillips and Balthazar (1979) reported the effects of long-term institutionalization on the language of severely and profoundly retarded persons. Two groups were observed at five-year intervals. One group was observed twice and another three times. Of the fifty-nine individuals observed twice, 5.1% exhibited no communication, 30.5% regressed, 20.3% were irregular, 25.4% were stable, and 18.6% made progress in their language development. Within the group of twenty who were observed three times, 5% had no communication, 30% regressed, 45% were irregular, 15% were stable, and only 5% progressed.

While this is a bleak picture, institutionalization cannot be considered the sole problem in the lack of language development for extremely low IQ individuals. Certainly central nervous system damage, which is more in evidence at lower levels of retardation, can be implicated. The problem is that any deficit due to physiological factors cannot be fully determined until whatever deficit due to environmental factors is ameliorated. Perhaps the trend toward keeping more profoundly retarded individuals in the home and the community and providing them with appropriate public school education will improve their language performance.

Reading

Like language, reading is a uniquely human characteristic. Most often, reading is considered to be an extension of verbal language that has two components: translating visual images into words and understanding the meaning of these words. Since language development of mentally retarded persons is generally delayed, we might expect that reading ability might be delayed just as much or perhaps more.

Many studies have addressed the issue of how well mentally retarded people can learn to read. Reviews of these studies have been written by Kirk (1964), Quay (1963), Cegelka and Cegelka (1970), Orlando (1973), and Dunn (1973). Most of the studies have been limited to mildly retarded students although a few have examined the reading potential of moderately retarded persons.

Reading and the mildly retarded individual. One of the most generalized findings is that educable or mildly retarded individuals do not read up to their MA expectancy level, usually falling one or more years below. In fact, reading is generally considered to be their weakest area of learning, especially reading comprehension. Comparatively, mildly retarded students tend to do better on reading words than on understanding what it is they have read.

There are two ways one can recognize the words they are trying to read. They can use an orthographic approach, sounding out the letters and letter combinations; or they can use a whole word or sight word approach, recognizing each word from rote memorization. Most mildly retarded students tend to use the latter approach perhaps because they have most often been taught this way (Orlando, 1973). Kirk (1964) concluded that the teaching method did not make much difference in terms of how well these students learned to read. Similarly, Dunn (1973) suggested that the method is probably not as important as the teacher.

Mildly retarded children make many errors during the word recognition process of oral reading. Sheperd (1967) analyzed the reading errors of poor, mildly retarded readers and found them weak on consonant and vowel sounds, blending skills, and substitution and omission errors. In an earlier study, Dunn (1956) compared mildly retarded boys and equal MA normal boys on several reading skills. He found the retarded boys to be below the normal boys on vowel sounds, omissions, using context clues, and auditory and visual acuity.

More recent research has attempted to discover some of the key problems related to reading difficulties experienced by mildly retarded persons. One of the main problems seems to be the reliance on a sight word approach and the use of contextual cues to identify words. The context of the word will help the normal individual. However, mentally retarded readers' reliance on sight word memory and context clues may hinder their efforts. Mason (1978) found that mildly retarded persons did well using a sight word strategy with high frequency words (those that are more common) but made more errors with low frequency (uncommon) words. The problem appeared to be that they had not memorized the less common words and could not decipher them using a letter-sound approach. In a similar study, Allington (1980) arrived at the same conclusion.

Reading comprehension is probably the lowest area of skill attainment by mildly retarded students. Even though they might learn to read a number of words, either orthographically or more commonly through a sight word approach, getting meaning from what they have read appears to be a more formidable task—one on which they do not perform very well. Hurley (1975) has pointed out that little research has been done in this area and teachers are at a loss as to what comprehension skills to teach, when they should teach them, and how they should be taught. Orlando (1973) noted that most reading programs for mildly retarded students have focused on basal readers and teaching sight words. Thus although the problem might be one of cognitive ability, perhaps an experiential deficit also exists.

Reading and the moderately retarded individual.   Until recently, little research appeared on the ability of moderately mentally retarded persons learning to read. Brown's (1973) report was probably among the first to demonstrate efforts in this area. He reviewed much of his own research that demonstrated the successful use of a behavioral, task-analytic approach to teach sight words to moderately retarded children. His efforts have been replicated by others. Folk and Campbell (1978) reported Down's syndrome children learning upwards of one hundred words. Sterick (1979) reported that some children classified as moderately retarded were able to learn up to 275 words and retained them for ten years. It should be noted, however, that many of Sterick's subjects were later found to be functioning at a level higher than moderate retardation.

Vandever and Stubbs (1977) studied moderately retarded students' ability to retain learned sight words and to generalize their reading skills to new words. From a list of 150 high frequency sight words, their twenty-one students learned a mean of 26.29 words during the first year. After the summer, they retained 20.95 words and after the second year had learned a mean total of 40.75 words. Using a second (different) list of thirty-two high-frequency words, they found some generalization occurred although it was slight.

There is little reported research on how successfully students at the moderate level can develop skills necessary to read new words by deciphering the letter sounds contained within the words. Some reports (e.g., Folk & Campbell, 1978; Hayden & Haring, 1976) have reported successful initial efforts in these areas. Rynders, Spiker, and Horrobin (1978) suggested the educability of Down's syndrome children had generally been underestimated due to methodological errors in the research. They pointed out that early intervention projects with Down's syndrome children show much promise for their potential in acquiring academic skills, including generalizable reading skills (Hayden & Haring, 1976; Rynders & Horrobin, 1975). As of now, the literature offers little insight into this area.

House, Hanley, and Magid (1980) reported a reading approach which, although uncommon, may offer some retarded individuals a way to read that will be easier and allow a more expanded vocabulary. In their approach, House et al. did not use words but logographic symbols (see Figure 6–4). They found that their subjects could readily learn the words associated with these symbols and comprehend them. When they put the symbols into sentence format, the students were able to demonstrate that they knew what the sentences said by manipulating objects. The authors

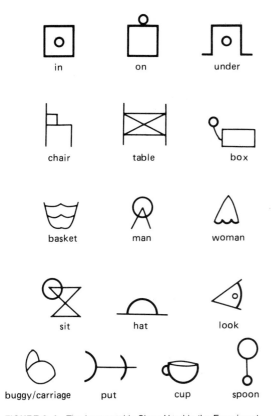

FIGURE 6–4   The Logographic Signs Used in the Experiment

From B. J. House, M. J. Hanley, and D. F. Magid, "Logographic reading by TMR adults." *American Journal of Mental Deficiency*, 1980, 85, 161–170. Reprinted by permission.

said that the symbols were easier to read than words and suggested their use in designing reading materials for retarded persons.

At this point we can conclude that some moderately retarded children can learn to read words. This has been demonstrated mostly through sight word reading. Using this approach, the number of words learned has been small and they have taken a great deal of time to learn, but when learned they have been retained at least to some degree.

The use of a traditional orthographic approach to teach reading to mildly and moderately retarded children lacks research. Attentional parameters and memory abilities may limit such learning but direct research can better answer this question. There is also a need for research in the area of reading comprehension. Currently it seems that this area has been sorely neglected in both research and practice.

Arithmetic

There are two types of arithmetic skills. One is the ability to compute numbers in appropriate ways (e.g., add, subtract, multiply, and divide); the second is selecting the kinds of computations needed to be done in certain situations. This is the ability to reason or use logic.

Arithmetic and the mildly retarded individual. The arithmetic performance of the mildly retarded is stronger in the first area mentioned above (Dunn, 1973; Kirk, 1964; Quay, 1963; Guskin & Spicker, 1968). Generally their ability level in arithmetic computation is commensurate with their mental age level. In the use of reasoning skills, however, Kirk (1964) pointed out that they were less able to select the relevant facts needed to solve specific problems. In other words, they are weak in solving problems but capable of learning the more mechanical tasks of adding and subtracting. The only problem with the latter skill is that often careless errors are made in the computational process (Dunn, 1973).

Piagetian researchers have often noted that quantitative concepts occur in normal children in a certain order. These same concepts tend to occur in mentally retarded children in the same order. Normally, at about seven or eight years of age, children reach the concrete operational stage of thought processes. Mildly retarded children reach this stage at a later age, somewhere between ten and fourteen years. Thus Vitello (1976) noted that at this age they *should* be capable of using the reasoning skills necessary for solving mathematical problems, thus going beyond mechanical computational processes. At this point in their lives, they should be able to use numerical rules and concepts to solve routine problems. Vitello suggested the problem has been an educative one in which stress has been placed more on computation than application.

Arithmetic and moderately retarded individuals. Research on the arithmetic learning ability of moderately retarded children is scant. The work that has been done has generally been of a fairly straightforward, applied nature (Brown, 1973). For example, Bellamy and Brown (1972) described a program for teaching moderately retarded students to add any two numbers that totaled to ten or less. They analyzed the task into the following steps:

1. label printed numerals (1–10)
2. write numerals from a verbal cue
3. count quantity of lines and report the total verbally
4. draw quantity of lines corresponding to printed numerals
5. count quantity of lines and write the total
6. complete two preaddition exercises involving stimulus fading

After 268 instructional trials, the children could calculate the sums. Thus, like mildly retarded persons, moderately retarded children can probably learn mechanical computational tasks although to a lesser degree of sophistication.

In order for moderately retarded persons to function more completely, certain skills will be useful. The most basic skills will include telling time (or following a time schedule), handling money, and measuring lengths and quantities. Fortunately, various studies have shown that some such specific skills can be taught through applied behavior analysis. Demonstrations of generalizing these skills, for example, using reasoning abilities, are still lacking.

CONCLUSION

Several general conclusions can be drawn from the literature reviewed in this chapter. People classified as being mentally retarded have demonstrated many and sundry deficits in development and learning. They tend to develop cognitively in the same order and direction as do average people but they do so at a much slower rate and never achieve the level of mental maturity reached by normal people. In various areas they demonstrate learning deficits. In attention, in organizing information, in using logic, and in remembering information, they are deficient; likewise, in language development, reading, and math. They are below par for their chronological age and seemingly, in at least some areas, they are below par for their mental age.

In a more positive vein, the cognitive development of retarded individuals continues for a longer period of time than is normally found. This gives them a slight edge that they otherwise might not have and holds implications for continuing education for the mentally retarded adult.

In many of the same areas that they have demonstrated learning deficits, they have demonstrated learning potential. Attention improves when relevant dimensions are identified; they benefit when someone shows them how to organize or cluster material; they can use rehearsal strategies and other retention tactics when they are taught to do so. Thus as Mercer and Snell (1977) pointed out, while researchers have studied structural learning deficits, they have found learning potential along the way.

Because of the efforts of many researchers we do indeed know more about mentally retarded persons than we would otherwise. Spitz (1979) suggested that there is a continuum of tasks requiring different levels of ability. The continuum ranges from tasks requiring stereotyped responses to complex reasoning and logic. Through research, it has been discovered how retarded people compare with normal people on different parts of this continuum. Knowing how retarded people learn and the degree of their learning is one important step toward their improvement in these areas. Knowing their limits in various areas clearly indicates additional steps are necessary.

STUDY QUESTIONS

1. What is the difference between cognitive development and learning?
2. Describe the mental age development of persons with different degrees of retardation.
3. What is the difference between "quantitative" and "qualitative" mental development?
4. To what degree do mentally retarded persons of various levels of intelligence proceed through Piaget's stages? What factors may affect their development?
5. In what way are retarded individuals limited in attention?
6. Describe the current consensus of the memory and rehearsal abilities of retarded persons.
7. How is the ability to organize information related to the use of logic by mentally retarded persons?
8. What has been the purpose of operant learning research with mentally retarded individuals? What are some general conclusions about the use of reinforcement with retarded persons?
9. What are some factors that may affect the observational learning ability of retarded individuals?
10. What is meant by incidental learning? What particular aspects of this type of learning present difficulties to retarded individuals?
11. What types of speech problems occur among mentally retarded persons, to what degree, and within what levels of retardation?
12. What are some typical language problems manifested by retarded individuals? Characterize the nature of their language development.
13. How do most mildly and moderately retarded persons learn to read? What is their best skill in this area? Their weakest?
14. What are the strengths and weaknesses of mentally retarded students in the area of arithmetic?

7

Personal and Social Characteristics

PRELIMINARY CONSIDERATIONS ABOUT PERSONAL
AND SOCIAL CHARACTERISTICS

Much variability exists in the personal and social behavior of individuals. This is no less true for mentally retarded persons, it may be even more so. An individual's personality and its manifestation in social situations depends on many factors, some identified, some unidentified, but all unique to that person. No two people, retarded or nonretarded, experience the same environmental conditions nor have the same biological constitution. It would thus be ludicrous to propose that totally generalizable truths exist about the personal-social development or learning of mentally retarded persons. The contents of this chapter should therefore not lead the reader to inviolate conclusions. What must be kept in mind is that the various theories and accounts presented have usually been drawn from studies of *groups* of mentally retarded persons and their specific applicability to one *individual* will not always be valid.

Given this limitation, it is still of value to study the theories and research in this area. One reason for this is that the information about personal and social characteristics gives us insight into the population though perhaps not so much into a specific person. Another reason is that it may help us in preparing to understand behaviors that sometimes occur. Of course, knowledge of these will not alone remedy them, but it may aid as we search for appropriate strategies.

PERSONALITY DIMENSIONS OF MENTALLY
RETARDED PERSONS

Various theories have been used to explain or describe personality. Some of these include type theory (introverts, extroverts), trait theory (honest, compulsive), need theory (warmth, acceptance), avoidance theory (projection, repression), and threat theory (anxiety, phobia). Cromwell (1967) suggested that these theories could be used as the basis for understanding the personal behavior of individuals who are mentally retarded (See Figure 7–1).

In Figure 7–1, the central section (c) represents the person (organism) as described by the type theory. To the far right of the figure (e) are needs or goals which particular individuals would approach based on their personality characteristics. Trait constructs are represented by the components (d) between the individuals and their goals. In other words, one or more of these traits would characterize the individual in terms of how the goal is approached.

To the left side of the figure are the constructs that would explain "moving away" behavior. Threat constructs or objects (a), such as the var-

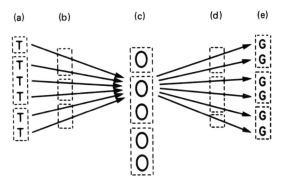

FIGURE 7-1 Threat avoidance and goal approach behavior as a basis for (a) threat constructs, (b) defense mechanism constructs, (c) typology constructs, (d) trait constructs, and (e) need constructs in personality theory

From R. L. Cromwell, "Personality evaluation," in A. A. Baumeister (Ed.), *Mental Retardation*. Chicago: Aldine, 1967.

ious phobias and fears, may impinge upon an individual and require the employment of some defense mechanism(s) (b). In sum, the individual's personality is described in terms of behavior as it is (at least theoretically) affected by these different constructs. The individual's personality is thus a *dynamic* phenomenon, moving away from some threat (a) via defense mechanisms (b), and/or toward some goal (e) via personality traits (d).

Cromwell (1967) suggested that personality be thought of as passing through different levels of development. Within the normal individual, these levels would be related to CA. Retarded persons would show different personality levels based on MA. Cromwell (1967) offered the following five levels to describe this sequence.

Basic boundary development. At this level, the individual can simply differentiate between himself or herself and various aspects of the environment. Threats and goals are differentiated as are other people. An individual deficient in basic boundary development would have difficulty in differentiating between himself or herself and various objects in the environment.

The intact hedonist. The person at this level is interested in immediate gratification of needs and avoidance of pain or discomfort.

The conceptual motivational system. This stage of development indicates more maturity than the previous two. At this level, the individual is able to respond to more conceptualized goals. Directional behavior occurs for the sake of achieving success and not simply for some immediate satisfaction of a need. The individual is capable of delaying gratification. Similarly, failure is avoided not because of punishment or pain but simply because it is failure. The individual is said to be task-oriented, not environmentally manipulated.

Development of interpersonal functioning. After the development of the conceptual motivational system, the individual attains the ability to see the situation as another sees it; that is, to conceptualize the feelings, attitudes, and motives of another. Sometimes this is referred to as "role taking," an element of "social intelligence." (See Greenspan, 1979, for a thorough review of this topic.)

Development of cultural functioning. This level is seen when people show concern for humankind or society in general, not just for specific persons.

Adhering to Cromwell's (1967) developmental scheme, many mildly retarded persons would probably approach the level of conceptual motivation or perhaps interpersonal functioning. Progressively lower retarded individuals such as the moderately and severely retarded would not advance as far in their development although they may attain certain characteristics of some levels. The profoundly retarded would generally not develop much beyond the first or second level.

While it is difficult to precisely relate level of IQ to development of personality, Cromwell's outline provides a foundation for exploring more discrete personality elements. In them we will see degrees of support and refutation of Cromwell's theory.

Approach and Avoidance[1]

Central to the issue of personality development is what motivates a person to act, behave, move, or respond. Rotter (1954, as discussed by Cromwell, 1963) presented a *Social Learning Theory* that attempted to explain individuals' behavior in terms of their expectancy for reinforcement in certain situations for specific behaviors. Expectancy is dictated by the person's experience in general or experience in the particular situation on previous occasions. If persons have generally been successful (attained goals, needs, etc.), chances are that they will act again to achieve the outcome. That is, they will continue to *approach success*. On the other hand, if they have more often failed (experienced some aversive consequence or not achieved the goal), they will more likely try to *avoid failure*. Since mentally retarded persons have a reduced intellectual ability, it might be assumed that they have had fewer successful experiences and more failure experiences than most individuals. They would therefore have a lower generalized expectancy for success. This would become most evident in situations following instances of failure. In such situations, it would be expected that mentally retarded persons would give up or not try as hard on subsequent occasions. That is, they would avoid future failure and be considered *failure avoiders*. On the other hand, persons with a general history of success would not have their efforts suppressed by an

---

[1]Most of the research in this area and in the areas subsequently discussed was conducted with institutionalized mildly retarded individuals. However, its applicability to lower level retarded persons may be inferred.

instance of failure but would instead attempt on subsequent occasions to try to achieve the success that had eluded them in their first attempt. Such individuals are referred to as *success strivers.*

Cromwell (1963) reviewed several studies, mostly employing mildly retarded persons, that indicated these individuals would more often be classified as failure avoiders rather than success strivers. In comparison to matched CA and/or MA normal children, the retarded children often terminated an activity following failure while the normal children would continue to work toward success.

It is most likely that this finding is a result of experience and is not a direct function of intelligence (Zigler, 1966; Balla & Zigler, 1979). Most retarded children at all levels have experienced failure and will be hesitant about striving for success in difficult situations. An implication is that many successful experiences should be provided. Such experience may alter individuals' status from failure avoiders to success strivers.

Locus of Control

Integrally related to the approach/avoidance concept is locus of control. It was noted by some researchers conducting the success-approach/failure-avoidance studies, that some retarded children did not particularly care whether or not they succeeded or failed. This led Bialer (1960, as cited by Cromwell, 1963), to conclude that some mentally retarded children were oblivious to failure. That is, it did not seem to matter to them if they failed or succeeded. Subsequently, it was suggested that success and failure had to be redefined into two levels. The first level was generally characteristic of early stages of development (i.e., the intact hedonist). At this level, the individual would tend to view their behavior as being externally controlled. They were therefore considered to have an "external locus of control" (ELC).

The second level was more truly success and failure as we consider it; that is, there is a perception that an outcome is based on our own efforts (a characteristic of the conceptual motivational system). An individual operating under the second system would demonstrate approach behavior "for the express goal of demonstrating behavioral effectiveness." At this level the individual considers himself or herself to be in control of his or her own behavior and the corresponding consequences. The person is thus said to have an "internal locus of control" (ILC) (Cromwell, 1963).

The locus of control concept has many implications. The ILC person would be able to delay gratification whereas the ELC person would desire more immediate satisfaction. The ILC individual would rely more on his/her own ability when attempting to achieve some task, whereas the ELC person would search the environment for cues when attempting to complete a task. The ILC person would generally demonstrate more self-control, whereas the ELC person would not.

In regard to mentally retarded persons, locus of control is thought to gradually shift from ELC toward ILC as mental age (MA) increases. Typically it does not reach the same level of ILC as is found with nonretarded individuals (Cromwell, 1963). Lawrence and Winschel (1975) discussed the application of the concept of locus of control for mildly retarded students. They hypothesized that five stages of locus of control existed and that mildly retarded persons probably clustered around the second and third stage. These are:

Stage II— Internality for success begins to emerge while externality for failure, though still evident, begins to fade.
Stage III— The maturing child becomes essentially internal, although this belief is principally evident in self-responsibility for success. (p. 487)

Lawrence and Winschel suggested that teachers should allow retarded children the opportunity to accept responsibility for their success and failure in order to improve their internal locus of control.

Positive and Negative Reaction Tendencies

Zigler's (1966) *positive-negative reaction tendency theory* had its basis in the form of a disagreement with the early work of Lewin (1936) and Kounin (1941a, b). The Lewin-Kounin formulation suggested mildly retarded individuals exhibited *cognitive rigidity*. This was based on their observation that often these persons did not shift to new tasks or terminate old tasks as readily as did nonretarded children. Their hypothesis was that a physiological pathology impaired their performance. Zigler (1966) reported and summarized a number of studies that suggested the Lewin-Kounin "rigidity" findings could be easily accounted for by motivational characteristics of mentally retarded individuals. His countering position was referred to as a "social deprivation" theory. The basic tenet of Zigler's position was that the difference in the responses of mentally retarded persons (they continued to respond long after the normal children were satiated) was due to their desire to please the experimenter, an adult, and thus gain his approval and affection. According to Zigler (1966), the reason the matched MA retarded children perseverated and the normal children did not was because the institutionalized retarded children had a greater history of social deprivation; that is, they had not received as much adult attention as had the normal children. Zigler (1966) cited much data to support his position. This tendency to please others because of previous social deprivation was referred to as a *positive reaction tendency*.

At times, however, it was noted that mentally retarded persons exhibited a wariness of individuals (Zigler, 1966; Balla & Zigler, 1979). This wariness was referred to as a *negative reaction tendency*. It was attributed to a history of failures and other negative experiences during interactions with adults. Balla and Zigler (1979) reported that negative interactions with adults would have a more depressing effect on retarded individuals than on normal individuals. Again, this was due to more depriving social histories.

Expectancy of Success and Failure

From the concept of locus of control, we might expect that many retarded individuals having an external locus of control would not accept personal responsibility for failure nor feel that they could control success. From Zigler's work (1966, Balla & Zigler, 1979), a different perspective was offered. In short, it was suggested that a history of failure, such as would produce a negative reaction tendency, would also result in an anticipation of future failure. Furthermore, the impact of a failure experience on future performance would be directly related to the responsiveness of the retarded person to adults in general and particularly to the adult involved in the task. This, of course, would be based on the individual's social history. In one study (Butterfield & Zigler, 1965), it was found that the degree of responsiveness of the child to the adult affected his or her reaction to failure and success. Highly responsive children, those most likely to benefit from adult attention (positive reaction tendency) reduced their performance when failure occurred. Children who were classified as having low responsiveness (negative reaction tendency) actually increased performance after initial failure. The adult reinforcement seemingly meant little to them. From this it could be concluded that if a retarded person has had some history of social deprivation, and if this person demonstrated a positve reaction tendency, then with the appropriate amount of social reinforcement, the individual would learn to work toward, and anticipate, success. On the negative side, failure for this person and the withdrawal of social approval could reduce subsequent efforts. A history of such experience could lead the person to anticipate failure and thus to avoid the failure. In turn, he or she would be less likely to work toward achieving success.

Outerdirectedness

The term *outerdirectedness* has been used to describe the common observation that many mentally retarded individuals search the environment (usually other people) for cues as to how to behave or respond (Zigler, 1966). Instead of studying the task itself (e.g. being task-oriented), they would observe how others deal with it or how others responded to them as they dealt with it. Zigler (1966) suggested that this searching behavior, or outerdirectedness, indicates retarded persons are less likely to trust their own abilities. They are thus not spontaneous or creative in their efforts but often quite sensitive to environmental models and prompts.

Balla and Zigler (1979) posited that three factors affected outerdirected behavior: the level of cognitive development; the relative amount of success achieved when being self-reliant as opposed to relying on others; and the extent of attachment to adults. They suggested that outerdirectedness is due mainly to the many experiences of failure, and this influences retarded individuals to rely more on the cues of others than on their own ability. When attending to what others do, they are more successful. Failure causes them to rely less on their own abilities. In one study (Turnure & Zigler, 1964), it was found that not only were retarded individuals more prone to imitate than were nonretarded individuals, but that their imitation (attention to others) increased *after* they experienced failure.

Self-control

Akin to the area of locus of control is the idea of self-control. When we say someone demonstrates self-control, basically we are saying that they regulate their own behavior, that is, external control shifts to internal control. Kurtz and Neisworth (1976) suggested that self-control implies three abilities: cue regulation, self-reinforcement, and self-observation. Typically we would not expect to find these abilities in most mentally retarded individuals, particularly those at moderate, severe, and profound levels. Cue regulation would require the individual to arrange his or her own environment in a way that would provide cues for certain behaviors. The cues may be physically or cognitively arranged. Self-reinforcement would require the person to select his own reinforcers and deliver them at the appropriate time. Self-reinforcement could only be appropriately executed if the person could monitor his or her own behaviors (Neisworth & Kurtz, 1976).

While the level of cognitive development would seemingly preclude retarded persons from making a complete shift from external control to self-control, some recent work by Litrownik and his associates indicate that possibilities exist for directly teaching self-control tactics to moderately and mildly retarded children. They found that several moderately retarded children would delay the delivery of reinforcement in order to earn a more desirable reinforcer (Franzini, Litrownik & Magy, 1978) and that learning time concepts would increase their willingness to delay reinforcement (Litrownik, Franzini, Geller & Geller, 1978). In additional studies, it was found that modeling could be used to teach moderately retarded children to monitor and signal the occurrence of specific behavior (Litrownik, Frietas & Franzini, 1978), to set standards for their own performance (Litrownik, Cleary, Leckliter & Franzini, 1978), and to increase the amount of time before reinforcement is delivered (Franzini, Litrownik & Magy, 1980).

This line of research provides important implications because it shows that modifiability exists for many behaviors often cast under the rubric of self-control. Given appropriate training, then, it may be erroneous to conclude that lack of self-control is immutably aligned with mental retardation as a personality characteristic.

Self-Concept

A commonly used construct in the discussion of personality characteristics is self-concept. Heber (1964) described self-concept (a term coined by Rogers, 1947) as the sum total of a person's characteristics and the positive and negative values attached to those characteristics by the person. Another way of putting it is that self-concept is a person's attitude toward himself or herself.

Actually, self-concept is measured through providing answers to questions about one's self. Self-concept pencil and paper instruments are often used although questions and answers may be orally exchanged. The use of several of these scales in studies to measure self-concept of mentally retarded children (usually mildly retarded) have been reviewed by Heber (1964), Lawrence and Winschel (1973), and Balla and Zigler (1979). A particularly difficult issue with the use of these tests with retarded persons has been their reliability, that is, their ability to test consistently from one time to another. Heber (1964) reported that the scores from these instruments tended to be less reliable than desirable. This, of course, would make any conclusions about the self-concepts of retarded persons questionable. In addition, Balla and Zigler (1979) pointed out that lack of verbal fluency and/or introspective skills of mentally retarded persons would impair their ability to relate an accurate self-concept.

Notwithstanding these limitations, a number of studies have been conducted that have produced some mixed results. Some have shown that mildly retarded children have lower self-concepts than equal CA normal children. Positive relationships have been found between self-concept scores and measured intelligence and self-concept and academic achievement (Lawrence & Winschel, 1973). On the other hand, Balla and Zigler (1979) reviewed several studies that did not find these correlations.

The position that lower intelligence leads to less success and thus a lower self-concept has been a popular one. However, not only has some research *not* supported this position, some has suggested that mildly retarded individuals *overestimate* their abilities. (There has been little research in this area with lower-functioning retarded people.) Balla and Zigler (1979) discussed the need to consider the disparity between an individual's ideal ability and true ability. A zero degree of disparity would indicate an accurate self-concept. From this perspective, Balla and Zigler reported studies indicating that self-concept is a developmental characteristic. We would therefore expect younger children and mentally retarded individuals to have a less accurate self-concept.

Obviously self-concept is a broad construct that may be accounted for by various factors. An individual's developmental level and experience will probably interact in some fashion to form his or her self-concept. Lawrence and Winschel (1973) suggested that it might be more beneficial to look at different components of the construct than to consider the global measure. For example, in an early study, Guthrie, Butler, and Gorlow (1962) factor-analyzed self-concept reports of mildly retarded institutionalized girls and found that they expressed seven general attitudes: there is nothing wrong with me; I do as well as others, I don't give trouble; I act hastily; I am shy and weak; I am useless; and nobody likes me. It would seem that each of these self-perceptions (and other views) would provide more information about retarded persons than a more general measure of self-concept.

Anxiety

Another major construct that has been considered in the study of personality is anxiety. Like self-concept measures, measures of anxiety are usually self-reports.

Generally mentally retarded persons tend to demonstrate more anxiety than do nonretarded persons at either the same CA or MA. This tends to be most true for the institutionalized retarded person (Balla & Zigler, 1979). However, the results of studies tend to be mixed with some showing no relationship between some groups of retarded and nonretarded persons and anxiety (Heber, 1964). Within groups of both retarded and nonretarded persons, there tends to be either a negative correlation or no correlation between IQ scores and anxiety. Thus it may be that any differences found between the two groups on this characteristic are due to some experiential factors rather than their intellectual level.

Conclusion

Various dimensions have been used to describe the personal behavior or characteristics of mentally retarded persons. Certainly the personality of many mentally retarded people is different from nonretarded people. The theoretical account of these differences cannot fully explain observed differences but they provide us with some possibilities. Zigler's theories and research regarding deprivation and motivation is very insightful. Although he presents it largely to account for the behavior of institutionalized mildly retarded persons, it may also help us understand other levels of retardation. At this time there seems to be little direct research on the personality development of more severely retarded persons. However, Cromwell's (1963, 1967) theories of personality development and the pain-avoidance/pleasure-approach motivational system provides a framework for some of their personal behavior.

We must not forget that the descriptions provided are typical trends seen in large groups of retarded persons. As such they are accurate accounts. We should also remember, however, that a great deal of variability exists among these individuals. With this in mind, stereotyped conclusions about the people within the population should not be drawn.

PERSONALITY DISORDERS AND ABNORMAL BEHAVIORS

In the last several sections, personality characteristics of retarded persons and the theories used to account for them were examined. The "normal" personality status of retarded persons was described within several dimensions. In this section we will discuss disorders of personality that have variously been referred to as behavior disorders, emotional disorders, and psychiatric disorders. These characteristics often overlay the individual's retarded mental development and, to say the least, compound the problem caused by the intellectual deficit. Additionally, abnormal behaviors often found among the severely and profoundly retarded are discussed in this section.

Personality Disorders

Personality disorders can range from quite severe (schizophrenia) to quite mild (various psychoneuroses). They can occur at different degrees of retardation and be manifested in different ways. At the lower levels of retardation, it is quite difficult to separate the influence of the severe intellectual deficiency and that caused by the personality disorder. It is also often sheer speculation as to which came first or what caused what. Most of the cases of personality disorders studied have been in the moderate to mild range of retardation.

Beier (1964), based on his review of research, reported that a greater percentage of institutionalized mentally retarded persons exhibited behavioral disorders than in the general population. Actual percentage estimates vary greatly, having ranged between 25% and 100% (Robinson & Robinson, 1976). The most severe form of disturbance in mental retardation, and the form most often studied is schizophrenia (Beier,

1964; Garfield, 1963; Heber, 1964). This form of disturbance (a type of psychosis) is quite rare and again the estimates vary with common figures being between about three to five children per 10,000 (Robinson & Robinson, 1976). These children often fall into the moderate to mild range of retardation and should be differentiated from many severely and profoundly retarded children who demonstrate bizarre behavioral patterns. Children who exhibit schizophrenic behavior tend to seem out of contact with their environment. They are noncommunicative; do not discriminate between animate and inanimate objects; and have little if any personal relationships with peers. Schroeder, Mulick, and Schroeder (1979) stated that the concern today with such personality disturbances and other behavior problems is more with management of the behavior and less with etiological diagnosis. The main reason for this, they say, is that differences in etiology have not led to differential treatment success.

A less severe form of personality disorder is psychoneurosis. Beier (1964) pointed out that the diagnosis of a neurosis is subjective and is more difficult to accurately assess than a severe form of psychosis such as schizophrenia. It is this factor that results in the wide range of prevalence estimates.

It seems to be generally agreed that mentally retarded children, particularly those at lower levels, are subject to more stress in childhood than are normal children. Often this is considered to result from rejection or overprotection. Coupled with this is the child's reduced level of intelligence that affects his or her capacity for dealing with various situations. In addition, these children can be expected to be slower in the development of typical family and societal standards of what is right and what is wrong (Beier, 1964).

Nihira, Mink, and Meyers (1981) examined the relation between the home environment of TMR children and their social adjustment in school. They reported that the "harmony and quality of parenting, stimulation through equipment, toys, etc. and stimulation of mature behavior, were most strongly related to TMR children's adjustment in school" (p. 13). Less important were the social climate, family values and traditional indices of family background such as SES status, mother's education, number of other children, and so on.

The etiology of such mild psychological problems as neurosis is not clear. It does not seem that low IQ directly results in such development but given a nonstimulating or nonsupportive environment, adjustment difficulties may arise.

Abnormal Behaviors

Various abnormal behaviors may be demonstrated by severely and profoundly retarded persons and seemingly more so with the latter group. Two general classes of abnormal behaviors are stereotyped behaviors (or stereotypy) and self-injurious behavior (SIB). The latter is sometimes considered to be a subclass of the former.

Stereotyped behaviors may take several different forms. Some of the most common include body rocking, head rolling, hand movements, and unusual limb posturing. Besides these, any repetitive, frequently occurring behavior that seems to serve no purpose may be considered a stereotype behavior (Baumeister & Forehand, 1973).

Self-injurious behaviors are more serious than simple stereotyped movements. SIBs are stereotyped, self-destructive movements that occur in about 9%–10% of the severely and profoundly retarded population. They may include head banging (the most common), eye gouging, self-biting, scratching, and other forms of behavior that result in physical damage to the individual (Baumeister & Rollings, 1976; Frankel & Simmons, 1976).

For years theorists have speculated about the source of stereotyped and self-injurious behaviors. Psychodynamic theories have been offered as one explanation. They suggest that the behaviors may be expressions of tension, frustrations, guilt, regression, and poor ego identity (Baumeister & Forehand, 1973; Baumeister & Rollings, 1976). In this framework the behavior is regarded as symbolic, such as a search for self-identity, suicidal behavior, displacement of anger, and so on. Baumeister and Rollings suggested that this type of theorizing was "unsubstantiated speculation" (p. 8).

Another view is the homeostatic theory that states an individual must receive a certain level of stimulation at a given time. Because of their sensory and intellectual deficits as well as their often understimulating living conditions, the severely or profoundly retarded individual may not receive enough stimulation and therefore will attempt to create some form of self-stimulation. The result is stereotypy or SIB.

In addition to the above, SIB has been considered in some cases to have an organic basis, i.e. a chemical or structural brain defect (Baumeister & Rollings, 1976). In support of this theory, it has been noted that lower IQ is associated both with more SIB and more organic involvement. Additionally, certain syndromes (Lesch-Nyhan and Cornelia De Lange) have much SIB associated with them. This would clearly indicate a physiological-behavioral relation.

Stereotyped and even self-injurious behaviors are sometimes seen in normally developing infants who display them for a period of time and then seem to grow out of them. It has been suggested that these behaviors can therefore be accounted for by developmental theory. According to this position, the retarded persons become fixed at an early level of development and do not outgrow the behavior.

Finally, operant learning has been suggested as an explanation for stereotypy and SIB. Here it is believed that environmental conditioning serves to maintain the behavior. One possibility is that stereotyped behavior occurs in the individual as part of normal development and is accidentally reinforced by the concerned attention of parents early in life. Subsequently, they are maintained by intermittent reinforcement. Another possibility under the operant theory is that the behaviors serve as a manner of avoiding or escaping undesirable conditions such as a high-demand situation or even conditioned fear (Baumeister & Rollings, 1976). According to operant learning theory, then, the behavior may either have been socially reinforced or serve as avoidance behavior (negatively reinforced).

The actual cause and continuation of these abnormal behaviors probably exists in one or more of these theories. It is also possible that different theories may account for different forms of stereotypy. However, as Schroeder et al. (1979) pointed out, the theoretical basis of the behavior has not had much effect on the success of various treatments.

Conclusion

The disorders discussed in this section can only be found in relatively few mentally retarded individuals. However, their occurrence is distressing for two reasons: one, they add an additional debilitating condition to an individual already handicapped by reduced intelligence; and two, little is known about why they occur. In all, these conditions further complicate the phenomenon of mental retardation.

SOCIAL CHARACTERISTICS

Whatever the particular personal characteristics of a mentally retarded person may be, they are ultimately displayed in relation to other individuals, that is, in social situations. Thus, not only can the individual be considered as a demonstrator of certain behavior, but that behavior is considered in light of different social contexts. A two-way relationship occurs. In one direction, the behavior of the person is judged in terms of the particular situation; in the other direction, we see the social situation as influencing the development and maintenance of behavior. In the following sections, we will consider the involvement of mentally retarded individuals in social contexts.

Mentally Retarded Individuals in Society

Within society, mentally retarded individuals are often cast into a category that discourages their involvement among nonretarded persons. Farber (1968) referred to retarded persons as a "surplus population" meaning they did not fit the needs of society or its members. Similarly,

Guskin (1963) noted that when social relations are formed, they generally occur between individuals of similar ability levels. This is supported not only by the fact that there is little association between retarded and non-retarded persons, but also that there is little between retarded individuals at different levels of mental development.

Despite this general lack of acceptance, it has been suggested that this "surplus population" has a specific role in society. It is not a role that is admired or desirable, but nonetheless it is a role that is understood. The role is defined by certain expectations and unfortunately these expectations may contribute to the problem of mental retardation. The expectations call for the retarded person to achieve only a minimal amount of learning, for removal from most of society, and for a certain degree of helplessness. In addition, stereotyped views develop about the population of retarded persons and thus about its individual members. Some of these views include the inability to hold a job, the inability to take care of personal needs, the inability to control sexual desires, and so on. The fact that the research indicates all of these and similar views to be incorrect does not really matter. They are expectations about mentally retarded people and they define the role of the mentally retarded person in society.

Social Behavior of Mentally Retarded Persons

Despite the dilemma of societal nonacceptance, most mentally retarded people are socially oriented. Various types of social behavior have been studied and a number of pertinent findings reported.

Peer relations. A number of researchers have been interested in how mentally retarded people function socially with each other. Strain and Shores (1977) reviewed the literature in the area of social reciprocity (the exchange of reinforcing behavior between two or more people in the same environment). Their conclusion was that some retarded children in educational settings are social isolates. They noted that individuals who reinforce other persons are often themselves reinforced and that a high correlation exists between social reinforcement given and a person's popularity. Many retarded children lag or do not develop such social relations with their peers. Strain and Shores emphasized the need to improve the social skills of retarded individuals in socially reciprocal situations.

A series of studies on social interactions of retarded adults were conducted by Berkson, Romer, and their associates. These studies used natural observation procedures to document the social behavior of people in community-based group-living facilities and in sheltered workshops.

One of their studies examined affiliation and friendship among retarded people (Landesman-Dwyer, Berkson & Romer, 1979). Moderately and mildly retarded people living in different community homes were observed. It was found the individuals spent about 28% of their time in close proximity to one or more other persons and about 35% in social contexts. Most social behavior occurred in pairs. Lower level individuals were the most socially isolated. The overall level of the individuals in the setting was the most important predictor of socialization. If the mean IQ for the house was high, individuals were more likely to be engaged in social activity much of the time. If it was low, there was less interaction. Sixteen peer friendships were found among the 208 persons studied. Generally the friends, like most people, shared common interests. They were often seen engaging in sports activities, games, grooming, handicrafts, studying, or working together.

Romer and Berkson (1981), in another study, analyzed different social behaviors across a number of settings. They found that more social activities occurred in sheltered workshops whereas more TV watching and social isolation existed at home. Additionally, higher IQ persons engaged in more conversation than those with lower IQs; women had more inactive relations and ate more; and older retarded people were less affectionate and had less conversation.

The researchers were particularly interested in the different relationships existing between people at different levels of intelligence. Therefore they analyzed interactions according to the degree of retardation and the particular kind of socialization demonstrated. In the area of communication, they found that low level individuals (severe) directed communication more at other low individuals; moderate level persons communicated more with the highest level (mildly retarded); and the mildly retarded communicated about the same with all levels. In the area of affection, low level persons directed it toward moderate and high levels; moderate individuals directed affection toward all levels; and high level persons mostly demonstrated affection with other high level individuals. Helping behavior was directed by the low toward the low; medium level people helped other medium level people; and high level people did not help hardly anyone. Aggression was manifested by the low against the low while the medium and high groups were not very aggressive.

From these studies, important conclusions can be drawn. Among themselves, mentally retarded people develop various kinds of peer relations. A particular individual's relations to some degree will be affected by his or her level of intelligence but probably just as much (if not more) by the sociability of those in the group. Social behavior will occur as a function of the setting with more socialization occurring in places such as workshops rather than in situations such as community homes where TV watching might detract from social interactions. It can be concluded then that among moderately and mildly retarded (and some severely retarded) persons, active social relations are possible.

Play and leisure activities.   While there have been various suggestions regarding the leisure and play needs of mentally retarded persons (e.g., Wehmen, 1976 a, b; Wehman & Schleien, 1980), there has been less research on what activities typically occur or when. Li (1981) reviewed the available research on the play activity of mentally retarded children and drew some tentative conclusions. In comparison to nonretarded children, retarded children seem to prefer more structured toys that have a self-prompting action (e.g., puzzles) as opposed to more flexible toys that require creativity in their use (e.g., blocks and clay). Likewise, retarded children are usually more narrow and less exploratory in their play. Interaction with toys was found to be less extensive and less complex and restricted to single toys as opposed to multiple toy use. Additionally, there was little symbolic play reported and little social play. Most often the children's play was solitary. Li concluded that "these studies indicate a restricted play repertoire, both in the use of play material, verbal language play, social child-to-child play as well as pretend symbolic play" (p. 122). Li (1981) suggested that play therapy be considered an important component of the educational process of these children.

As in various other areas, play behavior of mentally retarded children probably occurs in some line of developmental sequence. Odom (1981) studied the play behavior of moderately and severely retarded children at different age levels. He reported that the sophistication of cognitive and social play improved with the children's developmental level but was not associated with CA. In a similar study, Crawley and Chan (1982) noted that moderately and mildly retarded children at older ages increased their play behavior and decreased the time they spent as passive onlookers. Both solitary play and peer interaction was found to increase as the children grew older. However, peer interaction occurred considerably more often for the mildly retarded as compared to the moderately retarded. Of course, these studies do not indicate the potential of retarded children given systematic play instruction.

Like the area of play, there has not been much research on the inclination of older retarded persons toward specific leisure activities. Although leisure is an important area of development for most people and various leisure curricula have been suggested for mentally retarded students, we really know little about what mentally retarded people like to do when given the choice. This is important because it is freely choosing an activity that defines it as a leisure activity. One relevant study was found that examined this question.

Reiter and Levi (1981) asked sixteen moderately retarded and twenty-eight mildly retarded adults who lived at home what they did with their free time. Their answers were compared with those found in an earlier study of normal adults in terms of the percentage of respondents who participated in the various kinds of activities. The results are presented in Table 7–1. In comparison to the normal adults, the retarded adults tended to remain at home more and engage in more solitary activities such as a hobby or listening to the radio or record player. (The study was conducted in Israel where television is not very common.) Reiter and Levi found that the retarded adults did not go out much during the evening and did not socialize a great deal with friends.

Many factors may affect the enjoyment of free time by mentally retarded persons. At low MA levels, cognitive factors might be an impedance. At higher levels, opportunity and/or experience may be lacking. Additional research could provide more answers in this area.

Sexual relations.   The development of sexual relations places many mentally retarded persons in a precarious position. At least for the majority of these individuals, there is no reason to believe that their emotional or sexual desires are any different than those of anyone else (Heshusius, 1982). However, because of their intellectual status, sexual activity is affected (mostly precluded) both directly and indirectly.

In a direct sense, they often know little about sexual activity and its implications. Various studies (Edmondson & Wish, 1975; Edmondson, McCombs & Wish, 1979; Hall & Morris, 1976) have pointed out the limited knowledge mentally retarded people have about various aspects of sexual encounters. Indirectly, they are affected by parental concerns and attitudes (Dupras & Tremblay, 1976) as well as by those of caretakers when residing in institutions (Mitchell, Doctor, & Butler, 1978) or in com-

TABLE 7–1   Percentage of Retarded and Nonretarded Adults Who Participate in Various Activities

ACTIVITY	RETARDED	NONRETARDED	χ^2
Out of home activities			
Attending theatre several times per year	11	47	20.48***
Attending light entertainment within the past 3 months	18	50	15.95***
Attending cinema once a week or more	34	57	8.42**
At home activities			
Meeting friends weekly or more	32	81	28.65***
Listening to records	70	46	9.45**
Having a hobby	86	69	5.81**
Listening to the radio	100	90	6.72*

*$p < .01$.
**$p < .001$.
***$p < .0001$.

From S. Reiter, and A. M. Levi, "Leisure activities of mentally retarded adults," *American Journal of Mental Deficiency*, 1981, 86, 201-203. Reprinted by permission.

munity facilities (Adams, Tallon, & Alcorn, 1982). The problem, of course, is that sex outside of marriage is typically not openly condoned, and marriage and childrearing require mature social behavior. Tarjan (1973) referred to sexual relations of mentally retarded persons as presenting a tri-polar problem with the sources including the individuals themselves, their parents, and society.

Whether or not nonretarded people engage in sexual relations in a "responsible" manner, most realize the implications, particularly the potential for pregnancy or venereal disease. Many mentally retarded people do not have this benefit. Even if they had the opportunity to engage in a sexual relationship, they might not be aware of possible outcomes. Hall and Morris (1976) found that mildly retarded adolescents were knowledgeable about masturbation, menstruation, sexual intercourse, and pregnancy, but that most knew nothing about venereal disease, birth control, or sterilization. Edmondson and Wish (1976) presented moderately retarded male adolescents with pictures of different sexual activities and asked them to describe what was happening in the pictures. The most correctly interpreted picture was male masturbation, the most incorrect was the age of a newborn. Additionally, most of the subjects did not know how a man became a father or how a woman got pregnant. In a later study, Edmondson et al. (1979) found that moderately and severely retarded women knew more about menstruation, birth control, childbirth, and venereal disease than did the male subjects. Overall, the least amount of information was in the area of venereal disease and birth control.

Various sex education curricula for mentally retarded persons are available. However, sexual relations for retarded persons will remain a problem for some time. Most everyone expects people to engage in sexual activity either within or outside of marriage. However, few in our society would accept the explicit instruction that would be necessary for retarded persons to have normal sexual relations, especially if this were to occur out of wedlock. This is one of the greatest dilemmas faced by parents and professionals. Heshusius (1982) suggested that if we truly want to normalize the life-styles of many retarded persons, we will have to modify our attitudes toward sexual behavior.

Criminal activity.   Beier (1964) pointed out that early thoughts about mentally retarded persons almost inevitably linked them with delinquent and criminal behavior. Emerging from the field of moral psychology in the 1800s was the belief that retarded mental development, insanity, moral deficiency, criminal activity, and licentiousness all had the same source: inferior genetic material. Despite such beliefs, there was no substantial data to support this conclusion.

MacEachron (1979), in addition to her own research, provided an excellent review of the research on the prevalence and characteristics of mentally retarded offenders. She noted that research has shown a wide range in the prevalence figures of mentally retarded persons in prisons. These figures fall anywhere from about 4% to 40% of the state prison populations. MacEachron suggested that different factors may influence the variation in these figures. Some might include variations in regulations, prison reforms, and community service programs. In addition, types of intelligence tests given, when they were given, who they were given to, who gave them, and how they were scored may affect reported prevalence figures.

According to MacEachron's (1979) review, the literature characterizes most mentally retarded criminals as nonwhite school dropouts in their late twenties or early thirties. They usually possess second or third grade level academic skills, have poor job skills and a history of being on welfare. Their most common offenses are against persons and second most common are against property. She also pointed out that mentally retarded offenders tend to get long prison sentences and participate less in prison rehabilitation programs.

In her own study, MacEachron (1979) examined the prevalence of mentally retarded persons in the prisons of Maine and Massachusetts. She carefully examined prison records and calculated prevalence first based on an IQ score of 70 and then on a criterion of falling below a − 2 standard deviations from the mean on the test. (Since the two are not always synonymous, the latter criterion was expected to more correctly give the actual prevalence.) In addition to intelligence test data, MacEachron also examined various legal and social data. Her conclusions included the following:

> Prevalence figures were lower when only *some* scores were available as opposed to *all* being available.
>
> If an IQ of 70 was used as a criterion, prevalence figures were higher. If a − 2 standard deviations criterion was used, they were lower.
>
> Using the latter criterion, the proportion of prison populations that are mentally retarded were nearly the same as found in the general population.
>
> Social characteristics of the retarded offenders were similar to those previously reported in the literature.
>
> Most were in jail for serious offenses, most had been in jail before, and most showed a pattern of committing increasingly serious crimes.

An important finding was the low prevalence figure. MacEachron stated "these findings undermine the century-old supposition that mental retardation predisposes a person to criminality" (p. 171).

Conclusion

Mentally retarded people are members of two social systems. One is the large system in which we all live; the second is their own system. In the larger system, they are compared to nonretarded individuals and their performance lags developmentally in some areas. This can be seen in play, in leisure activities, and in sexual awareness. They are about the same as others in criminal activity, being proportionally no better or worse.

Within the social system of mentally retarded people, social activity parallels that of normal people in the larger system. They have social relations, interact and develop friendships. Two factors may affect their actions within this micro-system: their mental deficiency and the controls exerted over their activity in this system by the larger system. Because of their cognitive limitations, external control seems necessary. Unfortunately this control has not always been beneficial to the social functioning of mentally retarded people. In this area where their functioning is most obviously problematic, the influences of the larger system should be carefully considered and conducted in a fashion beneficial to better development.

STUDY QUESTIONS

1. Explain Cromwell's (1967) theory of personality development and how it is thought to relate to different degrees of mental retardation.
2. Why are mentally retarded persons sometimes referred to as "failure avoiders?" What does this term mean?
3. What is "internal" and "external locus of control?" What are their implications? How are they manifested by mentally retarded individuals?
4. How does Zigler's social deprivation theory explain positive reaction tendencies? Why do negative reaction tendencies sometimes occur?
5. What is "outerdirectedness?" What influences its occurrence?
6. What is meant by "self-control" and how well can we expect mentally retarded persons to demonstrate it?
7. Why is it difficult to analyze the self-concept of retarded individuals?
8. Why is it difficult to diagnose personality disorders among mentally retarded persons?
9. Describe some of the theories that have been used to explain stereotyped and self-injurious behaviors.
10. How can society's views of mentally retarded individuals affect their development?
11. Discuss some peer relation characteristics of mentally retarded individuals.
12. Describe the play and leisure activities of most mentally retarded individuals.
13. How might the sexual relations of mentally retarded persons best be described. What is their general level of sexual knowledge?
14. How does the criminal activity of retarded individuals compare with the general population?

Physical Characteristics and Related Disabilities

PHYSICAL PROBLEMS AND MENTAL RETARDATION

Mentally retarded individuals are defined as such by their intellectual and adaptive behavior abilities. In some cases, however, they will also exhibit physical characteristics that diverge from the norm. This is especially true for persons classified as moderately, severely, or profoundly retarded. Generally, the lower a retarded person's measured intelligence, the higher the probability that a physical anomaly will be present. This often requires additional considerations when developing instructional programs, such as the provision of physical and occupational therapy and the use of orthotic devices or wheelchairs.

Besides more serious physical disabilities, there will often be delays in basic motor functioning. Motor skills, of course, are important for nearly all phases of daily life including self-help skills, vocational skills, leisure activities, and so on. If a lag exists in an individual's motor development, it may hamper adequate functioning in these areas. For this reason it may be necessary to identify such a deficiency and focus training efforts in that direction.

The purpose of this chapter is to examine key physical problems, delays, and related disabilities sometimes associated with mental retardation. Most of the discussion will be pertinent to moderately, severely, and profoundly retarded persons although some segments will also apply to the mildly retarded. Besides the disabilities discussed, additional information will be reviewed on the use of drugs, dietary considerations, and body-behavior problems.

GENERAL PHYSICAL AND MOTOR CHARACTERISTICS OF MENTALLY RETARDED PERSONS

Lower functioning retarded people (moderate, severe, profound) are often quite fragile individuals. They are said to have a lower level of biological integrity (Berkson, 1963). One indication of this is their size which tends to be small for their chronological age. Their physical stature has been found to be directly related to their intellectual development (Mosier, Grossman & Dingman, 1965). This means that the lower an individual's intelligence, the smaller he or she will usually be (Bruininks, 1974; Hardman & Drew, 1977). It is likely that organic sources of brain impairment also affect growth impairment either directly or indirectly. Thus, while organically impaired individuals often have smaller than average bodies, cultural-familial mildly retarded individuals are usually about equal in size to their nonretarded chronological age peers.

In some cases, problems in the opposite direction occur; that is, the retarded person may be overweight for his or her height. Fox and Rotatori (1982) studied weight characteristics of 1,152 retarded adults and found many of them to be either overweight (weighing 11% to 19% above the standard range for their height) or obese (20% or more above the standard). Twenty-one percent of the women and 16% of the men were overweight, while 25% and 16% of the men and women respectively were obese. The weight problems were found to occur more often with mildly and moderately retarded persons than with the severely and profoundly retarded. Fox, Switzky, Rotatori, and Vitkus (1982) noted that in some rare syndromes (Praeder-Willi and Laurence-Moon-Biedl) weight control appears to be particularly difficult. In most cases, however, the problem has the same source as in the nonretarded population, that is, too much caloric intake in relation to physical activity. Fox et al. (1982) provided a behavior modification program that had been used effectively to help retarded persons lose weight.

Another characteristic of many moderately to profoundly retarded people is their susceptibility to different physical ailments. These tend to cut across many syndromes of retardation. Additionally, within specific syndromes, various unique disabilities will have a higher than average probability of occurring (see Carter, 1975, for an extensive listing). Down's syndrome serves as an example. Physical problems observed in some of these individuals include lack of muscle tone during infancy, hypoelasticity of the joints, thyroid dysfunction as an adult, diabetes mellitus, cardiac abnormalities, strabismus, leukemia, and respiratory problems (Isaacson & VanHartesveldt, 1978; Smith & Wilson, 1973). Obviously, such serious problems will compound the difficulties of Down's syndrome individuals as well as other retarded individuals who are affected by them.

A reflection of physical development is motor performance. How well a person can perform on different tasks requiring specific motor skills is generally considered to be a measure of the person's physical status. Even though an individual might not display problems such as those listed above, a reduced measure of physical fitness might indicate less than adequate physical development. Such is the case with many mentally retarded individuals including those in the mild range (Bruininks, 1974; Malpass, 1963). On various tasks of physical motor performance, mentally retarded persons have been found to score below their chronological-age nonretarded peers. Mildly retarded persons tend to lag behind about two to four years on motor skills and more severely retarded persons even more. Some common motor deficits include poor equilibrium and performance balance, locomotion, complex coordination, and manipulative dexterity. As the individuals grow older, motor skill differences between retarded and nonretarded individuals get larger. Fortunately, it has been found that highly structured diagnostic physical training programs can reduce this gap to some degree (Bruininks, 1974).

The normal development of motor skills depends on biological and experiential factors (Malpass, 1963). As with intelligence and learning, it is difficult to separate the influence of these sources. The fact that many retarded children show improvement in their motor skills with systematic training would lead one to believe that their deficits are at least partially due to a lack of experience. On the other hand, Molnar (1978) reported that many children of various levels of retardation exhibited significantly delayed postural adjustment reactions (reflexes) and subsequent motor milestones during infancy. For at least some, then, biological influences may be an impediment to later motor performance. This will more likely be true for moderately, severely, and profoundly retarded persons.

One final aspect of general physical development can be considered and that is the capacity for physical exertion. Coleman, Ayoub, and Friedrich (1976) studied the amount of exercise mildly and moderately retarded adult males could demonstrate before reaching a level of physical stress. All of the participants were free of physical disabilities. The exercise was performed on an ergometer (an exercise bicycle) and the stress was measured by physiological responses (i.e., pulse and oxygen uptake). The researchers discovered that their subjects performed 20% to 30% below the level of normal individuals before reaching the same level of physiological exertion. They suggested that improvement in physical conditioning would be necessary before many mildly or moderately retarded persons would be able to perform strenuous work activities.

In summary, mentally retarded people's general physical development appears to require attention as do other areas of development. Moderately, severely, and profoundly retarded people tend to be frail and small. And yet, a number of retarded individuals are overweight or even obese. Many are susceptible to a wide variety of diseases and physical problems. The lower the individual's intellectual level, the greater the probability that he or she will suffer from one or more physical ailments. Mildly retarded people are not as susceptible to chronic physical problems; but their physical condition, as judged by their motor performance, is usually not equal to that of normal persons. With intensive practice, they can improve upon these abilities. Structured physical education programs, or in some cases physical therapy, will be beneficial for many of the physical deficiencies of retarded persons. Sometimes continuing problems occur that require special treatment or consideration.

CEREBRAL PALSY

Cerebral palsy (CP) is a generic term referring to a number of motor disabilities that result from damage to the brain before, during, or after birth (Robinault & Denhoff, 1973). It is primarily characterized by a lack of control over the voluntary muscles of the arms, legs, mouth, tongue, and/or eyes. Other problems are often associated with cerebral palsy including convulsive disorders, behavior disorders of an organic origin, perceptual problems, sensory defects, and mental retardation.

The various causes of cerebral palsy are the same as many of the different organic causes of retardation. Anything that can do damage to the brain can result in CP just as it can result in mental retardation. Therefore, it should not be surprising that a good number of cerebral palsied individuals (though far from all) are also mentally retarded.

According to Denhoff and Robinault (1960), there are five major forms of CP although often combinations will occur. The major clinical forms include:

Spasticity: This is the most frequent form. It accounts for about 60% to 65% of all cases. Spasticity is characterized by the overcontraction of muscles resulting in extremely poor postural arrangement. This is the form of cerebral palsy seen most often in mentally retarded individuals, particularly the severely and profoundly retarded.

Athetosis: This form occurs in about 25% of the cases. It is characterized by a series of slow, recurring, involuntary movements of the hands, feet, and trunk. The movements are sometimes described as being "wormlike."

Ataxia: This form is indicated by a lack of coordination that affects postural control and walking. About 7% of the cases take this form.

Tremor: This is similar to athetosis but with coarser movements. It accounts for about 1% to 5% of the cases.

Rigidity: This is identified by the individual's resistance to a limb being moved and appears in about 7% of all cases of CP.

Various steps can be taken to reduce the impact of CP and generally the earlier these are taken, the better. Of primary concern is as much prevention of contraction and muscle deterioration as possible. CP is not a progressive disorder in the sense that the brain lesion gets worse. However, without intervention to the muscular needs of the individual, contractions may take a permanent form and postural improvement may be extremely difficult. Exercising, bracing, and/or surgery may all be necessary before three years of age. Medication for seizure control may also be necessary.

The relationship of cerebral palsy to mental retardation is not clear (Hardman & Drew, 1977). The safest statement to make is that mental retardation exits within the CP population to a relatively greater degree than it does within the nonCP population. One of the problems in determining the incidence of retardation among CP individuals is the difficulty caused by the CP individual's motor impairment. This may affect their

IQ score by impeding their performance in standardized test situations. It may also affect their performance by reducing the number of experiences that would normally promote intellectual development.

Based on their review of various prevalence statements, Hardman and Drew (1977) concluded that "programmatic research has not been implemented to any substantial degree" (p. 44). Probably the most agreed upon figures are that about 50% of the CP population score below 70 on intelligence tests; another 25% score between 70 and 90 points; while the last 25% score in the average or above average range.

We can also look at the CP–MR relationship from the other perspective; that is, within a certain range of mental retardation, what percent of the people will be cerebral palsied? While there does not appear to be a readily available answer to this question, it seems that the lower one moves on the continuum of retardation, the greater percent of cerebral palsied individuals are likely to be found. We know that more brain damage is found at lower levels and that this damage is more diffuse. It is logical, therefore, that a greater percent of the population at each successively lower level would have neuromuscular disorders due to brain damage.

EPILEPSY

Epilepsy, like cerebral palsy, results from a brain disorder. It has been characterized in several ways, but the most notable feature is the recurring seizures that the individual manifests from time to time. Barnes and Krasnoff (1973) defined it as a "chronic, episodic disturbance in function of the central nervous system which is characterized by one or more of the following usually transitory features: disruption of consciousness, convulsions, and alterations in sensory, motor, autonomic, cognitive, and affective status" (p. 259).

Seizures can take different forms. Gadow (1980) described the seizure as "a sudden attack, usually manifested by a complete or partial loss of consciousness and accompanied by involuntary muscle movement or a cessation of body movement" (p. 33). A single seizure would not necessarily indicate the presence of epilepsy. Seizures or convulsions are caused by an electrical discharge in the brain. This can happen to anyone if the right stimulus affects the electrochemical activity of the brain. Such stimuli could include infections, poisons, drugs, sudden oxygen deprivation, metabolic disturbances, head trauma, and various other sources. Only when the seizures continue over a period of time is the disorder referred to as epilepsy (Gadow, 1980; Spooner & Dykes, 1982).

Different schemes have been used to classify seizures. One scheme is concerned with cause, while another with the form of the seizure. In the first system, seizures are classified according to why they occur. Somewhere between one-half and three-fourths of the time, the cause of the seizure will be unknown. These are referred to as *idiopathic* seizures. Other times, seizures result because of some definite damage to the brain. These are referred to as *secondary, organic,* or *symptomatic* seizures (Barnes & Krasnoff, 1973; Gadow, 1980). Barnes and Krasnoff list eight general categories of symptomatic epilepsy. These include congenital: birth injuries, syphilis; degenerative: multiple sclerosis; inflammations: encephalitis, meningitis; vascular: arteriosclerosis, strokes; traumatic: head injuries; tumor: gliomas, meningioma; general somatic disease: acute fevers, hypoglycemia; and intoxications: botulism, alcohol, drugs.

The second common classification system categorizes epilepsy based on the type of seizure that occurs. The most common are grand mal seizures, petit mal seizures, and psychomotor (temporal lobe) seizures. A fourth category sometimes suggested is myoclonic seizures (Livingston, 1972). Table 8–1 describes the various seizures.

The most common seizures are the grand mal. They account for about 80% to 90% of all seizures. They are also the most common seizures experienced by retarded people who have seizures. Petit mal seizures are found in about 2% to 3% of the individuals with epilepsy and sometimes lead to grand mal seizures later in life. Psychomotor seizures rarely occur in children under six but may be demonstrated by 10% to 20% of the older children, adolescents, and adults who have seizures. Myoclonic seizures are rare and sometimes occur along with grand mal seizures. Livingston (1972) divides myoclonic seizures into two classes based on the age of the child (see Table 8–1).

The expression of the seizure is a direct result of the part of the brain that is affected. Sometimes only a part of the brain is involved and a *focal* seizure occurs. The result might be a twitching or tingling of a certain part of the body, but the rest of the body remains unaffected. A *generalized* seizure involves electrical activity affecting the entire brain. Sometimes a focal seizure will begin and will progress to a generalized seizure. When this occurs, it is called a *Jacksonian* seizure. The seizure may begin with the twitching of a finger on one hand, progress up the arm, affect the same side of the face, move down the same side of the body, and then move over to the other side of the body and thus become a generalized grand mal seizure (Livingston, 1972).

Four approaches have been used in the treatment of seizures (Spooner & Dykes, 1982). The most common is the use of anticonvulsant drugs. Another is neurosurgery or electrical treatment. This procedure focuses on the brain lesion responsible for the seizure activity. The third approach attempts to deal with seizures as operant behaviors and controls environmental aspects that may influence or inhibit them. For example, reinforcement may be delivered in the absence of seizures or aversive contingencies employed when seizures occur. The fourth tactic is not so much intended to inhibit the seizure as to reduce the possible physical damage that may result. Spooner and Dykes (1982) referred to this as "orthotic management." It consists of using helmets or arranging the environment in a way to prevent the person from being hurt during the seizure.

As with cerebral palsy, the estimates of the prevalence of epilepsy among mentally retarded persons vary. Certainly the prevalence is greater than in the nonretarded population. Tizard and Grad (1961) reported that 18% of mentally retarded persons had a history of seizures; Payne, Johnson, and Abelson (1969) reported that 31% of 23,000 residents of institutions in the western United States had seizures. Corbett, Harris, and Robinson (1975) and Spooner and Dykes (1982), based on their reviews, concluded that severely and profoundly retarded persons were more likely to have seizures than were higher level individuals.

In a recent study, Richardson, Koller, Katz, and McLaren (1981) examined the occurrence of epilepsy among 185 of the 221 individuals (88%) born in a city in Britain between 1951–55 who were identified as mentally retarded. The individuals were followed, up to the age of twenty-two. Based on interviews and agency records, the researchers analyzed various aspects of seizure activity.

They found that the degree of seizure impairment (major, intermediate, or minor) was similar across age stages with the exception of minor impairments. These occurred significantly more often during the preschool years. Totally, 94% of the studied sample reported some degree of seizure activity but only about 9% of the population had severe or moderate–severe seizure impairments. There were no statistically significant differences between males and females in regard to seizures; however, in the severe and moderate–severe categories, there were more males than females.

Richardson et al. also noted the occurrence of seizures according to level of retardation. They divided their sample into sub-50, 50–59, 60–69, and 70+ IQ groups. They reported that "of those with IQs less than 50, almost half had at least one seizure, and the odds of having one or more seizures were about three times as great for this group as those with IQs above 50." The occurrence of seizure activity became less and less in the higher IQ groups. Overall, in contrast to a comparison group of nonretarded persons, it was found that the odds of a retarded person having a history of seizures was forty times greater than that of a normal person. Although this is but one study, it provides a fairly clear picture of the susceptibility of mentally retarded persons to epilepsy.

TAELE 8–1 Characteristics of Various Types of Epilepsy

TYPE OF EPILEPSY	AGE AT ONSET	SEIZURE PATTERN	DURATION OF SEIZURE	FREQUENCY OF SEIZURES	EEG FINDINGS
Major Motor (grand mal)	May occur at any age	Generalized tonic-clonic tonic clonic atonic Focal	Variable: most commonly several to 5 minutes or so; however may last as long as one hour or longer	Variable	Nonspecific abnormalities; interseizure tracing may be normal
Petit Mal	Usually between 4 and 8 years; rarely before 3 or after 15	Simple staring (most frequent) Staring with clonic movements Staring with automatisms	Always brief (momentary)	Daily, frequently as many as 50 to 100 per day	Diffuse bilaterally synchronous spike and wave forms usually recurring at frequency of 3 per second
Psychomotor (temporal lobe)	Most commonly in older children and adults	Manifestations vary considerably: most commonly automatisms consisting of staring episodes with smacking of lips, chewing movements, mumbled speech, confused states: bizarre motor and/or psychic performances	Usually lasts several minutes or so	Daily in many patients	Epileptiform discharges usually spikes from the anterior temporal areas in most patients particularly in the older child and adult. In some patients, the EEG reveals other types of electrical abnormalities; occasionally interseizure tracing is normal

Myoclonic Infants	During the first year of life most commonly between 3 and 9 months	Flexor spasm of musculature resulting in massive myoclonic seizure in recumbent position and head dropping attack in sitting position; extensor spasm of musculature occurs less often	Individual spell very brief, several seconds or so; spells frequently recur in clusters lasting several minutes	Usually daily	Hypsarhythmia
Myoclonic Older Children	After 2 years of age, most commonly between 3 and 7 years	Flexor spasm of musculature resulting in head dropping attack when mild, and precipitous fall forward when severe; extensor spasm of musculature occurs less often	Very brief, several seconds or so	Daily, weekly	Modified hypsarhythmia

From S. Livingston, *Comprehensive management of epilepsy in infancy, childhood, and adolescence,* 1972. Courtesy of Charles C Thomas, Publisher, Springfield, Illinois.

VISUAL AND HEARING IMPAIRMENTS

In a recent analysis of Carter's (1975) *Handbook of Mental Retardation Syndromes*, it was found that over 140 of the syndromes listed could have some degree of visual impairment associated with their occurrence. Indeed, the occurrence of visual impairments (partially sighted and blind) among mentally retarded people is relatively high. D. Ellis (1979) recently provided a review of this area. Overall, visual impairments were found to range from about 5% to 11% of the population samples studied. Falbe-Hansen (1968), for example, reported that 11% of the individuals in a Danish institution for the mentally retarded had ocular anomalies; while Warburg (1970) reported that about 5% of institutionalized residents she studied were blind and 6% to 8% were partially sighted.

Various researchers have studied the causes of visual impairments among mentally retarded children. What has been found is that the clinical conditions are extremely heterogeneous. However, D. Ellis (1979) concluded that mentally retarded people are particularly susceptible to "cataracts, optic atrophy, perinatal damage related to prematurity, maternal infections, and genetic anomalies" (p. 501). No research was found reporting the incidence of visual impairments at different levels of retardation. Obviously, however, organically impaired children will have more visual problems than nonorganically impaired.

Several writers have noted the increased incidence of hearing impairment among mentally retarded persons as compared to the normal population. Lloyd (1970) reported that while about 4% of the normal population have some hearing loss, 10% to 15% of the retarded population does. Dibenedetto (1976) reviewed literature on the prevalence of hearing impairments and concluded that the mentally retarded population has three to four times as many hearing deficits as does the normal population. In their survey of 518 retarded persons residing in group homes, Reynolds and Reynolds (1979) found that 14.6% were reported to have some degree of hearing loss.

While assessment procedures and criteria used to determine hearing losses have varied (Lloyd, 1970), the data have indicated increased hearing impairment for the mentally retarded with the greater incidence of impairment occurring with lower level individuals. Dibenedetto (1976) stated that the organicity resulting in mental retardation also caused many hearing impairments. Reynolds and Reynolds (1979) found that 44% of their sample who were classified as severely or profoundly retarded had hearing losses as opposed to 24% of those classified as moderately or mildly retarded. They also found that those classified as profoundly retarded had more severe hearing losses than any other level. The percentage of individuals with severe losses decreased at each successively higher level of retardation.

Sensory deficits (visual impairments and hearing impairments) will certainly have a serious effect on the development of mentally retarded persons. As with CP, epilepsy, or various other disorders, these deficits will only serve to compound problems of the individual's adaption to his or her environment. The intellectual deficit the person has will be furthered by these conditions. Multiple handicapping conditions such as cerebral palsy and epilepsy or blindness and deafness are not uncommon, particularly in profoundly retarded individuals.

DRUG TREATMENT

Because of various physical and behavioral conditions, drugs are often used in education and treatment programs for mentally retarded persons. These drugs are varied and are used extensively in residential facilities (Silva, 1979) and in public schools (Gadow & Kalachik, 1981).

Two major categories of drugs are used: psychotropic drugs and antiepileptic or anticonvulsant drugs. Psychotropic drugs are generally used to alter mood, thought processes, or behaviors. They include *stimulants, major tranquilizers, minor tranquilizers, antidepressants, hypnotics,* and *sedatives.* The purpose of anticonvulsant drugs, as implied by their name, is to control seizures (See Table 8–2).

Psychotropic drugs

Stimulants such as Ritalin and Dexedrine are often used to control hyperactive behavior in children. More often they will be used for non-retarded children, but they may also be used with retarded children, especially those at higher intellectual levels. Ritalin is the most frequently used drug with children in general, being used primarily to control hyperactivity (Krager, Safer & Earhardt, 1977).

Stimulants are less likely to be used with moderately, severely, and profoundly retarded children and institutionalized individuals. More often tranquilizers will be used to control hyperactivity as well as other behavior problems. Aside from their use with retarded persons, the major tranquilizers are generally used with psychotic adults to control bizarre behavior. Sometimes they are referred to as antipsychotic agents. Besides hyperactivity, they will be used with retarded persons to control aggressive behavior, self-injurious behavior, stereotyped acts, and to facilitate general compliance. The major tranquilizers slow people down. They tend to become more detached, serene, and are not easily disturbed when under medication. Additionally, they tend to become more indifferent to people and express less emotion. Cognitive performance and learning ability may be dulled (Agran & Martin, 1982).

TABLE 8–2 Drugs Commonly Used With Mentally Retarded Individuals

	TRADE NAME	GENERIC NAME	PURPOSE
1. *Stimulants:*	Ritalin Cylert Dexedrine	Methylphenidate HCL Magnesium Penoline Dextroamphetimine	Used to control hyperactivity. Used more with nonretarded children but sometimes also with retarded children. Their effect is to reduce movement and allow the child to concentrate on the task. Tend to reduce behavior problems. Side effects may include changes in mood, headaches, stomach aches, nausea, insomnia, and loss of appetite.
2. *Major Tranquilizers:*	Mellaril Thorazine Haldol Stelazine	Thioridazine Chlorpromazine Haloperidol Trifluoperazine HCL	To control aggressive, self-abusive, stereotyped, and acting-out behavior, psychotic states. Minor side effects include dry mouth, constipation, drowsiness, increase in appetite. Major side effects include shaking of hands, shuffling walk, difficulty in speech, restlessness.
3. *Minor Tranquilizers:*	Valium Atarax Librium Vistaril	Diazepam Hydroxyzine HCL Chlordiazepoxide HCL Hydroxyzine Pamoate	May be used to calm mild agitation, anxiety, or tension. Also used as a muscle relaxant for cerebral palsied individuals. Will sometimes be used to control seizures in epileptic children and to induce sleep.
4. *Anticonvulsants:*	Dilantin Eskabarb Mebaral Mysoline Dyamox Zarontin Depakene Tegretol ACTH Corticosteroids	Phenytoin Phenobarbital Mephobarbital Primidone Acetazolamide Etaosuximide Valproic Acid Carbamazepine Corticotropin	Used primarily to control grand mal seizures. Used primarily to control petit mal seizures. Used to control psychomotor seizures. Sometimes used to try to control myoclonic seizures but relapse rate is high.

Breuning and Davidson (1981) studied the effects of psychotropic drugs and behavior modification on intelligence test performance of mentally retarded adults. Scores increased by an average of 7 IQ points when the individuals were not on their medication. When the no medication condition was modified by rewarding the individuals for correct answers, their IQs increased by an average of 30 points. In a related study Marholin, Touchette, and Stewart (1979) found that by withdrawing the administration of chlorpromazine, a psychotropic, their subjects' behaviors improved noticeably although there was variability between them. Some of the improvements were in social skills, sensitivity to directions and reprimands, vocational tasks, and the reduction of self-abusive behaviors.

Because of such examples as these, the use of major tranquilizers has been criticized. In contrast, however, Singh and Aman (1981) reported several slightly positive effects due to the administration of Mellaril (thiordazine). They compared individually prescribed dosages, standard dosages (generally lower than those individually prescribed) and a placebo on various measures. They found that weight increased under individual dosages but not the standard dosage and that heart rate and blood pressure were unaffected by either drug condition. Across conditions, they found no statistically significant differences on motor performance, the quality of eating, instruction following (although this was slightly better when on drugs), self-stimulation (also slightly improved on drugs), or social behavior (slightly improved while on drugs). Both standard and individualized dosages decreased hyperactivity and bizarre behaviors. Self-stimulation decreased more on standard doses than individualized doses. The effects of the drugs on cognitive performance were equivocal.

It has only been recently that well-controlled studies such as these have begun to ascertain the effects that drugs have on behavior. Up until this time, most of the conclusions about drugs have been based on clinical observations. Hopefully, more information will become available, especially for the major tranquilizers.

Minor tranquilizers (see Table 8–2) are used most often to control anxiety. They will also be used sometimes to control seizures and to reduce the muscular tension in cerebral palsy. Valium is used often in this latter capacity. Common side effects include lethargy, drowsiness, ataxia, depression, and nausea. Other psychotropic drugs may be prescribed for different reasons. Antidepressants will be used to control enuresis; sedatives will be used to reduce anxiety; and hypnotics will help people fall asleep. One group of hypnotics, the barbiturates, has anticonvulsant properties. Phenobarbital is an example. It is included with the other anticonvulsants.

Anticonvulsants

As seen in Table 8–2, a number of drugs are used to help control seizures. Only a few are listed in the table. Their effectiveness will vary from drug to drug and from person to person. Phenobarbital and Dilantin are the two most commonly used drugs to control grand mal seizures. Other drugs listed in Table 8–2 will be used if one of these is not effective or if undesirable side effects occur and cannot be controlled.

Zarontin is the most common drug used for petit mal seizures. Sometimes when these seizures occur, the child will be placed on phenobarbital initially and then later Zarontin. This is because petit mal seizures often precede grand mal seizures and the physician wants to avoid this. After about a month on the phenobarbital, the Zarontin will be introduced. If the petit mal seizures are not controlled, another anticonvulsant will be substituted (Livingston, 1972).

Psychomotor (temperal lobe) epilepsy is often treated with Tegretol. Sometimes, however, Dilantin and Mysoline will be used. ACTH and corticosteroids are used to treat myoclonic seizures, but this is the most difficult form of epilepsy to control. Even when these drugs are successful, there is a high relapse rate. Valium will also be used sometimes but again it is generally not effective in the long run. Livingston (1972) advocates attempts to control myoclonic seizures using the *ketogenic* diet. This diet requires a high fat to carbohydrate plus protein ratio.

The use of anticonvulsants with epileptic retarded children has not been subject to as much criticism as has the use of psychotropic drugs such as major tranquilizers. Recently, however, Kaufman and Katz-Garris (1979) studied the practice of using anticonvulsant drugs in one institution and reported some disheartening findings. Of the 127 individuals studied, forty-one were receiving some kind of anticonvulsant medication. Of the forty-one, however, only seventeen had ever shown any evidence of epilepsy. For the other twenty-four, there was no documented clinical evidence of seizure disorders or any other need for the medication; yet they were regularly administered the anticonvulsants. None of the forty-one individuals' charts contained pertinent information such as anticonvulsant blood levels, EEGs, and so on.

Use of Drugs with Mentally Retarded Persons

Several studies have documented the rather extensive use of drugs with mentally retarded people. Lipman (1970) found that 51% of the residents of state and private institutions surveyed had received psychotropic drugs at some time, mostly Mellaril and Thorizine. More recently, Sprague (1977) found the 66% of the residents in one institution and 65% in another received drug treatment. In both institutions, over half the people getting medicine were getting two or more kinds. In order, the most frequently administered medicines were Mellaril, Dilantin, and Phenobarbital.

Silva (1979) reported very similar findings. During a three month observation period, 65.8% of the residents in one institution received some medication while 56.2% were on continuing medication. Again, the most frequently prescribed were Mellaril, Dilantin, and Phenobarbital.

Less is known about the use of drugs by mentally retarded students in public school programs. Recently Gadow and Kalachnik (1981) shed some light on this area. Their study consisted of a survey of 325 teachers of 3,306 TMR students. In their results they reported that 84% of the teachers had at least one student receiving psychotropic and/or anticonvulsant drugs; 64% of the teachers had children with seizure disorders, and 42% had children with behavior disorders. Ten percent of the students were being treated for seizure disorders, 5% were treated for behavior disorders, and 1.8% were concurrently treated for both. The six most frequently prescribed drugs (and the percent of students receiving them) included Dilantin (6.9%), Phenobarbital (6.2%), Ritalin (2.7%), Mysoline (2.2%), Mellaril (1.5%), and Valium (1.4%). Dilantin and Phenobarbital were the most commonly used drugs for seizures and seizure-behavior disorders; Ritalin and Mellaril were the most commonly used for behavior disorders. Gadow and Kalachnik concluded that medications for seizures and behavior disorders, although used extensively, were prescribed less often for public school students than for institutionalized residents. The use of drugs in public school programs for retarded students presents teachers with an additional responsibility since they are the ones who usually administer them (Gadow, 1982; Courtnage, 1982).

The extensive and sometimes perhaps unwarranted use of drugs with mentally retarded people has been criticized (Agran & Martin, 1982). Currently, attempts are being made to correct the situation. Gadow (1980) reviewed several requirements imposed by recent court rulings (*Wyatt v. Stickey*, 1972; *New York ARC v. Rockefeller*, 1975) concerning the administration of drugs to retarded persons. These included:

> The right to be free from unnecessary or excessive medication
>
> Accurate medical records reviewed weekly by the attending physician
>
> No medication for purposes of punishment, for the convenience of the staff, or that interfere with habilitation or training programs
>
> The administration of drugs only by trained staff
>
> Written policies and procedures for the administration of drugs
>
> The reporting of errors in the administration of medication to the physician who ordered the drugs

Hopefully, these and similar guidelines will improve the appropriate use of medication with mentally retarded people.

DIETARY CONSIDERATIONS

Not discounting the various neurological and physical disorders of mentally retarded individuals that require drug intervention, some problems
may be improved with proper diets. Clearly one area would be the overweight conditions or obesity discussed earlier. Laidler (1976) noted that
often the diets of institutionalized mentally retarded persons lack some
basic ingredients to promote healthy bodily functioning. A common "minor" ailment among many institutionalized persons is constipation. Laidler (1976) pointed out that the meals served in institutions often consist
of concentrated and refined foods and lack in fiber and bulk. Such a diet
coupled with a lack of exercise impedes normal bowel movement activity.
Consequently, laxatives are often prescribed. Silva (1979) found in his
study that 10.4% of the residents were taking laxatives.

Another problem often seen is regurgitation. Sometimes this is attributed to psychological problems and is susceptible to behavior management techniques. Other times it may be attributable to food problems. If
it is a physiological response, a change in the diet may be beneficial. Laidler suggested that high carbohydrate foods may be helpful. He also suggested that eating six smaller meals a day would be preferable to three
larger ones.

Dietary intervention has also been recommended to control allergic
reactions (Feingold, 1974). Many foods as well as other substances may
act as allergens (see Table 8–3). Allergies can take many forms among
mentally retarded and nonretarded people including learning and behavior problems, hyperactivity, perceptual problems, and seizures (Knapczyk, 1979). Hall (1976) reported that 50% of the children with convulsive disorders have allergies that affect the frequency of their seizures.
Knapczyk (1979) suggested that teachers of severely handicapped children could probably safely assume that at least one of their students is
suffering from an undiagnosed allergy.

BODY-BEHAVIOR PROBLEMS

Mentally retarded people and other people whose physical appearance
connotes their disability suffer an impairment in addition to their diagnosed disability. This impairment is manifested sometimes when they
come into contact with other people. Meyerson (1971) referred to it as the
"somatopsychology" of a disability. The thrust of the problem is in the
reactions of others that must be encountered by the physically impaired
person. Along with the various intellectual, emotional, and physical problems that a mentally retarded person may have, he or she has the added
difficulty of existing in environments where adverse social reactions are

TABLE 8–3   Common Substances Which Can Cause an Allergic Reaction

- **Inhalants**
  pollen
  dust
  mold
  cosmetics
  fumes from glue, paints, and strong chemicals
  tobacco smoke
  animal dander

- **Ingestants**
  Almost any type of food substance, especially:
  wheat
  milk
  corn
  eggs
  cola
  salicylates (e.g., apricots, cherries, tomatoes)
  chocolates
  refined sugars
  spinach
  nuts
  citrus fruits
  Additives to foods including:
  colors
  flavors
  preservatives, residues
  Almost any type of drug or additive to drugs

- **Contactants**
  clothing dyes
  plastics
  cosmetics
  rubber
  poison ivy
  soap

- **Injectants**
  snake and insect bites
  injected medicines and vaccines

From D. R. Knapczyk, "The presence of allergies among severely handicapped persons," *AAESPH Review*, 1979, *4*, 354–363. Reprinted by permission.

common. At each step they are challenged with a new situation because they never know what form of human reaction to expect.

Most retarded people, by virtue of their intellectual status, are socially relegated to a position of relative isolation. When a physical mark such as CP, blindness, or any of the unique features common to the different syndromes brand them, their social plight becomes more difficult.

Neisworth, Jones, and Smith (1978) noted that the behavior of others is abnormally modified and this, of course, affects the behavior of the handicapped person. People with severe physical handicaps suffer more personal-emotional problems than those without them (Meyerson, 1971). Physically different children may be ridiculed, excluded, or patronized (Neisworth et al., 1978). Neisworth et al. suggested that in addition to educational and habilitation services, cosmetic prosthetics be used when possible to improve the normalcy of the person's appearance.

CONCLUSION

The student of mental retardation should be aware of the physical status of mentally retarded individuals. In mildly retarded persons, the deviation may be slight, perhaps only evidenced by minor lags in motor development. Among the moderately, severely, and profoundly retarded, more impeding conditions may occur. These can range from being physically smaller and more fragile to having cerebral palsy, epilepsy, or multiple debilitating conditions. In these cases, it is most clear that the treatment program provided, be it in the school, institutions, or home, incorporate the expertise of medical as well as educational personnel.

However, it must be understood by all that the individual's wellbeing is paramount. Drugs should be used only under carefully monitored situations because, in effect, they create a very restrictive environment. Other alternatives, such as dietary intervention, should always be given consideration.

There is more hope for mentally retarded people today than at any other time in history. As progress is made educationally and medically, this hope will grow and much of it will be realized.

STUDY QUESTIONS

1. What is the general relationship of physical status to mental retardation?
2. What are some physical problems sometimes associated with Down's syndrome?
3. What variables are normally related to motor development? What is the relationship of these variables to different levels of mental retardation?
4. Describe the relationship between the etiology and prevalence of mental retardation and cerebral palsy.
5. How are seizures in epilepsy classified? What are the most common seizures experienced by mentally retarded people who have them?
6. What treatment techniques have been used to help control seizures?
7. To what degree are mentally retarded persons affected by visual or hearing impairments?

8. What are the two major types of drugs used with mentally retarded individuals?
9. What are some effects of major tranquilizers?
10. What are the two most commonly used drugs to control grand mal seizures?
11. To what extent are drugs used in programs for mentally retarded individuals?
12. What is meant by the "somatopsychology" of a disability?

9

Public School Programs

OVERVIEW: EDUCATION, PL 94–142, AND THE LEAST RESTRICTIVE ENVIRONMENT

One of the greatest services of our modern society is a free public school education. Public school systems represent a major American institution designed not only to provide academic knowledge but to inculcate society's mores in its young people. The study of education shows a history of changing values that parallel those of society. It is a history filled with ideas, approaches, criticisms, changes, and new ideas.

Public school programs serve all children, including those who are mentally retarded. In fact, public school services are one of the most extensive services provided by society for mentally retarded individuals. Public Law 94–142, The Education for All Handicapped Children Act, passed in 1975, was the culmination of a long history of efforts to provide "free and appropriate" educational services to mentally retarded and other handicapped persons (Nazzaro, 1977).

In addition to its guarantee for a free and appropriate education, the law also required handicapped students be educated in the "least restrictive environment" possible. This seemingly simple dictum has produced a great deal of discussion and debate in the last several years. According to the U.S. Department of Education (1980):

> Public Law 94–142, Section 612(5)(B), requires that to the extent appropriate, handicapped children be placed with children who are not handicapped. Any special classes or other separation should be undertaken only when the nature or the severity of the handicap renders regular classes unsatisfactory even when supplementary services are provided. (p. 33)

Conflict resides in what some consider to be a disharmonious relationship between "appropriate" education and education in the "least restrictive environment" for many retarded students. On one hand it might be desirable for various reasons to place a mentally retarded child in a regular classroom with normal pupils, that is, the least restrictive environment. On the other hand, the law (and common sense) requires that an *appropriate* education be provided. While at a conceptual level the two may seem congruent, at a practical level difficulties often appear.

In the present chapter this issue and its complexities will be discussed. In doing so, it is important to separate concepts and practices in order to provide an understanding of both, as well as their interrelation.

THE DEVELOPMENT OF SPECIAL CLASSES

Special classes had their origin in Germany in the late 1800s after residential facilities for mentally retarded persons were already well established. As Kanner (1964) noted, following the development of institutions in the early and mid-1800s, "it must have occurred to many educators that after removal of those who were conspicuously defective, there were still pupils in their classrooms who could not apply themselves to the pre-scribed curriculum" (p. 112). Thus in different cities in Germany in the early 1860s, special classes started to emerge to serve individuals whom we would classify today as moderately to mildly retarded. It is interesting to note in light of today's mandate of "least restrictive environment" that in these German cities, part-time special classes had more support than segregated classes or schools. The model adopted in Germany was the "auxiliary class" which first appeared in Dresden in 1867 serving sixteen children. By 1905 there were 181 German cities with 583 such classes (Kanner, 1964).

The time and place of the first special class for mentally retarded children in the United States is not exactly clear. Kanner (1964) reported that some efforts in this direction may have occurred in Cleveland in the 1870s. He reported, however, that general agreement places the first class as opening in Providence, Rhode Island, on November 30, 1896. The idea was well accepted and most major cities developed similar programs quite rapidly. By 1911 over one hundred cities in the U.S. had special classes in their schools and many states were passing laws to provide spe-cial funding for these classes (Aiello, 1976).

The development of special classes in the United States probably re-ceived its impetus from different sources. One source was the compulsory school attendance laws (Aiello, 1976). These started in 1840 with Rhode Island and by the turn of the century nearly all states had such mandates. When some parents either could not or would not send their mildly re-tarded children to residential facilities, schools often provided a place for them and this place was either a special class or a special school. Nor-mally, it was not expected that the regular class teacher would tolerate these individuals nor would they be allowed to interfere with the learning of the other children.

The latter issue is an important point and was another major reason why special classes developed. These classes, sometimes called "opportu-nity classes," did not provide what might be considered quality education. This was really not their purpose. More truthfully, they were intended to segregate "problem" children. Not only did they house mentally retarded children, but also various other "troublemakers" that disrupted regular classes (Reynolds & Rosen, 1976).

After the turn of the century, two unrelated events occurred that swelled special classes and the number of children in them: intelligence tests were developed and later racial desegregation of the schools oc-curred. The combination of these events, although separated by several years, resulted in many minority children being formally classified as ed-ucable mentally retarded. In the late 1950s and throughout most of the

1960s, special classes for the mildly retarded increased dramatically as many minority children were placed in them.

Federal support became a major source of funding in the 1960s. In 1965, PL 89–10, the Elementary and Secondary Education Act (ESEA), through Title I, committed a great deal of money to programs for educationally disadvantaged children. In 1966, PL 89–750 amended ESEA and created the Bureau of Education for the Handicapped within the Office of Education. By the end of the 1960s, special classes for the mildly retarded were the predominant public school service available for these students.

THE DEVELOPMENT OF SPECIAL SCHOOLS

Just before special classes for EMR students hit their growth spurt in the late 1950s and 1960s, special schools, primarily for moderately retarded students, began to rapidly emerge. In the early 1950s times were ripe for special school programs to develop.

Between World War I and World War II, public school programs for trainable mentally retarded students were by and large limited. There were a few special schools but not nearly enough to provide needed services. Institutional placement was the standard service offered for these children, but many parents opted to keep them at home.

In the few years following World War II, three things happened which greatly influenced the creation of programs for moderately retarded students. First, the war resulted in many handicapped soldiers. The presence of these individuals in society raised our consciousness of handicapping conditions. To have a handicap was not as much of a stigma as it had been in earlier years. Federal resources were committed to solving some of the problems these people faced. It became politically astute to support handicapped war veterans and some of this concern and related technical innovations spilled over to handicapped children. In short, the results of the war helped ready society for the provision of public school services for lower functioning mentally retarded children.

Another catalyst was the influence provided by prominent people. Individuals such as the writer Pearl Buck, movie stars Roy Rogers and Dale Evans, and the Joseph P. Kennedy family, all with mentally retarded children themselves, spoke publicly on behalf of mentally retarded people. In 1946 the Joseph P. Kennedy, Jr. Foundation was founded to promote programs of care, training, treatment, and research for mentally retarded persons.

Finally, while politicians and celebrities were promoting programs and services, parent groups began organizing and expressing their concerns and desires. A most notable organization was the National Association for Retarded Children. (Currently this group is known as the National Association for Retarded Citizens.) Members of this group and other concerned parents did several things. They started private special day schools for their children, lobbied politicians, and awakened the country to the needs and rights of retarded individuals. Ultimately, they were most influential in the development of special public schools (Aiello, 1976; Mesibov, 1976b; Reynolds & Rosen, 1976) and many such schools began to flourish in the 1950s and 1960s.

Thus we came up almost to our current status. Only one important component was missing: education for the severely and profoundly retarded. Until the early 1970s education of the severely and profoundly retarded was hardly considered. Reviewing many professional journals before about 1973, few pages can be found devoted to this group. Then in the early 1970s things began to change. The federal courts mandated the changes. In 1971, in the case of *Wyatt v. Stickney*, it was ruled that institutionalized persons have a right to treatment. One year later, in 1972, in the case of *Pennsylvania Association for Retarded Citizens (PARC) v. The Commonwealth of Pennsylvania*, public school education became the right of even severely and profoundly retarded persons. Similar cases followed: in 1972 *New York State Association for Retarded Citizens v. Rockefeller*, in 1974 *Maryland Association for Retarded Citizens v. the State of Maryland*. Quite obviously, the Association for Retarded Citizens found a useful ally in the federal courts.

While some states during this era began to pass legislation for educating severely and profoundly retarded persons as a result of the court rulings, it was federal legislation in 1975, PL 94–142, that fully insured the right of *all* handicapped children in the United States to a free, appropriate public school education. But the dynamics of providing public school education for mentally retarded individuals did not stop. Concern was expressed about providing that education in the least restrictive environment.

MOVEMENT TOWARD EDUCATION IN THE LEAST RESTRICTIVE ENVIRONMENT

By the late 1960s, special education was a growing field. Local school districts, state education agencies, and most importantly, the federal government, were providing strong financial support for special education programs. This support included developing and improving direct service programs, training teachers and teacher educators in colleges and universities, and sponsoring basic and applied research.

This movement of concern and service to mentally retarded people was not occurring in a social vacuum. The 1960s and early 1970s were years of an even larger, more pervasive movement, that being the Civil Rights movement. It was in this context, in a time when individuals' rights as human beings and citizens were being shown a serious commitment by society's representatives, that mentally retarded citizens were also greatly benefitting.

Ironically, the civil rights movement also restricted (or perhaps redirected) some of the special education momentum. In 1968 Lloyd Dunn published one of the most oft-quoted articles to appear in the field. Referring to the article as his "swan song," Dunn (1968) wrote the following in reference to special class placement for mildly retarded students:

> Much of our past and present practices are morally and educationally wrong. We have to stop living at the mercy of general educators who have referred their problem children to us.
>
> Let us stop being pressured into continuing and expanding a special education program that we know now to be undesirable for many of the children we are dedicated to serve.
>
> A better education than special class placement is needed for socioculturally deprived children with mild learning problems who have been labeled educable mentally retarded.
>
> In my best judgment, about 60 to 80 percent of the pupils taught . . . are children from low status backgrounds.
>
> It is my thesis that we should stop labeling these deprived children as mentally retarded. Furthermore, we must stop segregating them by placing them into our allegedly special programs. (pp. 5–6)

Although others (e.g., Blatt, 1960; Johnson, 1962) had previously questioned special classes, Dunn's article moved the field tremendously. He had raised serious questions about the common approach to classifying and educating mildly retarded children. Shortly after Dunn's article, a number of other writers expressed their criticism of special classes and the placement of children in them (Budoff, 1972; Christoplos & Renz, 1969; Iano, 1972; Lilly, 1971; Reynolds & Balow, 1972). Much of their criticism was similar to Dunn's.

Besides the concern about a disproportionate number of minority students being placed in special classes, critics of special classes expressed a second source of discontent about these programs. A number of studies conducted over the years, collectively referred to as "efficacy studies," had indicated that children functioning at a level of mild retardation did no better academically in special classes than when they remained in regular classes. These studies have been reviewed by Kirk (1964), Guskin and Spicker (1968), and Kaufman and Alberto (1976). Of the various studies published, none found that special class participation resulted in better academic achievement than did regular class placement.

While some in the field were, and are, critical of special classes, others came to their defense (e.g., Bartlett, 1977; Kidd, 1970; Kolstoe, 1972,

1976; MacMillan, 1971; MacMillan, Jones & Meyers, 1976; Stainback & Stainback, 1975). For example, Kolstoe (1972), among other things, said there was no evidence to support the assumed harmful effects of labels and contended that regular educators were not prepared to meet the needs of mildly retarded children. He later wrote that special classes allowed for more individualized instruction, the use of concrete materials, and the development of vocational skills (Kolstoe, 1976). MacMillan et al. (1976), while acknowledging that the concept was perhaps good, also reiterated the problem of regular teacher attitudes and their ability to provide the appropriate curriculum. MacMillan and his co-authors called for the need to separate principle and practice and to avoid letting the first interfere with the quality of the second. Bartlett (1977) expressed concern about the ability of regular classes and resource rooms to provide for the total needs of the child. He also defended special class placement against the charges of racism that had been implied by some of its critics.

Regarding the efficacy studies, those defending special classes pointed to their methodological weaknesses. They argued that special classes were meant to do more than develop the academic skills that were measured in many of the studies. Also, a number of the efficacy studies that measured social adjustment and acceptance found that mildly retarded children in special classes did better in these areas than when in regular classes (e.g., Kern & Pfaeffle, 1962; Porter & Milazzo, 1958).

As the professionals were arguing among themselves regarding special classes for the mildly retarded, the courts were acting. The net effect was that serious restrictions were placed on the process for identifying and placing children in EMR classes. The special focus was on minority children. Ultimately, Pl 94–142, the federal law that guaranteed the right to education for all handicapped children, also guaranteed the right to due process in the placement of children in special classes (acknowledging potentially stigmatizing effects) and the right to appropriate education in the least restrictive environment.

THE CONCEPT OF EDUCATION IN THE LEAST RESTRICTIVE ENVIRONMENT

The terms "least restrictive environment" and "mainstreaming" have been used a great deal during the last several years. They have been used synonymously by some while others have seen them as different. Exceptional children, including mentally retarded children, are legally required to be educated in the least restrictive environment but the law, PL 94–142, never uses the word "mainstreaming." While least restrictive environment is somewhat of an ambiguous term, it generally is taken to mean an environment as close to that of normal students as possible. This does not necessarily mean with normal students all of the time (Dybwad, 1980) but, in fact, implementation of the concept often means placing a child in the mainstream for at least a portion of the day.

Mainstreaming refers to the "temporal, instructional, and social integration" of handicapped children with nonhandicapped children (Kaufman, Gottlieb, Agard & Kukik, 1975). While some have considered mainstreaming as a specific arrangement; for example integrating retarded children for at least 50% of the instructional day (MacMillan et al., 1976), others have felt mainstreaming should not be so narrowly defined (Council for Exceptional Children, 1975). In a rather explicit statement, the Council for Exceptional Children offered the following definition:

> Mainstreaming is . . .
> Providing the most appropriate education for each child in the least restrictive setting.
> Looking at the educational needs of children instead of clinical or diagnostic labels.
> Looking for and creating alternatives that will help general educators serve children with learning or adjustment problems in the regular setting.
> Uniting the skills of general education and special education so that all children may have an equal educational opportunity.
> Mainstreaming is not . . .
> Wholesale return of all exceptional children in special classes to regular classes.
> Permitting children with special needs to remain in regular classrooms without the support services they need.
> Ignoring the need of some children for a more specialized program than can be provided in the general educational setting.
> Less costly than serving children in special self-contained classes. (p. 174)

Kenneth Wyatt, a past president of CEC, in an interview (Thomas, 1979) stated that the least restrictive environment was generally a misunderstood concept. He dichotomized between it and mainstreaming and emphasized the need to consider each child individually. For some children the regular classroom may be appropriate for a portion of the day whereas for others it may be totally inappropriate. Like others (Kaufman et al., 1975; CEC, 1975), Wyatt stressed the need for an ongoing evaluation of the process.

Some of the proponents of education of the mentally retarded in the least restrictive environment, or in the mainstream, have considered it a sociomoral issue. Reynolds and Balow (1972) discussed the rising revulsion in society against all forms of "simplistic categorization" of human beings. Reynolds and Rosen (1976) argued on behalf of the rights of the individual. Such rights, they suggested, are paramount, being more important than traditional societal institutions. To them the traditional indiscriminate placement of a child in a special class is a violation of these rights. Burton Blatt, a long-time proponent for the civil rights of mentally retarded people, defended mainstreaming for its goodness. "Living in a normal world is simply thought to be good for retarded children, as we think it's good for us" (Blatt, 1979, p. 304).

While the least restrictive environment developed as a concept pertinent mainly to the mildly retarded, some writers in recent years have expanded its implication to include lower functioning retarded persons (Brown, Branston-McClean, Baumgart, Vincent, Falvey & Schroeder, 1979; Brown, Pumpian, Baumgart, Vandeventer, Ford, Nisbet, Schroeder & Grunewald, 1981; Baumgart, Brown, Pumpian, Nisbet, Ford, Sweet, Messina & Schroeder, 1982; Hamre-Nietupski, Nietupski, Bates & Maurer, 1982). According to these writers, and others, severely handicapped persons (including the moderately, severely, and profoundly retarded) should receive their educational programs in regular schools along with nonhandicapped children to the degree possible. They have further suggested that as much of the education as possible should occur outside of the school in community settings in order that functional skills may be learned. Major criticism has been directed toward segregated educational environments that teach nonfunctional skills using techniques not found in the normal environment. (Brown et al, 1979; 1981; Baumgart et al, 1982). Brown and his co-authors have suggested that even though full integration may not be feasible, *partial participation* using *individualized adaptions* would be preferable to many current practices (i.e. segregated special schools).

PUBLIC SCHOOL ARRANGEMENTS FOR TEACHING MENTALLY RETARDED CHILDREN

In order to allow the practical and the conceptual aspects of the least restrictive environment concept to coincide, it is necessary that we be able to offer a continuum of alternatives (see Figure 9–1). These alternatives are considered to range from being least restrictive to most restrictive. They have often been referred to as a cascade or hierarchy of services (Reynolds, 1962; Deno, 1970). The idea is for the child to be placed in an environment which is appropriate to his or her needs and yet be as least restrictive as possible (as far toward the bottom of Figure 9–1 as possible). Under the plan, the child is to be regularly evaluated and moved toward the bottom of the model whenever possible. Generally, the instructional arrangements from bottom to top include the following.

Plan 1: The Regular Classroom

The mildly retarded child might be placed in the regular classroom and be fully integrated with nonretarded peers. In that this is the setting

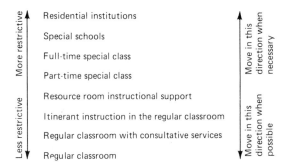

FIGURE 9–1 Cascade or Hierarchy of Services

From "A framework for considering some issues in special education" by M. C. Reynolds, *Exceptional Children, 28,* 1962, 367–370. Copyright 1962 by The Council for Exceptional Children. Reprinted with permission.

that most people in school are found, it may be considered the least restrictive. A child spending all or some part of his or her time in the regular classroom is mainstreamed. In this setting, the most visible aspect of special instructional variation may be some form of special instructional materials or equipment. Otherwise, the child would be as physically integrated as nonretarded children.

Plan 2: The Regular Classroom With Consultative Services

One step away from the norm is providing the regular class teacher with consultative services. This model assumes that the child needs slightly more than the regular classroom teacher can provide. Therefore, an arrangement is made for someone to help the teacher deal with the child's special needs. In both this arrangement and the one above, the regular class teacher, not a special educator, provides direct instruction to the child. All of the child's instruction takes place in the regular classroom.

Plan 3: Itinerant Instruction In the Regular Classroom

Under this plan the child would continue to remain in the regular classroom but would receive some form of direct instruction from an itinerant, special teacher while there. Of course, the special teacher would utilize special instructional materials.

Plan 4: Resource Room Instructional Support

Under this arrangement the mildly retarded child leaves the regular classroom for a brief period of time each day and goes to a resource room for special instruction in a specific area or areas, for example, reading and math. The resource room teacher cooperates with the regular class teacher in the planning of instructional areas and activities. The regular class teacher generally retains primary control over the child's curriculum. The resource room teacher's role is one of filling in the gaps in specific skill areas, not in planning and implementing a total curriculum.

The resource room approach has been strongly promoted and is probably the most widely used model in attempts to mainstream mildly retarded children. Several proponents of the resource room have written about its merits (Hammill & Weiderholt, 1972; Jenkins & Mayhall, 1973; Reger, 1973; Reger & Koppmann, 1971; Sabatino, 1972). Some of these include:

> children do not have to be categorized or labeled to be served;
> most of the child's time can be spent in the mainstream;
> appropriate instructional techniques can be used;
> it may provide preventative services for some young children with potential problems;
> it can serve more children than can be served in a special self-contained class;
> diagnosis and prescriptive education can be provided by the resource room teacher;
> each child's entry and exit can be flexibly arranged;
> the resource room teacher may serve as a consultant to the regular teachers.

Critics of the resource room approach for mildly retarded children feel that its approach to specific academic problems is too limited. Childs (1979) pointed out that the traditional EMR curriculum focuses on social, vocational, and survival skills. He contended that a purely academic curriculum was devoid of important elements for the total development of the child. Bartlett's (1977) position was essentially the same: special education for the mildly retarded should be developmental in nature, not remedial. Gresham (1982) summarized relevant research and noted the need especially for social skills training which is usually not offered in the resource room. The basic suggestion of these writers is that resource rooms may be fine for improving some specific skill areas for other handicapped learners, such as those with learning disabilities, but the mildly retarded require a more comprehensive educational approach to deal with their more comprehensive deficits.

Plan 5: Part-Time Special Class

If a resource room does not provide enough service, the child may be placed in a special classroom for about one-half of the school day. Usually, under this plan, the special class teacher is responsible for the student's curriculum. Integration with nonretarded children is often restricted to nonacademic areas such as music, art, and physical education.

The orientation of the curriculum in a part-time special class is usually different than in a resource room. In the latter, the special teacher's role is to attempt to remediate or compensate for certain academic deficits. In the special class, the curriculum is usually more developmental and functionally oriented. The student focuses on functional academics, career education, prevocational training, and social skills development.

Plan 6: Full-Time Special Class

This plan is the same as the part-time special class model except the children spend their entire school day here. In essence, it functions like a regular class in a traditional school setting except that all of the students are usually classified as mildly retarded. They come in the morning and stay the entire day. The special education teacher, of course, determines the curriculum and provides all of the instruction.

While part-time and full-time special classes are considered to be more restrictive, many of their critics tend to acknowledge their necessity, agreeing that some children will continue to need such services. The heaviest criticism has been about their role of harboring, and thus stigmatizing, minority children. With the implementation of laws to alleviate this situation, they tend now to serve children who truly fare less well in the regular classrooms. Gottlieb (1982) and MacMillan and Borthwick (1980) contended that the exclusion of many minority students from the ranks of the mildly retarded in recent years resulted in those left in special classes being more difficult to mainstream.

Plan 7: Special Schools

While the resource rooms and special classes in regular schools are most commonly used to serve the mildly retarded in the United States, special schools are usually provided for moderately, severely, and more recently profoundly retarded students (McGrew, 1977). On the continuum of arrangements (Figure 9–1), special schools obviously fall toward the more restrictive end. These schools are completely self-contained and the children attend them instead of going to regular schools.

Special schools are usually designed with their clientele in mind. Since many of the students have physical as well as mental handicaps, the schools are built to accommodate their needs (Litton, 1978). Bathrooms are arranged with toilets (and often bathtubs) that are readily accessible. Tables, doorways, and hallways are designed to allow easy access for those in wheelchairs. Various room sizes exist so that suitable environments are available for individual, small group, and large group instruction. In other respects, they are similar to regular schools having cafetoriums, gymnasiums, physical education and recreation fields, and sometimes even swimming pools. Within the schools, classes may be self-contained, departmentalized, or a team teaching approach may be used (Tetzlaff & Sedlak, 1978).

Most critics of restrictive environments have directed their criticism at special classes, not at special schools for moderately, severely, and profoundly retarded persons (Reynolds & Balow, 1972; Reynolds & Rosen, 1976). Some, however, have suggested that even at this level of retardation, integration should be promoted (Baumgart et al., 1982; Brown et al., 1979; Brown et al., 1981; Certo, Brown, Belmore & Crowner, 1977; Thomason & Arkell, 1980). The model for integration might place special classes for these students in regular schools.

Plan 8: Residential Institutions

Although more mentally retarded children now live in the community, a number of severely and profoundly handicapped children remain in residential institutions. During the school-age years, these individuals retain the right to a free, appropriate education in the public school system. They may either be taken out of the residential facility for this service or in some cases, the service may be brought in. Residential institutions are discussed in Chapter 10.

EVALUATION OF EDUCATIONAL MODELS

Programs for Mildly Retarded Students

If we accept the position that education in the least restrictive environment is a desirable goal, we must ask "how well does it work?" Put another way, if a mildly retarded child is placed in a regular classroom for at least a portion of the day, does he or she benefit from being placed in that setting? If there is little benefit, it might have to be acknowledged that we haven't really put the child in a "less restrictive environment" but only an environment containing nonhandicapped children. In some ways, this arrangement may actually be more restricting in its ability to provide an appropriate education. The law is clearly written and school districts must comply. However, a balance must be found between adhering to the concepts of least restrictive environment and appropriate education (USDE, 1980). As Thurman (1981) wrote:

> The philosophical strength of principles like the least restrictive alternative coupled with the existing legal mandates often results in a headlong plunge into policies and procedures which overlook the particular needs of individual children. (p. 69)

We cannot objectively evaluate the concept of education in the least restrictive environment; we can only evaluate a specific implementation of it. The most common implementation is placing the mildly retarded child in a classroom with other children for at least a portion of the day. In evaluating this arrangement, MacMillan and Semmel (1977) advised that the impact of the model be determined for four groups of children: those returned to the mainstream from the special class; those never placed in special classes but who, under traditional conditions, would have been placed; those children not yet of school age who would have been considered mildly retarded when they got into the school; and normal regular class students with whom the mildly retarded children would be placed. Additionally, they suggested that a thorough evaluation would have to include an ongoing assessment of the curriculum (Is the child being taught the appropriate content to meet his or her needs?), an assessment of instructional personnel (Are regular and special educators cooperating? Are adequate support persons available for the regular classroom?), and an assessment of whether or not the child is learning (Are academic, social, vocational, and other necessary skills being adequately learned?).

Studies in recent years have compared different degrees of integration and segregation along the continuum of placement possibilities. Corman and Gottlieb (1978) and Gottlieb (1981) have provided reviews of studies of mainstreaming practices.

Academic. Carroll (1967) found that integrated students made greater gains in reading but no differences were found for spelling and arithmetic between them and segregated students. Walker (1974) found mildly retarded students in regular classes who had resource room support had greater gains in reading than did special class students but found no differences in arithmetic gains. Bradfield, Brown, Kaplan, Rickert, and Stannard (1973) reported that EMR children in regular classes learned more in reading and arithmetic than did special class children when precision teaching methods were used in the regular classroom. Budoff and Gottlieb (1976) found no difference in the academic achievement of integrated and segregated students.

Meyers, MacMillan, and Yosida (1978), in a large study of former EMR children who had been reassigned to regular classes in California, found that these children did worse academically than the lowest achieving nonEMR students in the regular class but better than the EMR students remaining in special classes. In a similar study in Florida, Mascari and Forgnone (1982) followed 120 mildly retarded students who had been decertified as such. Four years following their placement from special to regular classes, seventy (58%) of the original 120 had been re-referred for special education. Of these seventy, thirty-two were reclassified as learning disabled, seventeen were again classified as EMR, twelve were designated as emotionally handicapped, and nine were found not to be eligible for placement.

In general, studies support the ability of integrated programs to do at least as well and sometimes better than special class programs in the development of academic skills by EMR children. However, two points should be made. First, the resulting effects are more likely due to teaching methods and the focus of instructional attention than *where* the child is placed (Corman & Gottlieb, 1978). Second, *no* program—integrated or segregated—has done an outstanding job in teaching academic skills. For example, Semmel, Gottlieb, and Robinson (1979) pointed out that no study has been able to report a mean grade reading level for EMR children above 3.8. This goes for both mainstreaming and special class arrangements. Gottlieb (1981) stated that "If these reading achievement data are used as evidence regarding the appropriateness of education, they suggest strongly that an appropriate education for mentally retarded children has not yet been developed" (p. 118).

Social adjustment.   Of course, academic gains are but one standard of judgment. At least as important, if not more so, is social adjustment. How well are mildly retarded children accepted by nonretarded children in the regular classroom? Several years ago when integration of mildly retarded students was just becoming an issue, Christoplos and Renz (1969) wrote that "Familiarization with deviation, via inclusion of deviates in regular classrooms, should minimize undesirable attitudes on the part of the 'normal' population" (p. 378). Unfortunately, this has been one of the least substantiated results of integration of mildly retarded children. Not only are EMR students less accepted and more often rejected than normal students (Goodman, Gottlieb & Harrison, 1972; Iano, Ayres, Heller, McGettigan & Walker, 1974; Reese-Dukes & Stokes, 1978), but they are also more rejected when they are integrated than they are when segregated in special classes (Goodman, Gottlieb & Harrison, 1972; Gottlieb & Budoff, 1973; Gottlieb, Cohen & Goldstein, 1974). Corman and Gottlieb (1978) were forced to conclude that "greater contact between retarded and nonretarded children is not accompanied by an increase in the social acceptance of retarded children" (p. 260).

In this generally bleak picture there are a few bright spots. First of all, there are some studies which contradict the general findings to some degree. Sheare (1974) reported favorable findings of nonretarded children's attitudes toward mildly retarded children who were integrated into junior high school classes. Bruininks, Rynders, and Gross (1974) found that while integrated mildly retarded children were not rated well in suburban school settings, in urban schools they were actually rated higher than the nonretarded children. Additionally, even in studies where mean sociometric status ratings are lower for retarded children, the difference is usually about one standard deviation. This means that about one-sixth of the sample of retarded persons is rated as high as the average for the nonretarded children. In other words, a portion are accepted (Gottlieb, 1981).

A second encouraging point is that while most sociometric status (pencil and paper) studies indicate a low level of acceptance, a couple of studies using direct observation of actual behavior indicate positive social behaviors exist between mildly retarded and nonretarded students in integrated settings (Gampel, Gottlieb & Harrison, 1974; Dunlop, Stoneman & Cantrell, 1980).

Finally, even though integration sometimes tends to result in negative social attitudes expressed toward mildly retarded students, there is some evidence that these attitudes can be improved (Ballard, Corman, Gottlieb & Kaufman, 1977; Gottlieb, 1980; Leyser & Gottlieb, 1980). But this modification of attitudes does not come automatically with integration. Specific activities such as group discussions (Gottlieb, 1980) must be employed. Also, the continuation of more positive attitudes after initial improvement will have to be monitored. Long-term bias is usually not turned into long-term acceptance through short-term intervention.

Self-concept. A third measure for evaluating what education in the least restrictive environment is supposed to do is an assessment of the mildly retarded child's opinion of himself or herself. Some investigators have thus compared the self-concept of children in integrated and segregated settings. The findings have been mixed. Carroll (1967) found that EMR children attending regular classes had better self-concepts and were less self-derogatory, but Walker (1974) found no differences between such children and those solely in special classes on self-concept and self-derogation measures. Budoff and Gottlieb (1976) reported that after one year, integrated students expressed greater internal locus of control, had more positive attitudes toward school, and were more positive about themselves as students than were segregated children in the comparison sample.

Overall, Corman and Gottlieb (1978) drew three important conclusions from the research literature:

1. Research on academic achievement is mixed. The trend is in favor of integrated settings, but there have been no efforts to control for the effects of different teaching methods. Definitive conclusions are not possible.
2. Regarding social status and development, the bulk of the research indicates that mildly retarded children are not as well liked as nonretarded children. There is also evidence to support the position that the more visible the EMR student, the less accepted he or she will be. Integrated students tend to be less accepted than segregated students.
3. Although there have been some inconsistencies, integrated students tend to have better self-attitudes than their segregated counterparts.

Gottlieb (1981) felt that mainstreaming had not done what it set out to do. To him, it seemed that too much emphasis had been placed on physical arrangements with much less on education. He wrote: "At this point in time, special educators are more involved with *placing* children in the least restrictive environment than with *educating* them in the least restrictive environment" (p. 122, italics added). His advice was to go beyond the court and legal mandates and proceed with the business of providing quality education.

Programs for Moderately and Severely Retarded Students

Like public school programs for mildly retarded students, programs for moderate and severe level individuals have also been evaluated to determine their effectiveness. Most of these efficacy studies took place after the establishment of public school programs and were designed to decide whether or not the programs were beneficial. Unlike the early studies comparing regular class and special class placement for EMR students, these studies compared programs and no programs (Kaufman & Alberto, 1976).

After the big push in the 1950s by the National Association for Retarded Children to develop TMR programs, some in the field of special education questioned their efficacy. Dr. Ignacy Goldberg and Dr. William Cruickshank (1958) debated as to whether or not the public schools should be responsbile for TMR programs. Goldberg, a consultant for the NARC, defended the need for programs and the children's right to them. Cruickshank, a long-time professional in the field, felt that children of this developmental level were unable to benefit from education and would not return to society what it cost to provide them with public school education. In the 1950s and '60s the TMR efficacy studies started to appear. Some of these studies have been reviewed by Kirk (1964) and by Kaufman and Alberto (1976). They are summarized here.

Reynolds, Ellis, and Kiland (1953) surveyed parents and teachers of TMR children in Minnesota. They found that socialization and self-care skills had improved due to the programs but academics had not; higher IQ children profited more than lower IQ children; and parent expectancies decreased over the duration of the programs. Goldstein (1956), in Illinois, evaluated moderately retarded children over a two-year period. Using rating scales and psychometric instruments, he found greater gains in the first year than in the second year in adaptive behavior. Many children with IQs below 35 were excluded from the programs because of disruptive behavior. He also reported that parents came to realize their children would not be independent.

In New York, Johnson and Capobianco (1957) and Johnson, Capobianco, and Blake (1960) compared children attending day schools with others living in residential institutions over a two-year period. Overall, the social quotient (SQ) on the Vineland Social Maturity Scale did not change over the two-year period. Children with IQs less than 30 tended to decrease on SQ; those with above 30 IQs tended to increase. Some differences were found between the institutionalized and the day school students. The latter tended to increase in tenacity and friendliness and showed a reduction in competition; the institutionalized children increased in conformity and decreased in gregariousness.

In Tennessee, Hottel (1958) compared children in special programs with some who remained at home receiving no special education. Over a one year period, he found no differences between the groups on changes in mental age, IQ, SQ, social age (SA), or parent ratings. High IQ (40–50) special class children showed gains in IQ but not SA or SQ.

Peck (1960) and Peck and Sexton (1961) compared TMR children in four settings in Texas. Totally, thirty children were evaluated: nine in a public school program, six in a private program, eight in an institution, and seven living at home receiving no special training. Over a two-year period, none of the groups showed any significant changes in IQ or SQ. However, the three groups receiving formal training showed significant improvement on a behavior rating scale.

In California, Cain and Levine (1963) also compared four groups of children. These included moderately retarded children in a special day class; some in a special class in an institution; others in an institution without being in a special class; and some living at home. Performance measures were taken at the beginning and end of a two-year period using a measure of social competence designed for the study. The scale measured self-help, social skills, communication and initiative, and responsibility. Generally, children in the community did better regardless of whether they were in school or not. Both school and nonschool children in the institution decreased in social competence.

Obviously, these studies were not extremely supportive of the efficacy of public school programs for TMR children. However, there were many methodological difficulties similar to those found in the EMR efficacy studies and hasty conclusions should not be drawn. Some of the problems were that sample sizes were small, the training periods were very short, and the measurement instruments were not very sensitive. It can also be pointed out that most of these programs were new, the teaching methods and curriculum were not well developed or detailed, and there was no control for the quality of teaching provided. Now that most of these programs have been around for about twenty or thirty years, it might be good to reassess their efficacy.

To what degree can the concept of least restrictive environment be applied to the moderate and severe population? Recently Brown and his colleagues (Baumgart et al., 1982) as well as others, have called for the implementation of *partial participation* for severely handicapped students.

According to this principle, students who would most likely be placed in special schools would be given the opportunity to function at least in part in lesser restrictive environments (e.g. regular schools) and in nonschool settings. In order to do so, individualized adaptions to the environment would be necessary such as the use of special devices or the provision of personal assistance. Presumably such provisions would be beneficial because the severely handicapped students would be perceived as more valuable, productive, contributing participants in their environment.

While this form of integration may in some ways be advantageous, it also may not be. If this is to become a commonly used approach, carefully controlled research is called for. This research should go beyond the traditional measures of personal development and also look at interactions between handicapped and nonhandicapped students since this is an area of critical significance.

ISSUES RELATED TO PUBLIC SCHOOL PROGRAMS FOR PROFOUNDLY MENTALLY RETARDED STUDENTS

Unlike those discussed above, no studies documenting the efficacy of public school programs for profoundly retarded students have yet been reported. These programs are still relatively new and the focus of effort seems to be more on what and how to teach them rather than where to teach them. For the most part, PMR students will be placed into special schools as are TMR students. This in itself will be a less restrictive environment for many such individuals. Because of the serious physical conditions of many profoundly retarded individuals, it can be expected that public school programs will have to provide not only educational services but will also oversee many medical services. Much dispersion of this population would make these services difficult.

While programs have yet to be formally evaluated, some professionals are already questioning the benefit of formal training for many extremely low functioning children (Bailey, 1981; Baumeister, 1981; Ellis, 1981) while others, of course, are defending them (Menolascino & McGee, 1981; Roos, 1979). At this point in time it may be too early to judge the efficacy of programs for PMR students. Because many of these programs are relatively new, several variables need to be examined and controlled before judgment is passed. Looking back at the efficacy studies of programs for EMR and TMR students, the field may learn from some of its mistakes. Peck and Semmel (1982) suggested that the least restrictive environment for severely handicapped children be determined through empirical analyses and that instructional settings be examined regarding their effect on students' development, the validation of goals and outcomes, and the impact on other children. Specific questions should be addressed including ones such as the following:

> What types of programmatic arrangements might succeed in integrated settings?
>
> What types of interventions might be useful in different settings?
>
> How might social interactions be best achieved if integrated programs are provided?

These and additional questions should be answered before more global evaluative studies can be meaningfully interpreted.

EXTENDED SCHOOL YEAR PROGRAMS

A recent development in the provision of public school services is the judicial ruling requiring extended school year programs for some severely handicapped students. Extended programs are those in which students attend school in excess of the 180 days normally provided by state and local education agencies. Such programs have developed in some areas because of court rulings (*Kline v. Armstrong*, 1979; *Scanlon v. Battle*, 1981) that have determined that an "appropriate" education for some students cannot be delivered if restricted to the typical 180-day period. In other words, a student's individual educational plan may require nearly year-round public school education (Leonard, 1981).

As of the present, the extended year program applies only to more severely handicapped persons including the severely and profoundly mentally retarded and those who are severely emotionally disturbed. The rationale for the practice is that many of these students experience a "regression-recoupment" disability following longitudinal gaps (e.g. summer vacation) in their educational programs (Larsen, Goodman & Glean, 1981). As Leonard (1981) stated: they experience a "substantial loss of skills . . . during substantial interruptions in educational programming." Because of this, parents petitioned the federal courts to require the schools to continue providing programs during the summer. They pointed out that the extended interruptions resulted in:

> A need for relearning after summer break
>
> An inability to rely on the end-of-the-year assessment by the previous teacher
>
> Greater cost of residential placement because of a lack of community programs
>
> Loss of family and community support during periods of summer institutionalization
>
> Loss of ability to maximize the most critical time for learning (Leonard, 1981)

Not all students will be eligible for extended year programs. The main criterion, in addition to being severely handicapped, is that the student demonstrate a loss if not included. Recently McMahon (1983) studied the benefits of an extended year for twenty-six students. He found that following vacant periods of instruction, notable regression in key skill areas occurred. In contrast, extended periods of instruction were characterized by increased performance.

CONCLUSION

The history of special education for mentally retarded persons is less than 200 years old. Compared to other professions (e.g., general education, law, medicine), we are still in our infancy—or at least in the toddler stage. Currently we are being directed by litigation and legislation to provide the best education in the least restrictive environment. Most of the emphasis has been on the latter; the former needs much more attention. Special education technology is growing rapidly. This technology should be fully employed in public school systems and more sophisticated measurement techniques should be used to document its effectiveness. The early efficacy studies are out of date. If special educators can put as much effort into honoring the intention of their own profession as they have in meeting the requirements of the legal profession, there will be no difficulty in achieving the successes that the various efficacy studies have failed to show.

Quality education should be our first target; where it's provided should be our second. Mainstream education can undoubtedly work for many retarded children and other children with academic difficulties who today are not covered by a formal categorical label. To place first and derive educational strategies later is an excellent example of the classical disarrangement of the horse and the cart. We should decide what the child needs to be taught before we decide where to teach him. If the child is to be placed in the regular class, at the very least a close analysis must be made not only of the child to be integrated, but also of the regular classroom environment including the teacher. Studies have shown that some teachers are simply not responsive to having mildly retarded or other handicapped children placed in their classroom (Gickling & Theobald, 1975; Shotel, Iano & McGettigan, 1972). This is unfortunate but it is one of those facts that cannot be ignored. What is fortunate, however, is that some teacher perceptions may change for the better, given adequate information and knowledge (Hudson, Reisberg & Wolf, 1983). The important point is an honest appraisal of the situation must be made before the child is placed into it. This will help determine the degree of its restrictiveness. Of course, other problems may continue, such as the appropriateness of the curriculum, teaching methods, and so on. But these might be capable of modification if the teacher is honestly willing to cooperate.

There is also need for special educators to cooperate. Dybwad (1980) suggested that mainstreaming is sometimes considered to be an attack on the field of special education. Such views, if they exist, should be corrected by special educators. Any form of mainstreaming will require superior special education services. Public schools that have the most successful mainstreaming programs will also have a strong special education faculty. Mainstreaming doesn't require less special education if it's done right. It is a complex process that requires much support.

STUDY QUESTIONS

1. When and where did special classes first appear? When and where were the first special classes in the United States and what was their purpose?

2. What influenced the development of special schools for TMR students? How were services first brought about for severely and profoundly retarded individuals?

3. In what social context did concern about education in the least restrictive environment emerge? What basic positions were taken by Dunn (1968) and others in regard to special classes for the mildly retarded? What defense was offered in support of special classes?

4. What is meant by the term "least restrictive environment?" How does it relate to "mainstreaming?"

5. On a continuum of public school arrangements, which are considered to be most restrictive? Which are least restrictive?

6. What type of child is most likely to be served in the regular classroom? the resource room? the special school? Briefly describe the operation of these facilities.

7. What has been the effect of mainstreaming mildly retarded students in the areas of academic development, social adjustment (acceptance), and self-concept?

8. What were some results of the early efficacy studies of programs for TMR students? What were some of the limitations of these studies?

9. What is the purpose of the extended school year program? Who are most likely to be served in such programs?

10

Community and Public Residential Facilities

TRENDS IN RESIDENTIAL ARRANGEMENTS: OVERVIEW

During the last one hundred years, public residential facilities (PRFs) represented the major source of formal services for mentally retarded individuals. In fact, not until after World War II did public school programs begin serving more school-age retarded children than were being housed in institutions (Lakin, Krantz, Bruininks, Clumper & Hill, 1982). Since that time, and especially during the last fifteen years, dramatic changes have occurred. Today fewer retarded people are living in PRFs as more are remaining in their natural homes or moving into community residential facilities (CRFs). These facilities, besides being in the community, are smaller in size, provide more of a home-like environment, and promote life-styles more like those experienced by nonretarded persons.

A major philosophical thrust toward deinstitutionalization and community living was provided by the concept of "normalization." Normalization promotes the idea that mentally retarded individuals should have the opportunity to have life experiences like most other persons. Since the late 60s the normalization concept has been the primary force affecting policy, administrative, and programming decisions related to lifestyles and living conditions of mentally retarded persons.

In the present chapter, attention is given to PRFs, CRFs, and the concept and practice of normalization. The discussion will procede along a chronological order; first addressing public residential facilities, then the concept of normalization and practice of deinstitutionalization, and finally CRFs which may be seen as a concrete embodiment of the normalization principle.

PUBLIC RESIDENTIAL FACILITIES (PRFs)

Early Development of Institutions

When public residential facilities or institutions were started in Europe and the United States in the early to mid-1800s, their primary goal was education and habilitation. They were considered to be residential schools and their purpose was to educate retarded persons to a level of normalcy. This goal changed toward the end of the nineteenth century and the beginning of the present century for two reasons. First, it was realized that the goal of achieving normalcy was not attainable. Second, a eugenics scare developed a nearly universal paranoia that lasted through about the first two decades of the present century. The net effect of these influences was to de-emphasize the role of the institution as a school and concomitantly to consider it as a long-term custodial care facility. Concern for education and training was replaced by perhaps an even greater concern for protecting society from mental retardation. Baumeister (1970) characterized residential institutions from 1900 throughout the first half of the present century in the following way:

1. The number of institutions increased.
2. Institutions grew larger.
3. Institutions became custodial rather than educational.
4. The medical model was widely adopted, with most institutions organized in terms of a "hospital" hierarchy.
5. Institutions became self-sustaining and managed as economically as possible.
6. New institutions were constructed in rural areas to provide farming opportunities and remove the defective as far as possible from the populace. (Apparently, the rule of thumb was one acre per inmate.)
7. Inmates were completely segregated by sex, age, and ability level.
8. Institutional architecture became very distinct, with the emphasis on highly specialized and sturdy buildings. Large dormitories were the rule, constructed with the intention of economically housing as many residents as possible.
9. The number of professionals employed became generally inadequate to carry on meaningful treatment and rehabilitation programs. Moreover, quality of professional services was typically very poor relative to other types of exceptionality.
10. Increasing emphasis was placed on legal aspects of commitment and release.
11. The residents were dehumanized, deprived of any legal rights, frequently subjected to physical and psychological abuse and personal indignity, and their welfare generally neglected. (pp. 14–15)

Fortunately there have been some important changes in PRFs in the last fifteen or twenty years. Many of these changes have been documented and reported in the research literature (cf: Butterfield, 1969; Best-Sigford, Bruininks, Lakin, Hill & Heal, 1982; Colombatto, Isett, Roszkowski, Spreat, D'Onofrio & Alderfer, 1982; Lakin, Krantz, Bruininks, Clumper & Hill, 1982; Scheerenberger, 1976, 1978, 1982). A summary of these findings are reported below.

Number of PRFs

Scheerenberger (1978) reported that as of June 30, 1976, 237 PRFs existed in the United States. In an updated study, Scheerenberger (1982) reported that 282 PRFs were in operation during the period of July 1, 1980, to June 30, 1981. This represents an increase of 16% in the number of PRFs in the five year period between 1975–76 and 1980–81.

Number of Persons in PRFs

While the number of PRFs increased slightly, the number of persons residing in them decreased. In 1975–76, Scheerenberger (1978) reported that 154,856 persons were in PRFs, while in his later study (1982), he reported an average daily population of 125,799 persons. Given that the number of institutions *increased* while the number of residents *decreased*, the obvious effect was that fewer residents were housed in each institution. In 1980–81, the median number of residents per PRF was 309 with a range between nine and 2,232 (Scheerenberger, 1982). Only 10% (n = 27) of the institutions contained more than 1,000 people.

These figures represent the lowest number of total persons in institutions and the lowest number of residents per institution ever reported. They also represent a continuing trend in deinstitutionalization of mentally retarded persons that is readily apparent in Figures 10–1 and 10–2. These figures (Lakin et al., 1982) indicate that from the late 1800s to the late 1960s the number of persons in institutions grew steadily. This growth in the institutional population hit a high point of 194,650 in 1967. (Butterfield, 1969 estimated that at this time there were probably another 20,000 individuals in private facilities.) Since that time there has been a sharp decline in the number of institutionalized persons.

The downward trend occurred for several reasons. PRF placements began to occur only after less restrictive alternatives were not found satisfactory; placements were made for the shortest duration possible; and more community alternatives became available (Scheerenberger, 1978).

Another difference in institutions today is that those more recently built were built smaller and for fewer residents. Scheerenberger (1978) contrasted PRFs built before 1964 (n = 135) and those built after (n = 102). He found the former to have a median bed capacity of 1,037 and the latter to have a median capacity of only 260 beds. In his latest report, Scheerenberger (1982) found the median bed capacity for *all* institutions to be 393.

FIGURE 10–1   Total Populations of Retarded People in Public Institutions from 1880 to 1978

From K. C. Lakin, G. C. Krantz, R. H. Bruininks, J. L. Clumper, and B. K. Hill, "One hundred years of data on populations of public residential facilities for mentally retarded people," *American Journal of Mental Deficiency*, 1982, 87, 1–8. Reprinted by permission.

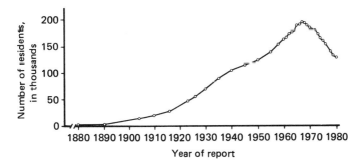

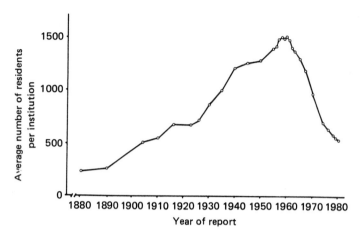

FIGURE 10–2   Average Number of Residents per Public Institution for Retarded Individuals from 1880 to 1978

From K. C. Lakin, G. C. Krantz, R. H. Bruininks, J. L. Clumper, and B. K. Hill, "One hundred years of data on populations of public residential facilities for mentally retarded people," *American Journal of Mental Deficiency*, 1982, 87, 1–8. Reprinted by permission.

Characteristics of Residents of PRFs

Besides size, and perhaps more important, the nature of the population has been gradually changing in public residential facilities. On the average, institutions are housing lower functioning retarded persons and older retarded persons (Scheerenberger, 1978, 1982). In his 1976 report, Scheerenberger found 71.2% of the residential population to be severely or profoundly retarded. In 1978, he reported 72.8% in these combined categories. In their 1982 survey, Colombatto et al. found 76% of the residential population to be severely or profoundly retarded while Scheerenberger (1982) found 80% to be at this level. Conversely, in these same reports, the percent of mildly retarded persons was reported to be 8.1%, 7.9%, 7.0%, and 7.1% respectively, indicating a steady decrease of mildly retarded persons in institutions, over recent years.

At the same time this shift has been occurring, there has also been a gradual increase in the age of the residents. In 1976 Scheerenberger found the 3–21 age group comprised 42.0% of the population, but in 1978 only 36.3% were in this range. Simultaneously the 22–61 age group increased their representation from 52.8% to 58.5%. This age group increased again in 1980–81 (Scheerenberger, 1982). Accordingly, the individual most likely to be found today in a residential institution is either severely or profoundly retarded and/or is an adult. It is also likely that this person will have multiple handicaps; that is, one or more handicaps in addition to being mentally retarded (Scheerenberger, 1976, 1978,

1982). An additional perspective of the population can be gained by examining their behavioral abilities. Scheerenberger (1982) found that based on data reported by 180 PRFs (n = 83,898 residents), 74.4% of the sample could walk, 46.2% could dress themselves, 65.3% could feed themselves, 76.1% understood when spoken to, 50.6% could communicate verbally, and 61.4% were toilet trained.

PRF Staff

Large residential facilities are staffed by many people. Because of their 24-hour-a-day self-contained nature, they must employ a wide range of professional and nonprofessional workers. While Colombatto et al. (1982) found an average of 587 residents per institution, the number of persons employed per institution averaged 870. Scheerenberger's (1982) data were similar with 282 PRFs employing approximately 217,200 persons to serve 125,799 clients. These figures indicate that for every one resident, there is approximately 1.4 to 1.7 persons employed within an institution. These ratios represent drastic declines from those reported in earlier years (see Figure 10–3).

The largest number of employees is the direct service providers or those who staff the living units. The fact that three shifts of these workers must be employed accounts partially for the large ratio of staff to residents. Institutions also employ their own medical staff, dentists, psychologists, social workers, various therapists, special education teachers, and chaplains. In addition, they will have a large kitchen staff, custodians, a

FIGURE 10–3 Ratio of Patients to Staff (Number of Patients Per One Staff Member) in Public Institutions for Retarded Individuals for the Years 1915 to 1978

From K. C. Lakin, G. C. Krantz, R. H. Bruininks, J. L. Clumper, and B. K. Hill, "One hundred years of data on populations of public residential facilities for mentally retarded people," *American Journal of Mental Deficiency*, 1982, *87*, 1–8. Reprinted by permission.

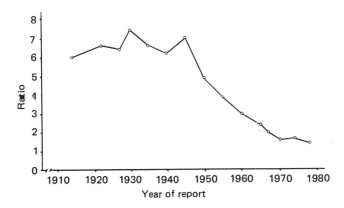

maintenance staff, grounds keepers, bus drivers, secretaries, clerks, and administrators.

Cost of PRFs

Not surprisingly, the cost of operating a PRF is quite high. The total annual operational budget for the 282 institutions in Scheerenberger's latest (1982) report was almost $3.6 billion or $12.4 million per institution. Eighty-two percent of this was for salaries while the remaining money went to general operational costs. It was estimated that another $271 million was spent on construction and major renovations. The $3.6 billion figure was $1.6 billion more than was spent in 1975–76.

In terms of cost per resident per day, figures in 1980–81 ranged from $25.61 to $213.00 with a mean of $77.99 ($28,466 per year per person). This figure represented a 117% increase over the cost of 1975–76 and a 615% increase over 1970–71. The dramatic increase in costs is somewhat due to inflation but even in terms of 1967 dollar values, the increases are formidable (see Figure 10–4).

Activities within PRFs

Scheerenberger (1978) reported that active training and development programs had increased in recent years in PRFs and even the lowest

FIGURE 10–4   Annual Cost Per Resident of Care in Public Institutions for Retarded Individuals for 1915 to 1978

From K. C. Lakin, G. C. Krantz, R. H. Bruininks, J. L. Clumper, and B. K. Hill, "One hundred years of data on populations of public residential facilities for mentally retarded people," *American Journal of Mental Deficiency*, 1982, 87, 1–8. Reprinted by permission.

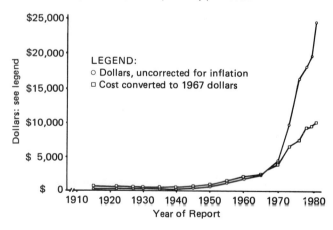

functioning individuals were participating in them. This same finding held true in his later report (Scheerenberger, 1982). Of course, school-age residents would spend a portion of their time enrolled in public school facilities. Other "off-campus" activities (e.g., sheltered workshop employment) were also available. Within their own physical structures, the institutions surveyed by Scheerenberger (1976, 1978, 1982) reported a variety of categories of treatment. Some included formal education and training, language and speech therapy, behavior management, work activities, motor training, self-help training (toileting and self-feeding) and recreation. Eighty-nine percent of the institutions analyzed for Scheerenberger's (1978) report stated that they had developed individual habilitation plans for their residents. The remainder were working toward that goal and were not completely satisfied that they were serving all needs when polled later (Scheerenberger, 1982).

Factors Affecting the Decision to Institutionalize

Obviously only a relatively small number of mentally retarded persons are placed in residential institutions. Many others remain in their homes and later live independently or in community-based facilities. Why are some individuals institutionalized and others not? During about the last twenty years this question generated a considerable amount of research. Some of this research dealt with different family characteristics while other investigations were concerned with the individual's characteristics. For example, several studies reported that lower socioeconomic families were more likely to institutionalize their children (Appell & Tisdall, 1968; Eyman, Dingman & Sabagh, 1966; Farber, Jenne & Toigo, 1960; Saenger, 1960), as were single parent families (Appell & Tisdall, 1968; Farber, 1968; Hobbs, 1964; Saenger, 1960; Shellhaas & Nihira, 1969). A child was also likely to be placed in an institution if the parents felt that his or her presence in the home would be an impediment to the other children's development (Farber, 1959, 1968; Farber et al., 1960). Saenger (1960) reported that Catholic and Protestant families were more likely to institutionalize than were Jewish families. Finally, several studies reported that families in which there was more stress and maladjustment were more likely to seek institutionalization (Fotheringham, Skelton & Hoddinolt, 1971; Graliker, Koch & Henderson, 1965; Kershner, 1970; Mercer, 1966).

Studies of variables related to the children showed that those with lower IQs were higher probability candidates for institutionalization than were others with higher IQs (Eyman et al., 1966; Graliker et al., 1965; Sabagh, Lei, & Eyman, 1972; Saenger, 1960). They were also more likely to be placed if there was a physical handicap in addition to their mental handicap (Edgerton, Eyman & Silverstein, 1975; Eyman, O'Connor, Tarjan & Justice, 1972; Sabagh et al., 1972) and if there was more of a deficiency in adaptive behavior and greater problems with maladaptive behaviors (Campbell, Smith & Wool, 1982; Eyman et al., 1972; Maney, Pace & Morrison, 1964; Shellhaas & Nihira, 1969).

Quality of Care within PRFs

Historically, criticisms of large PRFs have included charges that they are regimented, poorly staffed, offer a low quality of care, and often border on providing inhumane living conditions. Another criticism has been that institutional living has a negative effect on intellectual and behavioral development. Blatt and Kaplan (1966) in their well-known photographic description of institutions, portrayed a miserable existence for the individuals who occupied these facilities.

Some researchers, however, have questioned the idea that institutions are all bad and have proposed a more objective analysis of institutional effects. Their approach was not to consider institutionalization as a unitary variable, but to look within institutions for different physical and psychological variables that could affect development (Balla, 1976; McCormick, Balla & Zigler, 1975; Zigler & Balla, 1977). They considered two main variables: size of the institution and "quality of care."

The effect of size was analyzed by Balla (1976). He reviewed the available research and concluded that size was not a critical factor. Differences were found between PRFs and CRFs in the quality of care provided with community facilities generally being better (O'Connor, 1976); but within the different types of facilities (PRFs and CRFs) a great deal of variation was found. In other words, the quality of care was, on the average, better in smaller facilities but this did not hold true in all instances. More important than the overall size of the facility was the size of the living units. A smaller unit within a PRF might offer a better quality of resident care than a group living home with many persons. Zigler and Balla (1977) suggested that large institutions tend to have other specific variables associated with them that might be more important than overall size. Variables such as high employee turnover, low cost per resident, low ratio of aides per resident, low ratio of professional staff to residents and more "institutional oriented" practices are examples of such variables.

The position taken by Zigler and his colleagues (see Zigler and Balla, 1977 for a review) is that large institutions are not inherently bad. When considering a person's development in an institution, they feel that the institution itself can only be considered as one variable and that within the institution many subvariables, such as resident-care practices, should be considered. It would be possible to modify such practices without necessarily eliminating the traditional institution.

NORMALIZATION AND DEINSTITUTIONALIZATION

What is Meant by Normalization and Deinstitutionalization

Even though a defense of institutions has been cogently presented, and despite the opinion that there are no substantial data to support massive social policy change (Balla, 1976; Zigler & Balla, 1977), this is exactly what has been happening in the last several years.

Normalization had its origin in the Scandinavian countries. N. E. Bank-Mikkelsen from Denmark and Bengt Nirje and Karl Grunewald, both of Sweden, wrote key chapters in Kugel and Wolfensberger's monograph published by the President's Committee on Mental Retardation in 1969. This publication is often considered a landmark in the promulgation of the normalization principle in the United States. Later Wolfensberger (1972) expanded on this work in his own noteworthy publication.

Nirje's (1969) chapter provided the clearest explanation and characteristics of the concept. He wrote "thus, as I see it, the normalization principle means making available to the mentally retarded patterns and conditions of everyday life which are as close as possible to the norms and patterns of the mainstream of society" (p. 181).

Normalization is not so much an expectation as it is an ideology. As Wolfensberger (1972) explains, empiricism is modified by ideology. The ideology on which normalization is based is that human life, all human life, is valuable. This value surpasses economic restrictions. Normalization principles are not implemented because they save money or cost money but because they are considered by their advocates to be morally right. They are based on human ideals, not necessarily realism. As Blatt, Bogdan, Bilken, and Taylor (1977) phrased it: ". . . there has been far too much realism and far too little idealism in the past" (p. 41).

Wolfensberger (1972) interpreted the normalization principle as a directing source for both means and ends. He stated that normalization is the "utilization of means which are as culturally normal as possible, in order to establish and/or maintain personal behaviors and characteristics which are as culturally normative as possible." Basically he means that we should try to influence the retarded person to be as much like others as we can and we should use special techniques only to the degree necessary. This idea expands on Nirje's thoughts. Whereas Nirje primarily looked at normalization as a lifestyle, Wolfensberger viewed it as a foundation to education and treatment as well as living conditions. Both positions have important implications for deinstitutionalization.

The Law and the Normalization Movement

As with public school education, appropriate treatment for the mentally retarded in the least restrictive residential environment has some basis in litigation and legislation. One of the most often cited cases is *Wyatt v. Stickney*. Cavalier and McCarver (1981) reviewed the details of this federal case. Basically, Judge Frank M. Johnson ruled that several deficiencies existed in Partlow, a residential facility for mentally retarded persons in Alabama. Three main problems included the lack of an adequate humane physical and psychological environment, the lack of qualified staff, and the lack of individual habilitation plans. The *Wyatt* case was the first in which a federal judge mandated a set of standards for an institution. It should be noted that several professionals spoke on behalf of the institution. Their position primarily was that some mentally retarded persons function at such a low level as to preclude any benefit from active educational programs or deinstitutionalization. Instead, they felt that these persons should receive more of an enrichment program (Ellis, Balla, Estes, Warren, Meyers, Hollis, Isaacson, Palk & Siegel, 1981). Still, they agreed with many of the judge's recommendations.

One recent ruling by the U.S. Supreme Court has been viewed as somewhat a deceleration of the deinstitutionalization process. Previously many lower courts required attempted placements in community settings before allowing placements in residential facilities. Based on the Developmentally Disabled Assistance and Bill of Rights Act, advocates were able to preclude the placement of persons in traditional institutions (Coval, Gilhool & Laski, 1977). But in the case of *Pennhurst State School v. Halderman,* the Supreme Court on April 20, 1981, ruled that the states were *not obligated* by the Disabilities Act but *only encouraged* to make community placements (Education of the Handicapped, 1981). Therefore the Pennhurst institution plaintiffs lost their right to mandatory community facilities.

Another ruling by the Supreme Court in the case of *Youngberg v. Romeo,* however, affirmed the Constitutional rights of retarded persons in institutions to liberty, habilitation, and freedom from undue restraints (J. W. Ellis, 1982; Menolascino, McGee & Casey, 1982; H. R. Turnbull, 1982). In this case, the Court unanimously ruled that an involuntarily committed person had the right to more than food, shelter, and medical care. This represented the first full ruling on the substantive constitutional rights of institutionalized retarded persons (J. W. Ellis, 1982).

While *Romeo* did not guarantee deinstitutionalization would occur, according to Turnbull (1982) it began to dismantle a dual system of law and placed retarded persons on the same constitutional footing as nonretarded persons.

Criticism of the Normalization/Deinstitutionalization Movement

Normalization and deinstitutionalization seem to encompass such admirable goals that it would seem few could be critical of them. But indeed the deinstitutionalization/normalization movement has drawn some criticism and it is worthy of our attention.

Among the antagonists to deinstitutionalization are some parents. Meyers (1980) surveyed a group of parents of individuals living in an institution and found that 83% of them thought their offspring should remain in an institution as opposed to moving into a group living home or semi-independent living facility. The parents' main concern was that the availability and quality of care in the community would not equal that in the institution. Payne (1976) reported similar findings. Parents responding to his survey felt that the institutions had more experts, allowed retarded persons to be with others like themselves, protected retarded persons from the "stress of community life," and was the "tried and tested" way of providing services. (It should be noted that in the Meyers' study, only 50.7% of the questionnaires were returned and in the Payne study less than one-third were returned. While the low return rates tend to reduce the generalizability of these studies, the findings cannot be disregarded.)

A concern expressed by some writers is that mentally retarded persons may not be able to handle the stress and rigors of community living. Schwartz (1977) noted that our society is highly industrialized and complicated. She felt that in such a setting, the competitive pressure would preclude many retarded persons from achieving a normal lifestyle that should include self-esteem, emotional and sexual gratification, and a satisfactory level of achievement. Beckman-Brindley and Tavormina (1978) added that accepting responsibility is very much a part of a normal lifestyle. Not making retarded persons accept responsibility for their actions would be an infraction upon the principle of normalization. For this reason they felt that implementation of the normalization principle should be both individualized and judicious.

Another problem associated with deinstitutionalization is community acceptance. PRF superintendents surveyed by Colombatto et al. (1982) expressed this concern. Eighty-three percent of them did not think retarded persons would be well accepted by their neighbors. Sandler and Robinson (1981) reviewed some of the literature on community acceptance and reported that the bulk of it was not positive. The main concern expressed by community members was a lack of supervision for the retarded persons.

Another concern sometimes voiced is that placement of a CRF in a neighborhood would lower property values. Weiner, Anderson, and Nietupski (1982), however, along with other researchers found that this was not true. In fact, in some cases homes in neighborhoods with CRFs actually increased in value in comparison to other homes in similar neighborhoods. In a related study, Margolis and Charitonidis (1981) found most landlords were willing to rent rooms or apartments to retarded adults.

Criticism has been aimed at the normalization principle as well as deinstitutionalization. Basically, critics have pointed out that mentally retarded people are retarded, not normal. The criticism is mainly directed toward the aspect of normalization that calls for learning and development to occur in a fashion as normal as possible (Wolfensberger, 1972). Some have taken the position that the ends (goal) component of the concept is fine but the means (normal instruction and training) component is virtually impossible (Keith, 1979; Mesibov, 1976a; Throne, 1975, 1979). According to these writers, if retarded persons learned normally they would not be retarded. Since they do not, then they need specialized and more intense learning procedures. The most commonly suggested procedure is the operant training approach. From this point of view, normalization represents the right ends but the wrong means.

COMMUNITY RESIDENTIAL FACILITIES (CRFs)

The Development of CRFs

In the late 1960s and early 1970s, as the populations in PRFs were beginning to decline, placement in community facilities began to increase. This was a result of the normalization/deinstitutionalization movement but had been earlier foreshadowed as institutions began to be built smaller and became more regionalized.

There is no such thing as a typical CRF any more than there is a typical home. They are a diverse group of facilities having only the commonality of being based in the community and generally being smaller than PRFs. The following sections provide a general picture of the current status of these facilities.

Number of CRFs

Exactly how many CRFs exist is not clear. Using a number of registries, Bruininks, Hauber, and Kudla (1980) developed a list of 5503 community residential facilities in the U.S. Their definition of a CRF was:

Any community based living quarter(s) which provides 24-hour, 7-days-a-week responsibility for room, board, and supervision of mentally retarded persons with the exceptions of: (a) single family homes providing services to a relative; (b) nursing homes, boarding homes, and foster homes that are not formally state licensed or contracted as mental retardation service providers; and (c) independent living (apartment) programs which have no staff residing in the same facility. (p. 471)

In a similar, more recent study, Janicki, Mayeda & Epple (1983) found that as of January 1, 1982, 6,302 group living homes could be identified within the fifty states and the District of Columbia. Their definition of a group home was:

A community-based, group living residence for mentally retarded or otherwise developmentally disabled children or adults, providing a home-like environment on a long-term or transitional basis and staffed by either live-in or shift employees on a 24-hour basis. Not included in this category were specially licensed foster family care homes. (p. 46)

More important than the specific number of these facilities is their general rate of development. As Figure 10–5 depicts, a sharp increase in the opening of new CRFs occurred after 1967. This was the same time when PRF populations began to decrease.

Number of Persons in CRFs

Of the 5503 CRFs surveyed by Bruininks et al. (1980), 4,427 (88%) responded. Within this group of respondents, it was found that 76,250 retarded individuals were being housed in CRFs. Janicki and his colleagues (1983) found in their survey of group living homes that 57,494 residents were being served. The difference in these figures is probably due to the fact that the Bruininks study employed a wider range of facility types than did Janicki et al. (the latter being restricted to group living homes) even though their actual number was fewer. At this time it is difficult to state precisely how many retarded persons reside in CRFs because, unlike PRFs, there is not a universally accepted CRF standard. However, with the fairly rapid rate of release of residents from PRFs (Best-Sigford et al., 1982), it would not be surprising if the number of persons in CRFs soon equalled or surpassed the number in PRFs.

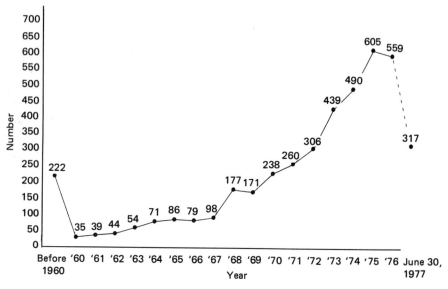

FIGURE 10–5   Year of Opening for 4,290 Community Residential Facilities in the United States in 1977 (87 Percent Reporting)

From R. H. Bruininks, F. A. Hauber, and J. J. Kudla, "National survey of community residential facilities: A profile of facilities and residents in 1977," *American Journal of Mental Deficiency,* 1980, *84,* 470–478. Reprinted by permission.

Characteristics of CRFs

A variety of CRFs may be found. Bruininks et al. (1980) found the facilities to operate under a number of different names and licensure categories. Typical references were to group homes, boarding homes, community residences, residential centers, and sheltered living homes. They found no standard classification system.

A CRF may be located in either rural or urban areas and may range in physical dimensions from individual apartments to small family-like facilities with as few as three to four residents to larger facilities, almost mini-institutions, with thirty or more persons (Butler and Bjaanes, 1977). In their survey, Bruininks et al. found that 73% of the facilities questioned had ten or fewer residents and 88% had twenty or less. On the other hand, they found that a small number of community facilities housed a large number of residents. Over half the residents living in the CRFs they polled were living with thirty-one or more housemates. In her study of deinstitutionalized individuals, Gollay (1977) found that 47.5% of them lived in facilities called group living homes, 17.8% were in foster homes, 13.9% were in their natural or adoptive homes, 10.9% were living independently, and 10% were in semi-independent facilities.

Ownership and management of CRFs is largely dominated by private, nonprofit agencies such as local Associations for Retarded Citizens. Janicki et al. (1983) found that 68% of the group living homes in their study were so controlled while 18.5% were operated by proprietary agencies (for profit) and 13.5% were operated by state or local governments. This represents a major distinction between CRFs and PRFs as the latter are always operated by state governments. The move toward CRFs is thus also a move away from government managed programs. (Of course, state and federal governments will continue as a major funding and regulating source for CRFs.) Fiorelli (1982) recently speculated that as funds become more restricted and more CRFs are needed, there will be an increase in more professionally operated facilities by proprietary businesses and a decrease in those operated by the nonprofit agencies.

The Residents of CRFs

Different CRFs will house individuals of different ages and functional levels. By far, higher functioning retarded persons (mild–moderate) are most likely to be found living in the community. In her study of deinstitutionalized persons, Gollay (1977) found only about one-fourth of them were classified as severely or profoundly retarded with the rest being in the mild–moderate range of retardation. Similarly, O'Connor (1976) in an extensive national survey of CRFs found only about 20% of the persons were in the severe–profound range. According to Bruininks et al. (1980), however, 55% of the facilities surveyed would accept persons who were severely or profoundly retarded. In the future, CRFs may accept more retarded persons of all levels. This possibility is given credence by the fact that institutional demographic patterns are showing a greater increase in the number of severely and profoundly retarded persons being released. Best-Sigford et al. (1982) reported that 46% of the released persons in their study were at this level (severe or profound). Although a number of them were placed in other PRFs, some went into CRFs.

In addition to being higher level persons, most community residents are apt to be young adults. This is probably as much a function of the newness of the facilities as it is anything else. Bruininks et al. found that 55% of their respondents accepted persons only eighteen years of age or older. Actual counts indicated that 62% were at least twenty-two years old whereas 36% were between five and twenty-one years. Gollay (1977) reported an age range of community residents of five to sixty-six years with a mean of 26.6 years; only 19% were under eighteen years of age. O'Connor (1976) and Baker, Seltzer, and Seltzer (1974) found that most CRF residents were between the ages of sixteen and thirty years.

Activities in CRFs

The whole idea of living in the community is to have a lifestyle like other community residents. Recalling Nirje's (1969) urging, the daily lives of retarded persons should be similar to nonretarded persons. In some cases, this occurs but in other cases it does not.

Since most community residents are young adults, it might be expected that they would be employed. In fact, many of them are. Gollay (1977) reported that 48% of the persons she studied were employed in either sheltered workshops or in competitive jobs while another 25% were in activity centers. O'Connor's (1976) findings were similar: 10% were competitively employed and 48% were employed in sheltered workshops. Both studies reported that about one-third of the residents they studied were attending school. O'Connor reported that only about 4% of the residents were without some form of productive daytime activity. In Gollay's study, the figure was a little higher, about 11%.

But work (and school) is only a part of life. In an earlier chapter we saw that recreational and leisure activities of retarded persons tend to be limited. Gollay's study reiterated this finding: most spare time was spent watching TV and listening to the radio. What is more unfortunate is that one of the greatest advantages of living in the community—community involvement—does not often occur at a level that might be hoped. Butler and Bjaanes (1977) found that there was often little use of community services or participation in community activities.

Probably the most common type of out-of-home activity for the community resident is a trip to a local park, movie, church, or store (Heal et al., 1978). But even such simple outings as these may decrease over time. Birenbaum and Re (1979) conducted a follow-up study of moderately and mildly retarded persons who had been in the community for four years and analyzed their findings in light of earlier research with the same group. With the passage of time, they found a sharp reduction in the number of extra-home activities in which the individuals participated. They also found that the residents had settled into a more or less uneventful pattern of sleeping, working, and at-home passive recreation. This was similar to the Butler and Bjaanes (1977) report. Butler and Bjaanes pessimistically concluded that community living does not necessarily mean normal living. Ironically, Birenbaum and Re drew a different conclusion. They felt that the subjects of their study had entered into a "comfortable and conventional" lifestyle that was not terribly different from that of most citizens.

Problems in Community Living

Community living for mentally retarded persons may present a special group of problems. At the top of the list is the availability of necessary services and interagency coordination; for example, medical, dental, psychological, and transportation. In the traditional PRF, all needs were readily met by the residential staff. Getting services in the community is not always so easy. O'Connor (1976) found that 90% of her respondents were unable to get access to one or more community services. Butler and Bjaanes (1977) echoed this finding. This is an important concern for two reasons. Number one, and most obviously, retarded persons need the same, and often more extensive, services as do other people. Two, if the community cannot (or will not) provide these services, the traditional institution will have to. This will be done by either bringing the person back to the PRF or making the CRF into a self-contained facility, in other words a small institution.

As far as the residents are concerned, the most common problems are finding and keeping a job, getting along with others, and achieving even more of an independent living arrangement (Birenbaum & Re, 1979; Gollay, 1977; Scheerenberger & Felsenthal, 1977). Additional personal concerns can also be found at times within a community home (Scheerenberger & Felsenthal, 1977). These take the form of personal limitations similar to those found in the larger residential institutions. For example, in different settings, travel in or around the community may occur only when the residents are accompanied by a staff member. Another example is that the individual has little to say about the job he or she is given. As stated earlier, the job is usually within a sheltered workshop and what the person does there is typically not by choice. Another concern of the residents is that around the home there may be strict rules that also reduce an individual's decision-making and thus the normality of the environment. A good example of this would be a staunchly enforced lights-out rule.

Finally, there may be problems associated simply with the move from a traditional facility to a community residence, at least for the severely and profoundly retarded. Several researchers have indicated that a "relocation syndrome" exists (Carsrud, Carsrud, Henderson, Alisch & Fowler, 1979; Cochran, Sran & Varano, 1977; Cohen, Conroy, Frazen, Snelbecker & Spreat, 1977). This malady sometimes occurs following a move from one setting to another. It may be characterized by depression, loss of appetite, crying, loss of body weight, and sometimes pneumonia or other respiratory ailments. Additionally, there may be a decline in adaptive behavior performance and death may even occur (Cochran et al., 1977).

Satisfaction and Quality of Life in CRFs

Despite the problems and concerns outlined above, mentally retarded persons would rather live in a community setting than in an institution. Those who have been in both express a strong preference for the community placement. No report was found that indicated a person would like to move from the community into an institution. Even when there are expressed problems about community living, the bottom line always seems to be the desire to remain in the community.

In their study, Scheerenberger and Felsenthal (1977) explored some of the attitudes of mentally retarded people who were formerly institutionalized. At the time of the study, these people were living in foster homes, group homes, or adult homes. The following was found:

> All of the persons preferred community living.
> Many had formed new friendships both within and outside the home.
> Most were pleased with the quality and quantity of food.
> They could decorate their rooms as they wished.
> They could go outside when they wanted.
> They could select their own clothing.
> They had spending money and could spend it as they wished.
> Most had a boyfriend or a girlfriend and could express affection.
> They could go places but usually had to be accompanied.
> Most had jobs and received their earnings.
> Many were in educational programs they enjoyed.

In some cases, deinstitutionalized persons do not live in CRFs but live independently in the community. Most often these individuals are mildly retarded or higher (some would be placed in the borderline category; i.e. IQs from about 70–85). In recent years some intriguing follow-up studies have been conducted with a number of these persons (Edgerton, 1967; Edgerton & Bercovici, 1976; McDevitt, Smith, Schmidt & Rosen, 1978). Edgerton's (1967) early book, *The Cloak of Competence,* is considered to be a classic.

How do these people do? All in all they do well. They tend to become marginal participants in society, but they survive and they are generally pleased with their ability to do so. Many find unskilled or semi-skilled jobs although others receive welfare payments. Some develop savings accounts and even become good credit risks although most rely on cash. Many get around the community freely through the use of public transportation. Less positively, social involvement is usually limited with most leisure activities being alone or with one or two other people. Functional academic skills are usually deficient. Activities requiring reading or arithmetic are usually limited although many learn to compensate for these deficits. Often advocates or benefactors (e.g., social workers, employers) will help out in difficult times (Edgerton, 1967; McDevitt et al., 1978).

Effects of Community Placement on Development

Some researchers have sought to determine if living in community settings affects behavioral and/or intellectual development. Consequently there has been some recent research in this area (Eyman & Arndt, 1982; Eyman, Borthwick & Miller, 1981; Eyman, Demaine & Lei, 1979; Eyman, Silverstein, McLain & Miller, 1977; Sandler & Thurman, 1981; Thompson & Carey, 1980). Overall, the findings have been encouraging although not conclusive.

In one of the most complete reports, Eyman and Arndt (1982) examined changes in adaptive behavior over a four-year period of persons living in institutions (n = 3,457) and in different community settings (n = 312). They also evaluated the quality of care provided by the facilities. Both institutionalized persons and community persons showed increases in adaptive behavior over the four-year period. The patterns of growth were similar for persons of similar IQs regardless of placement. However, community residents tended to have higher adaptive behavior scores. More importantly, older community persons tended to increase in adaptive behavior whereas older institutional residents tended to decrease over the four years on their adaptive behavior scores. It was also found that the quality of care measured in the institutions was not significantly associated with changes in adaptive behavior. On the other hand, in another study Eyman et al. (1979) found a relationship between the quality of care provided in community environments and the degree of improvement in adaptive behavior. Based on the PASS 3 instrument (Wolfensberger & Glenn, 1975) which measures conformity to the normalization principle, community facilities that had higher scores (were more normal) produced more gains in adaptive behavior than did community homes with lower scores.

Thompson and Carey's (1980) study also demonstrated development to occur in community settings. They examined the progress of four severely retarded and four profoundly retarded persons who had been living in a group home for two years. Prior to their placement, they had been in an institution for an average of almost seventeen years. When they moved into the community setting, they had a mean IQ of 24 and various inappropriate skills; for example, they were not toilet trained, had temper tantrums, and so on. Systematic training programs were provided during the day at a training center and at home during the evening and weekend. After two years, Thompson and Carey reported an average increase in IQs of 16 points. Adaptive behavior scores increased an average of 16.7% with major improvements occurring in language, social skills, domestic skills, and leisure skills.

Together these studies indicate that community facilities produce positive changes in behavior. But we should not hastily conclude that placement alone will bring about changes. Eyman et al. (1977) and Sandler and Thurman (1981) noted that these changes are associated with what is *done* in the facility, and not just the fact that the facility is located in the community. Another way to put it is that if settings *work* toward normalization, improvement will probably occur. On the other hand, a CFR that becomes only a small PRF will probably not effect any more change than a large PRF.

Success and Failure in the Community

Not all retarded persons will be successful living in community settings. Some will not show progress and others will be returned to residential institutions. Conversely, many will be successful and remain in the community. What affects the success or failure of an individual? There is no single correct answer. Two broad classes of variables have been studied: personal variables and environmental variables. The first deals with a number of individual factors such as age, IQ, and adaptive behavior. The second looks at such factors as the type of facility the person is in, the amount of training provided, the skills of the service provider, and so on.

McCarver and Craig (1974), in their review, found that few personal factors predicted success in the community. Most of what they found could only be described as tentative. Among these, age seemed to be mildly associated with community success with older persons tending to succeed more often than younger ones. The findings on IQ were also mixed. Many early studies found that IQ was not really associated with how someone did in the community. However, most of these studies were looking at mildly retarded persons and difference in IQ points did not much matter. As more retarded persons of all IQ levels move into the community, the significance of IQ may become more important (Heal et al., 1978; Landesman-Dwyer, 1981). Certainly, for some aspects of community living; e.g., community awareness, IQ will prove to be an important asset (Hull & Thompson, 1980).

More important than IQ or age will be a person's personal competence and social skills (McCarver & Craig, 1974). In a recent series of studies, Shalock and his associates (Shalock & Harper, 1978; Shalock, Harper & Carver, 1981; Shalock, Harper & Genung, 1981) investigated personalogical variables associated with progressing through a systematic program of community reintegration. More successful individuals were found to have better language skills, better sensorimotor and auditory functions, more vocational skills, and more training experiences (Shalock & Harper, 1978). They also demonstrated more appropriate social and emotional behaviors and had more skills in the areas of personal maintenance such as clothing care and use, community utilization, and functional academics (Shalock, Harper & Carver, 1981; Shalock, Harper & Genung, 1981).

When failure in the community is attributed to personal factors, the culprit is almost always a demonstration of maladaptive behavior by the resident (Heal et al., 1978; Landesman-Dwyer, 1981; McCarver & Craig, 1974). Several studies have documented reasons for the return of some mentally retarded individuals from their community placements back to public residential facilities. Thiel (1981) reported a high degree of general social maladaption. More specifically, Shalock, Harper, and Genung (1981) identified abuse of others, self-abuse, defiance, destruction of property, and aberrant sexual behavior as being critical factors. Similar behaviors were reported by Sutter, Tadashi, Call, Yanagi, and Yee (1980). Obviously such behavior will be difficult to accept particularly in community settings where social behavior must be closer to normal.

Certainly the success of retarded persons in the community will depend, at least to some degree, on the amount of support the community and their environment offers. Landesman-Dwyer (1981) suggested that environmental variables may better predict success than personal variables. Although the evidence is not complete, it is most probable that communities that are not accepting and in which resources are poor will result in an inordinate number of failures (Heal et al., 1978). It may also be hypothesized that what goes on within the community facility will be at least as important as the characteristics of the people there. Hull and Thompson (1980) measured individuals' abilities using an "Adaptive Functioning Index." This was to provide a measure of their functioning within the community. Better performance scores were associated with higher IQs but were even more associated with more normalized environments.

While the data are scant, there is indication that the environment plays an important role in predicting the success of community residents. What the research virtually ignores is the possibility that certain types of residences may be more appropriate or less appropriate for certain individuals. Studies of key environmental variables are just getting underway. Ultimately these may be fully investigated and the results may be useful in matching persons and settings (Heal et al., 1978). As Landesman-Dwyer (1981) pointed out, "Given the right program, most individuals will show beneficial growth regardless of their degree of impairment" (p. 228).

CONCLUSION

In the last fifteen or twenty years, residential programs for the mentally retarded have come the full swing. Starting out as schools in the mid-1800s, they later became custodial warehouses. After maintaining this status for over fifty years they again began to assume a role of education and habilitation for the mentally retarded instead of protection for society. An important part of the habilitative process has been a move away from large, central, self-contained facilities to smaller regional facilities and community based homes. Not only is this move a part of habilitation, it is an attempt to provide a better quality of life, a more normal life. There is some support that retarded persons do better in community settings. But the smaller size and home style of the building is no more likely to influence this development than is a large facility likely to depress it. In the final analysis, it will be the quality of the programs offered and the people who offer them that make any difference.

Heal et al. (1978) have suggested cautious proceedings. They note a parallel between today's enthusiasm and that of the mid-1800s. They state: "Hopes are high; 'cures' are being oversold; empirical investigation is lacking" (p. 214). In the mid-1800s the unrestrained enthusiasm led to disillusionment and then pessimism as institutions changed from residential schools to custodial warehouses. We should not make the same mistakes in judgment. A mentally retarded person will not become normal. With a more normal lifestyle, however, functioning may improve and life should certainly be happier. The latter may be enough in and of itself. We should hope for this and then we should work toward making the effects of the normalization more obvious.

STUDY QUESTIONS

1. For what purpose were public residential facilities originally developed? What were some of the characteristics of PRFs during the first part of the twentieth century?

2. Describe the historical trend of the number of mentally retarded persons living in PRFs.

3. What type of person is most likely to be found today in a PRF?

4. What is the approximate ratio of institutional employees to institutional residents? What is the average cost per year for a person to live in a PRF?

5. Describe some of the activities and services available in PRFs.

6. What criticisms have been directed toward large PRFs?

7. What specific characteristics of large institutions may affect a mentally retarded person's development?

8. Briefly summarize what is meant by "normalization." Where did the normalization principle originate? What is the relationship between normalization and deinstitutionalization?

9. What type of criticism has been directed toward the normalization (deinstitutionalization) movement?

10. Describe the recent trend in the number of CRFs and the number of persons residing in them.

11. What characteristics are most likely to be found of residents within CRFs? What types of activities occur?

12. What are some typical problems that may occur because of residence within CRFs? What is the overall satisfaction level of the residents?

13. What conclusions can be drawn about the effect of CRFs on individual development?

14. What personal and environmental factors may be associated with the success or failure of living in the community?

11

Teaching Approaches

THE PROCESS OF TEACHING RETARDED INDIVIDUALS:
AN OVERVIEW

Professionals have been formally teaching mentally retarded individuals for almost 200 years. Because of their teaching, the lives of mentally retarded individuals have often improved substantially. Teaching retarded persons, or anyone else, requires two basic components. First, it must be decided *what* is to be taught. Learning *goals* or *objectives* are developed that are to be achieved by the learner. When goals and objectives are grouped together they are referred to as a curriculum.

The second component of teaching requires deciding *how* to teach what is to be learned; in other words, how to best allow the person to achieve the objectives and/or goals contained within a curriculum. Typically, teachers employ various *methods* and *instructional materials* to get their students to learn what they need to learn. The instructional approaches used to teach retarded as well as nonretarded persons are many and varied. Sometimes a particular instructional technique is paired with a particular goal or objective in a curriculum. Sometimes the same technique can be used for different learning targets. In other situations, different instructional methods and/or materials can be used to achieve similar outcomes. Matching instructional goals and teaching methods can provide almost an infinite array of ways to foster learning.

The obvious question is: Is there a best way to teach a specific skill or bit of knowledge to retarded persons? The answer is definite: There is not. If there were, we could use it exclusively without hesitation or concern. Unfortunately we do not have such a wonder method and never will. What we have are various individuals who have different learning needs and who respond differently to a variety of instructional approaches.

Mentally retarded individuals demonstrate various learning problems. These include attending to relevant dimensions of stimuli, using reasoning skills, remembering, generalizing, incidental learning, and applying learned concepts. Such problems as these affect both how and what we teach retarded persons. It is the purpose of this chapter to examine some of the important approaches related to teaching mentally retarded people. As we examine these, various philosophies will emerge as to the *best* way to teach retarded persons and the *most* important things to teach them. As students of mental retardation, we should study these positions and learn from them. But we should also realize that professional opinions on these topics vary a great deal. It is not the purpose of this chapter to convince you of a particular philosophy or approach, only to inform you.

To achieve this goal, the present chapter is presented in three sections. First, we will briefly examine some historical approaches used in early education and training programs for the mentally retarded. Even though these strategies are considered "historical," they should not necessarily be dismissed as passé. Many of these practices, or variations of them, are still being used.

Second, an overview of some recent trends and practices will be discussed. Practices will be reviewed that have been widely adopted and adapted in special education for mentally retarded students at various levels. Third, major curricular elements and issues for different levels of retardation will be outlined.

HISTORICAL APPROACHES

Systematic special education for retarded persons began in the early 1800s. While earlier concern for care had been expressed, it was not until the nineteenth century that purposeful efforts to educate or train retarded persons were initiated. These first attempts at special education have been reviewed by Kirk and Johnson (1951), Wallin (1955), Dunn (1973), and Anderson, Zia, Springfield, and Greer (1977).

Itard's Instruction of Victor

Jean Marc Gaspard Itard was influenced by the school of sensationalism. The philosophy of learning was that man had essentially unlimited learning abilities and that learning occurred when the environment sufficiently stimulated the senses. In his approach to educating Victor, Itard used a series of stimulations and discrimination tasks that required Victor to use his senses. Itard's belief was that Victor's sensory abilities had been dulled due to a lack of exercise. He therefore attempted to activate the nervous system through educating the senses.

Itard developed activities to stimulate vision, hearing, taste, touch, temperature, and smelling abilities. He would present items that were in great contrast to each other in order to better assure that Victor could "sense" the difference. Then Itard would gradually decrease the differences between the stimuli and thus require finer discrimination. At times Itard would blindfold Victor in an attempt to get him to improve his hearing. Later he worked on auditory discrimination of various vowel sounds. In visual training, Itard contrasted different size objects and later went on to teach the discrimination of printed words. Imitation training was used in an attempt to teach speech but Victor never learned to talk. Itard also tried to create intelligent behavior by training Victor to make associations between printed words and objects but the success of this was limited. Victor was never able to generalize the associations he had learned.

Seguin's Physiological Method

Edouard O. Seguin was a student of Itard and was influenced by him. In his book *Idiocy: And its treatment by the physiological method* Seguin (1866) presented a method for training mentally retarded persons that was based on his neurophysiological theory that retardation resulted from a damaged or weakened peripheral or central nervous system. Accordingly, Seguin's treatment was similar to Itard's. He attempted to use sensory training to strengthen sensory receptors and thus allow stimulation to reach the central nervous system. He also stressed motor coordination. His approach called for the student to initially learn total gross bodily movements and then finer, more specific movements. Proper eye-hand coordination was a major goal. He considered the sense of touch to be very important and used stimuli that varied in shape, size, texture, temperature, and weight to refine tactile discrimination.

Seguin felt that learning should be of interest to the learner and thus appeal to his or her needs and desires. Various play activities were used to coordinate the senses and movement. Many different materials were employed that were of interest and were common to everyday life. In all activities, Seguin believed it was most important for the child to be actively involved in the learning process. The physical handling of materials was encouraged. He also encouraged teachers to develop a good rapport with their students and to consider the educational process as an integrated approach. All learning was to be related, not isolated.

The work of Itard and especially Seguin greatly influenced many latter day perceptual motor theorists. Some of these theorists (e.g., Strauss & Lehtinen, 1947; Kephart, 1960; Barsch, 1965) devised similar tactics to educate "brain-damaged" children classified as either mentally retarded, slow learners, or learning disabled. Many classrooms today for trainable and educable mentally retarded students, as well as those for learning disabled students, contain materials similar to those originally developed by Seguin for stimulating and educating the senses and motor abilities of handicapped students (Anderson et al., 1977).

Montessori's Auto-teaching Methods

Like Itard and Seguin, Maria Montessori was a physician turned educator. It was the medical background of Itard and Seguin that influenced them to consider mental retardation primarily as a sensory and physiological deficit. In this regard, Montessori disagreed with her predecessors. While she studied their work and employed many of their physical-sensory training tactics, Montessori considered mental retardation to be mainly a pedagogical problem, not a medical problem.

Her best known contribution, later used and made famous with normal preschool children, was her didactic auto-teaching materials. These materials were designed for children to use independently to improve their sensorimotor abilities. The teacher's role was reduced to that of an unobtrusive observer who would simply provide the materials for the child to learn. The materials were intended to be self-correcting so that when used, the child knew immediately if he or she had performed the activity correctly. Montessori claimed to instruct all the senses except smell and taste using these materials.

Dr. B. Decroly and Alice Descoeudres

The overwhelming characteristic of the approaches by Itard, Seguin, and Montessori was their strong attention to sensorimotor development. Early in the twentieth century, Dr. B. Decroly of Belgium and his student Alice Descoeudres started to bridge the gap between the sensorimotor training emphasis and training children in more applied areas. Working at the Polytechnic Hospital in Brussels, Decroly focused on the development of games to be used as instructional activities in areas such as reading and arithmetic. The lotto game format was developed for use in matching and discrimination activities and also for teaching reading and numbers.

Descoeudres later expanded on the work of her mentor and developed several principles she felt to be important when working with mentally retarded children. She stressed the need for learning through natural activities pleasant to children. John Dewey's philosophy of learning by doing was particularly important. This led to the practice of "correlating" or "concentrating" subject matter around a particular theme. She also felt that learning should be practical and applicable to the students' immediate needs.

Descoeudres stressed the need for learning activities for mentally retarded persons to be concrete and within the child's level of comprehension. The object lesson was a forerunner of the "units of experience" approach developed by Ingram. This procedure provided the child with some activity and experience and then incorporated various academic subject matter around the activity.

Christine Ingram's Unit of Instruction Approach

In the 1920s and '30s, Christine Ingram more fully implemented the Dewey philosophy with retarded students and became a well-known advocate of the activity method of instruction. This procedure has variously been referred to as the project method, the unit of instruction method, the correlation method, or the experience method. All learning, primarily academics, was to center around a particular area of interest.

Units included such topics as the home, the city, the food market, the telephone, money, trees, and so on.

Although Ingram felt that the unit plan could not be used for teaching all subject matter, she felt it was particularly important for practicing such skills in an applied fashion. Her influence is apparent today as many teachers continue to incorporate teaching specific skills around central themes.

Annie Innskeep's Watered-down Curriculum

Although units of instruction were praised, according to Kirk and Johnson (1951), they did not gain widespread acceptance. Instead, in most classes for the mildly retarded, a lower level academic curriculum was often used. A primary developer of this approach, which was tagged the "watered-down" curriculum, was Annie Innskeep. Her curriculum was divided into the traditional academic areas of reading, language, spelling, arithmetic, and similar areas typically included in an elementary curriculum. This curriculum has often been criticized for its lack of relevance to mentally retarded learners.

John Duncan's Project Method

Duncan, in England during the 1940s, suggested a curriculum for mildly retarded and slow learning students that was based on the hypothesis that these individuals were more efficient in the use of concrete intelligence than in abstract intelligence. Duncan suggested that teaching mentally retarded persons should occur through a medium that could be seen, touched, handled, and manipulated. Approaches that were too verbal or too abstract were to be avoided.

Duncan's approach, referred to as the project method, was designed to provide students with tasks in an organized sequence that would systematically allow them to observe relationships and promote thinking. Handwork and crafts, paper and cardboard work, woodwork, needlework, cooking, and similar activities were included in the curriculum. Academic subjects were incorporated into the manual tasks.

Richard Hungerford and Occupational Education

In the 1940s, considerable interest developed in the adult occupational adjustment of mentally retarded persons. Commensurate with this interest was the role of education in the preparation of retarded persons for participation in the world of work. Occupational education was born and Richard Hungerford was one of the main leaders in its delivery.

Hungerford was the director of the Bureau for Children with Retarded Mental Development in New York City. To him, occupational education was not simply training retarded persons in job skills, but the entire process of special education. He wrote:

> The whole program for the mentally retarded must be built around the achieving of vocational and social competence, for here, if anywhere, the retarded will most nearly approach normalcy. This different developmental program is called Occupational Education. (Hungerford, DeProspo & Rosenzweig, 1948, as cited in Kirk & Johnson, 1951)

Occupational education was concerned with developing attitudes and habits related to obtaining and maintaining a job. It emphasized wage earning as a privilege that required certain responsibilities and obligations. Focus was placed on those aspects of jobs common to various occupations. Social skills were also taught.

Alfred Strauss and Laura Lehtinen's Approach to Teaching the Brain-damaged Child

Strauss and Lehtinen (1947) are credited for developing special educational techniques for a segment of the mentally retarded population they classified as "brain-injured." Characterized by their behavior more than by actual identified physiological disorders, these children were considered to be in need of well-structured, nonstimulating environmental controls in order for them to use their intact mental abilities to the greatest degree possible. Some of the characteristics displayed by these children included attention to details rather than the whole stimulus, a disintegration of the visual-perceptual field, perseveration, a high degree of distractibility, a high degree of sensitivity to extraneous stimuli, thinking disorders, and various behavior disorders.

In their educational plan, Strauss and Lehtinen (1947) had as their goal the organization of mental processes in the child so that learning would occur more like the learning of a nonbrain-injured child. To accomplish this, they suggested that education occur in an environment devoid of much stimulation. Materials not in use were to be removed in order to minimize distractibility. Instruction was to occur in isolated parts of the room away from visual and auditory stimuli. Windows, brightly decorated walls, flashy clothes, and other children were to be minimized.

Tasks were to be used that required the child's participation and attention. These included cutting, sorting, and manipulating objects and instructional materials. Visual-perceptual training stressing part-whole relations were considered to be of importance. Visual cues were exaggerated in order to provide saliency and thus improve attention to them. Specific skills were to be taught. The unit method was not considered appropriate for these children because such an approach would produce too much stimulation at one time.

Synthesis

The early development of educational programs for mentally retarded students provided us with a foundation for more recent educational strategies. It seems interesting that initially the focus was on *how* to teach. This was a necessary consideration because before Itard's time, purposeful learning by mentally retarded persons was not considered a possibility. Concerned individuals theorized that retarded persons would learn best through sensory stimulation and expended much energy exploring this teaching process. The outcome of the learning process was not given much attention except for the general idea to improve sensory and thus intellectual functioning. Itard, Seguin, Montessori, and later Strauss and Lehtinen, were essentially process-oriented educators. Most of their efforts were guided by their belief that the learners lacked a basic, efficient learning ability.

Decroly and Descoeudres, Ingram, Innskeep, Duncan, and Hungerford were also concerned with effective learning and appropriate teaching methods. But they started to give more consideration to what was being learned. In other words, they were hopeful that some *practical* benefit would result from the learning process. There was a shifting away from a sensory-process orientation of training.

CONTEMPORARY PRACTICES

There can be no doubt that the efforts of the special education pioneers influence many of our practices today. Yet the field has expanded tremendously and additional approaches have been developed. Many factors have contributed to this expansion. We are, for example, providing services today to all levels of mentally retarded people, mild to profound. We are starting our intervention with younger individuals and continuing longer with older ones. We are individualizing instruction and being held accountable for providing an appropriate education. We are witnessing a variety of philosophies that support the significance of such areas as career education, age-appropriate education, and leisure education; not to mention the more traditional ones of academics, social skills, vocational skills, and daily living skills.

New instructional methods, materials, and technology have also emerged. A clearly dominating influence has been applied behavior analysis with its emphasis on specifying behavioral targets, systematic environmental control, and the precise measurement of behavior. There are instructional materials designed for every approach, every need, every philosophy, and more. There are so many instructional materials commercially available today that a teacher can be familiar with only a fraction of them. National, regional, state, and local materials dissemination networks have been established to facilitate the link between consumer and producer.

The age of technology has not bypassed special education for the mentally retarded. From the most basic audio-visual equipment, to programmed instructional machines, to microcomputers, special educators have been given access to educational approaches that did not, could not, exist before.

Clearly there are too many elements embodying special education for the mentally retarded today for each to be given just consideration. However, in a text of this nature, it is important for the reader to at least become familiar with some of the more salient trends. Three of these trends seem to cut across all levels of mental retardation and, to one degree or another, affect the education or training of every mentally retarded student. These include individual educational programs, instructional materials and technology, and applied behavior analysis.

Individual Educational Plans

Individual educational programs or plans (IEPs) are required by PL 94–142 for all children identified as needing special education services in the public schools. A standard is required in the law for what they must include. These are:

1. Current level of performance
2. Annual goals and short-term objectives
3. Special education and related services and the extent of participation in the regular classroom
4. Projected date for the initiation and duration of services
5. Evaluation procedures for measuring behaviors on at least an annual basis. (Turnbull, Strickland & Brantley, 1978, p. 135)

By requiring teachers to develop IEPs, the federal law attempted to insure accountability in the educational process. Even before PL 94–142, this trend was becoming evident in regular and special education (Jones, 1973). The requirement of the IEP formalized it and provided a mechanism for monitoring it.

What is important to realize is that simply providing special education to mentally retarded persons is not acceptable within accountability models. The education must be meaningful. It must be shown that learning has occurred or at least demonstrate that there was a plan for learning to occur.

The first step of this process is determining what is to be learned. This will vary a great deal per individual. Additionally it may be affected by the philosophy of the teacher, the parent, or the educational system. Formal and informal assessment will be used in fulfilling the first two elements of the IEP; that is, determining current performance skills and needed skills. Often used in this process is criterion-referenced assessment (Duffey & Fedner, 1978; Howell, Kaplan & O'Connell, 1979), which allows the teacher to diagnose specific learning needs of the student.

The third and fourth requirements of the IEP stipulate *no* particular placement (special school, special class, regular class), but do require that thought be given and plans be made to educate the child in the least restrictive requirement (Hayes & Higgins, 1978). They also do not allow this to be an ongoing, forgotten process, but require that specific starting and ending dates for the special services be indicated.

The fifth requirement of the IEP is another step toward accountability. Most often the same tests used initially to determine instructional objectives will be used to determine if the objectives have been achieved. This end of the year evaluation completes a pretest/posttest paradigm. It allows parents and advocates to have an answer to the question, "What have you done for this student?" The law does not specify what may ensue if the answer is not satisfactory, but it does at least provide for the question (Hayes & Higgins, 1978).

The IEP clearly adds a new dimension to the education of mentally retarded students and requires participation by key individuals in its formulation. The following persons must participate:

1. The student's teacher (regular and/or special)
2. A person other than the child's teacher who is responsible for providing or supervising special education
3. The student's parent(s)
4. The student, if appropriate
5. The person conducting the student's evaluation or a person knowledgeable in the interpretation of the test data. (Turnbull, et al., 1978, p. 125)

Other persons may also be involved if their presence will contribute to a more complete IEP. They may include health personnel, social workers, therapists, vocational rehabilitation specialists, or physical education specialists (Turnbull, et al., 1978). Turnbull, Strickland, and Goldstein (1978) have noted the need for training both parents and professionals in order to insure their fullest participation in the IEP development process. Such training seems to be of importance as full participation does not always occur (Goldstein, Strickland, Turnbull & Curry, 1980).

Certainly the development of IEPs places an additional burden on all involved in the student's education. Price and Goodman (1980) found that teachers spent an average of six and a half hours developing each IEP. Sixty-eight percent of this time was in school and the rest was personal time. But what must be considered is the quality of education that occurs as a result of the IEP. It is intended that the improvement in quality will more than compensate for the additional time requirement.

Instructional Materials and Technology

In about the last twenty years, there has developed a substantial growth in instructional materials for mentally retarded and other handicapped students. More recently we have seen sophisticated products, such as microcomputers and automated teaching devices, intended to facilitate the instructional process. The emergence of various materials has created a market that is both respectable in private industry and influential in special educational tactics. As a result, today's special educators must attend not only to developing individual programs, but must search the myriad of catalogs, listings, and advertisements seeking the most suitable products to meet their budgets and needs.

The availability and use of instructional materials. The range and extent of materials available today could not be presented in this chapter, this book, or several books of this length. In fact, the market is so broad that in the mid-60s, the federal government began to develop *Instructional Materials Centers* (IMC). The IMCs were regionally located facilities that gathered many of the materials on the market and made them available to the special education community. Teachers were given the opportunity to borrow materials, learn about their use, evaluate them, and make decisions regarding their pertinence (McCarthy, 1968). Today a much expanded version of the original system exists. It includes a National Center on Educational Media and Materials for the Handicapped (NCEMMH), four Special Offices (SO), and thirteen Area Learning Resource Centers (ALRC) (Anderson et al, 1977; Ashcroft, 1977). The NCEMMH/SO/ALRC network supports state and local school district centers.

Instructional media usually constitute the core of special teachers' tools for conducting learning activities. The most commonly used pieces of equipment include models, slide projectors, filmstrip projectors, overhead transparency projectors, film projectors, record players, audio tape players, and chalkboards. Many classrooms may also have automatic teaching machines such as Systems 80 and Language Master. In addition to these, and probably more effective for many areas of instruction with mentally retarded students, are actual objects such as money, telephones, vending machines, kitchen utensils, furniture, and so on. Because generalizing or transferring from the abstract to the real is difficult for retarded learners, using real items that the person will ultimately operate is preferable when possible.

Prosthetic and support devices.   The appearance of severely and profoundly retarded individuals in public schools has required many teachers to become familiar with the availability and construction of several prosthetic and support devices. Because many of these students also have physical impairments, specially designed equipment is necessary. These products serve two functions. They prevent the physical impairments from worsening and they aid in the individual's ability to perform certain tasks (Campbell, Green & Carlson, 1977). Campbell et al. described some commonly used devices that can be individually constructed for each child while Robinault (1976) provided an extensive catalog of many commercially produced physical-assist devices. One important rule must be kept in mind about this equipment. Its use must be individually prescribed by a physical or occupational therapist. Teachers should not take it upon themselves to use any of these devices unless they have been advised by an appropriate professional. However, the teacher's role is important. Once the equipment has become available, he or she must use it in the way it was intended based on the therapist's directions. Teachers will also be in a key position to point out other support devices the student may need.

Microcomputers.   Probably the most rapidly expanding technology in our society today involves microcomputers. The development of the microcomputer in recent years has placed this technology at the fingertips of even those among us who have difficulty operating a transistor radio. These devices have the same capabilities of larger main-frame computers but operate with a more limited memory storage capacity. Their limits, however, are compensated by their portability and versatility (Hofmeister, 1982). What is more important to their use in special education is the systems that have been developed to allow interactions to occur between people and machines. These systems allow the machine to present graphic displays on their video screens and even to present synthetic voices to tell the student what to do and then whether or not what was done was correct (Stallard, 1982).

Thornkildson (in an interview with Thomas, 1981) described a process in which students listened to an audio command and then simply touched the video screen where the correct item appeared. The computer indicated whether their response was correct or whether they should try again. Such an arrangement has been shown to be simple enough to teach mildly, moderately, and severely retarded students time telling, coin values, arithmetic skills, budgeting, shopping, and reading functional sight words, among other things (Brebner, Hallworth & Brown, 1977; Lally, 1981).

In a project described by Crawford, McMahon, Conklin, Giordano, Alexander, and Kadyszewski (1980), microcomputers provided teachers with individual student profiles that included performance in a variety of skill areas and the level of assistance necessary for the student to complete the task. The main feature of the computer in such a program is that it never forgets. It will store a great deal of information and be extremely reliable in its presentation. Similarly, the computer can be counted on to deliver the instructional stimuli in a very consistent fashion.

These examples of the uses of microcomputers only hint at their potential. Lance (1977) pointed out several aspects of today's special education practices that call for computers' capabilities; for example, mainstreaming, IEPs, teaching the profoundly handicapped, and the need to teach all retarded persons more. Additionally, Budoff and Hutton (1982) suggested that certain features (nonthreatening, failure-free, reinforcing capabilities) made microcomputers desirable for special education instruction. They also noted, however, that much work remained to be done, specifically in the development of software (the instructional program). Given the rapid rate of development in this field, we can well expect the potential of these devices to be realized in the very near future.

Applied Behavior Analysis[1]

One of the most pervasive strategies used in educational practices with individuals at all levels of retardation has been referred to as operant conditioning, behavior management, behavior modification, or applied behavior analysis. Generally, the approach considers a behavior or operant to occur as a direct function of environmental influence. Because mentally retarded persons are characteristically deficient in their behavioral repertoires (Bijou, 1963), many practitioners have considered the purpose of education and training to be to develop and strengthen new behaviors. To do this they have turned to the tools provided by behavior analysis that are discussed below.

The strongest aspect of the environment that can affect the occurrence of behavior is the consequence of the behavior. Positive reinforcement is the presentation of a stimulus following a behavior that increases the probability that the behavior will occur more often. Negative reinforcement is the cessation of an aversive stimulus following the occurrence of a behavior. It also increases the probability that the behavior will recur. Both positive and negative reinforcement are presented *contingent* on the demonstration of the behavior. In other words, the reinforcer is delivered if and only if the behavior occurs. Thus the term *contingency management* is sometimes used.

If undesirable behaviors are manifested such as aggression or self-injurious acts, another kind of consequence will be used. This will be a form of punishment or extinction. Punishment presents an aversive (painful) stimulus when the behavior occurs. Extinction inhibits any type of reinforcement following the behavior. A common extinction practice is called time-out. Time-out removes the individual from a presumably reinforcing environment in order to prevent the undesirable behavior from being reinforced. Both punishment and extinction are intended to have the same effect: to decrease or eliminate the occurrence of a behavior.

When certain behaviors do not exist (and therefore cannot be increased or decreased), it is necessary for the behavioral practitioner to first create the behavior before modifying its rate of occurrence. A number of tactics are available for developing behaviors. The most direct methods include modeling or verbally directing the learner. If the student cannot comprehend either of these, a relatively more concrete tactic such as physical guidance or prompting can be used. Regardless of the cue used, when the behavior occurs, it is reinforced. Ultimately the behavior will be learned.

Successive approximation is also useful for developing new behaviors. This tactic requires that the learner demonstrate some "rough" form of the behavior. The teacher looks for closer approximations to the correct topography of the behavior. Each time the behavior is closer to normal than on previous occasions, it is reinforced.

Chaining is used to link several simple behaviors into more complex acts. Sometimes there is a situation that requires the student to demonstrate a series of behaviors in a certain order. The student may be able to perform the simple behaviors independently. The teacher's job, then, is to cue the learner to perform them in a certain order. Ultimately the completion of each behavior in the chain becomes a cue for the next behavior to occur. The chain may either be taught in its natural order (forward chaining) or by working backward from the last behavior in the chain to the first (backward or reverse chaining).

As can be seen, behavior analysts have several tactics available to modify behavior. In addition to these tactics, a direct measure of the behavior will usually be taken. This is usually done by counting how many times the behavior occurs within a period of time. The resulting measure is called frequency (the number of behaviors divided by the amount of time). Frequency measures are often taken daily and charted on some type of graph paper. (Koorland & Martin, 1975; Pennypacker, Koenig & Lindsley, 1972). By charting frequencies daily and examining the charts on a regular basis, the teacher can observe trends in the data such as whether the behavior is increasing, decreasing, or remaining the same. Changes in tactics can thus be made based on individual need rather than on subjective impressions.

Probably because of the relative consistency of success, behavior analysis and modification procedures have become widely used by individuals working with every level of retardation. There is hardly a special class, special school, institution, or community-based facility that does not, in one form or another, practice some of the principles of behavior management with their students and clients. Table 11–1 lists some of the areas reported in the literature in which applied behavior analysis has been used successfully with mentally retarded individuals. While the list is far from complete, it does provide the reader with an idea of the universal employment of behavior analysis tactics.

CURRICULA FOR MENTALLY RETARDED PERSONS

General Considerations

Ideally, what we teach a mentally retarded student should depend on what the student needs. But what does a mentally retarded person need? The spectrum of curricular possibilities is almost unlimited. But since even people of average or above average intelligence cannot learn all there is to learn, common sense tells us that mentally retarded people can learn even less. Although IEPs, teaching materials and equipment, behavior analysis, and various other approaches provide us with a framework for the instructional process, they do not tell us what is to be taught.

There are at least three questions that must be addressed before the curriculum for any student, retarded or nonretarded, can be planned. These are:

1. What skills will the person need to function as an adult?
2. How much time is there to teach the skills?
3. In what sequence should the skills be taught in order to maximize the learning process or, put another way, which skills are prerequisite to other skills?

The first question is most difficult. What exactly does "function" mean? Are there different standards for functioning by a retarded adult vis à vis a nonretarded one? As a matter of fact, there are. As a matter of potential, we cannot be certain because, given the most appropriate education, we do not know the potential of a retarded individual. Most of the

TABLE 11–1   Examples of Areas of Learning in Which Applied Behavior Analysis Has Been Used Successfully with Mentally Retarded Persons

AREA OF LEARNING	REFERENCES
Reading	Brown, Huppler, Pierce, York & Sontag, 1974 Brown & Perlmutter, 1971 Domnie & Brown, 1977
Arithmetic	Allyon, Garber & Pisor, 1976 Borakove & Cuvo, 1976 Broome & Wambold, 1977 Wheeler, Ford, Nietupski, Loomis & Brown, 1980
Language Development and Use	Baer & Guess, 1975 Hobson & Duncan, 1979 Nelson, Peoples, Hay, Johnson & Hay, 1976 Reid & Hurlbut, 1977 Salisbury, Wambold & Walter, 1978
Self-Feeding	Azrin & Armstrong, 1973 Berkowitz, Sherry & Davis, 1971 O'Brien, Bugle & Azrin, 1972
Toileting	Azrin & Foxx, 1971 Azrin, Sneed & Foxx, 1974 Mahoney, Van Wagenen & Meyerson, 1971
Dressing	Azrin, Schaeffer & Wesolowski, 1976 Martin, Kehoe, Bird, Jensen & Darbyshire, 1971
Toothbrushing	Abramson & Wunderlich, 1972 Horner & Keilitz, 1975
Grooming and Bodily Care	Hamilton, Allen, Stephens & Davall, 1969 Teffrey, Martin, Samels & Watson, 1970
Social Skills	Bates, 1980 Gable, Hendrickson & Strain, 1978 Stokes, Baer & Jackson, 1974 Whitman, Mercurio & Caponigri, 1970
Motor Skills	Hill, 1980 Murphy & Doughty, 1977 O'Brien, Azrin & Bugle, 1972
Vocational Skills	Cuvo, Leaf & Borakove, 1978 Gold, 1974; 1976 Katz, Goldberg & Shurka, 1977 Sowers, Rush, Connis & Cummings, 1980

curricular elements for mentally retarded students, however, assume that as adults, they will function as other retarded adults have.

In traditional public school education, the time allowed for a student to learn particular skills is fixed. Since retarded people learn slower than nonretarded persons, the fixed amount of time available for instruction becomes an important issue. What is selected to be taught will have to be what is most critical or functional.

A curriculum should also provide a sequentially appropriate teaching order. One skill or bit of information should be learned in order that it will make other skills easier to learn. Usually we think of the former skills as prerequisites to the latter ones. Often, however, it is not easy to determine what should be a prerequisite to what. Again, because of the time issue, we want to provide our instruction in the most important areas. If a skill is really not a prerequisite and is not functional, it should not be taught.

In the following sections, we will consider curricular elements for mildly, moderately, severely, and profoundly retarded students. One thing to remember is that classification does not necessarily dictate what a person can learn to do. Nor does it always imply what a person should learn to do. Learning goals for a student in one category may often be suitable as goals for another student in a tangential category.

Curriculum for Mildly Retarded Students

General curriculum content. Education for mildly retarded students has traditionally included learning goals and objectives designed to prepare the person for independent living as an adult. To reach this state of development, comprehensive curriculum plans have been established that include functional content areas with an emphasis on specific learning areas varying from the preschool years through the secondary school years. Basic readiness and practical academics tend to be heavily emphasized during the preschool and elementary years as do communication, oral language, and cognitive development. As the individual gets older, greater emphasis is placed on prevocational and vocational development, and housekeeping. Throughout the school years a suitable amount of time is allotted to socialization, family living, self-care, recreation, and personality development.

While the relative weight of each area changes from year to year, each curricular area is included at every level of schooling. However, as the retarded student comes closer to the time of leaving school, traditional academic areas (e.g., reading, arithmetic) decrease in intensity and more critical skills for independent living (e.g., vocational, domestic) increase. This arrangement reflects a concern with the questions presented earlier. It includes skills important to the adult, provides a realistic time framework for developing the skills, and suggests a temporal order for teaching the skills.

Although there is no one standard EMR curriculum, most of those available reflect the elements outlined above (Kolstoe, 1976; Kirk & Johnson, 1951). Nearly every state and many school districts have produced their own curriculum guides. Based on his review of the literature, Kolstoe (1976) recommended the elements listed in Table 11–2 as minimum essentials in programs for EMR students.

TABLE 11–2   Essential Elements of a Curriculum For Educable Mentally Retarded Students

Intellectual characteristics:
1. Academic achievement above the 2.5 grade level in reading, language arts, and arithmetic
2. Thought processes at least at the level of grouping and ordering by more than one dimension, and command of the concept of evaluation
3. Oral language and listening skills sufficient to give and/or follow uncomplicated directions

Personal characteristics:
1. Acceptable habits of cleanliness, grooming, and health
2. Ability to inhibit reactions to stimuli to stem inappropriate outbursts
3. Self-management skills enabling appropriate choices based on probable consequences
4. Acceptable values involving loyalty, honesty, truthfulness, and dependability

Social characteristics:
1. Ability to get along with peers
2. Ability to accept supervision
3. Ability to resist social pressure
4. Cheerfulness
5. Ability to maintain oneself in a living situation

Motor skills:
1. Adequate strength, speed, and coordination for unskilled and semiskilled work

Vocational skills:
1. Persistence or perseverance
2. Ability to work under pressure or distraction
3. Pacing
4. Evaluation of own work
5. Initiative
6. Judgment in the care of materials and property

Home management:
1. Budgeting and buying
2. Maintenance of property and clothes
3. Meal planning and preparation
4. Child care and family living

Vocational/career education. An important direction pursued by many special educators is the training of prevocational and vocational skills. In this pursuit there is evidence of concern for the student as an adult. As we saw, Hungerford was a pioneer in developing the philosophy and practice of providing vocational education. Others have continued promoting the importance of this learning area (Kolstoe & Frey, 1965; Brolin, 1976; Brolin & Brolin, 1979; Kokaska, 1968). Brolin and Brolin (1979) outlined the elements they considered to be important to a model vocational education program. The process begins with an initial assessment and continues through the process of placing the individual on a job, conducting follow-up, and evaluating the program. Kolstoe and Frey's (1965) overview of a work-study program offered a sequential strategy for training. Their plan called for the student to start a prevocational evaluation phase in the ninth grade and then, during the last three years of public school education, to spend a gradually increasing amount of time in on-the-job training (OJT). Real OJT is seen to be critical, as opposed to pencil, paper, and book learning because it provides the individual with concrete rather than abstract experiences. Any academic learning (e.g., reading, Schilit & Caldwell, 1980) is only presented as it relates to vocational activity.

In the last decade or so, the concept of vocational education has been expanded into the concept of career education. The two are not the same. While the former has generally been limited to training actual job skills during the secondary school years, the latter has been seen as a more comprehensive framework that spans the entire school experience (Brolin, 1973; 1977; Brolin, Cegelka, Jackson & Wrobel, 1977; Brolin & D'Alonzo, 1979; Brolin & Kokaska, 1979; Cegelka, 1977; 1979; Sitlington, 1981). Writing the official policy statement on career education for the Council for Exceptional Children, Brolin et al. (1977) stated:

> Career education must not be viewed separately from the total curriculum. Rather, career education permeates the entire school program and even extends beyond it. It should be an infusion throughout the curriculum by knowledgeable teachers who modify the curriculum to integrate career development goals with current subject matter, goals, and content. It should prepare the individual for several life roles which make up an individual's career. These life roles may include an economic role, a community role, a home role, an avocational role, a religious or moral role, and an asthetic role. Thus, career education is concerned with the total person and his/her adjustment for community working and living.

Clinical teaching. The traditional curriculum for mildly retarded students has downplayed academics. Except for those skills considered to be functional or critical to adult living, the three R's have generally not been emphasized by many curriculum planners. There is a logical basis for this position, that is, limited time of the program and cognitive ability of the students (Heller, 1979). Some, however, have challenged this position. They have posited that given the proper techniques, children classified as mildly retarded (or learning disabled or behaviorally disordered) can learn academic skills to a greater extent than is generally believed. Their approach is not based on traditional categorical models, but on behavioral skills, abilities, and deficiencies. The foundation of their approach for educating the mildly handicapped is to diagnose the learning problem and then to remediate it.

Given this common foundation, two divergent approaches with similar intentions have been used. These approaches include the *process or ability model* and the *precision teaching* model. Several important differences exist between the two approaches with the most important being their respective theoretical underpinnings. Raschke and Young (1975) compared the models on several characteristics. Three of the major features are presented in Table 11–3.

Both clinical teaching methods have their proponents, their apostles, and their critics. Despite the differences, the systems have several characteristics in common. They are both individually based; they both attempt to diagnose the student's learning needs and they both attempt to provide instruction based on these needs. In addition, both represent an alternative to the nonacademic orientation of most EMR curricula.

TABLE 11–3   A Comparison of the Process-Ability Model and Precision Teaching Model Used in the Instruction of Mildly Retarded Students

	Process-Ability	Precision Teaching
1. Assumptions about learning	Learning strengths and weaknesses can be identified; are internal cognitive processes.	Learning depends on environmental events.
2. Assumptions about teaching	Appropriate teaching consists of matching the learning style with the appropriate mode of instruction.	Appropriate teaching consists of seeking suitable environmental arrangements.
3. Assessment	The learner's unique learning process must be identified through perceptual-motor and/or psycho-linguistic assessment.	The learner's skill needs must be identified through criterion-referenced assessment.

One of the major criticisms of these approaches is that they are re-medial in nature as opposed to being developmental. That is, they focus attention on specific academic disabilities and do not attend to the broader needs of the student, for example, social and vocational skills. As such they are considered nonfunctional (Cronis, Smith & Forgnone, 1983) and should give way to such a model as presented by Kolstoe (see Table 11–2). Cronis et al. (1983) wrote:

> Regular and remedial curriculums will not address the special needs of these (mentally retarded) persons. The primary, significant service special educators can offer the mildly retarded is a functional curriculum that has meaning, purpose, and value to the learner. (p. 2)

Curriculum for Moderately Retarded Students

General curriculum content.   When programs for moderately mentally retarded students were started in the 1950s, there was little available in-formation or philosophy on what these individual students should be taught. Some of the teaching efforts were influenced by the work of Itard and Seguin. However, many of the teachers had no background in special education and were more influenced by progressive educational theories. Kindergarten activities and group play were major components of their programs (Dunn, 1973).

From this starting point, educational planners developed curricula that corresponded more to the needs of trainable retarded individuals. Many curriculum guides and teaching manuals were developed (e.g., Baumgartner, 1960; Perry, 1960; Rosenzweig & Long, 1960; McDowell, 1964; Frankel, Happ & Smith, 1966; Molloy, 1972; Alpern & Boll, 1971; Bensberg, 1965; D'Amelio, 1971; Stephens, 1971; Waite, 1972; Litton, 1978). As these publications and various state and district plans emerged, a definite educational structure evolved. Major learning areas included: self-help, basic readiness, and independent living; communication, oral language, and cognitive development; socialization and personality devel-opment; and vocational, recreational, and leisure skills. Similar to the plan outlined previously for mildly retarded students, the educational program for the TMR individual re-orients its focus as the years pass. The major change is the decrease in time allotted to more basic life skills and the increase in vocational, recreational, and leisure skills instruction.

Because of their relatively greater cognitive deficiency, TMR stu-dents will necessarily have to focus on more basic, functional skills. This was indicated in a study by Geiger, Brownsmith, and Forgnone (1978). These investigators surveyed 122 teachers of TMR students to determine the relative importance of various curricular components. The teachers were asked to rate the significance of 550 specific skills and twenty-six major skill areas. Tables 11–4, 11–5, and 11–6 report their major find-

TABLE 11–4 25 Most Important Skills as Ranked by Teachers of TMR Students

SKILLS	N[a]	MEAN	SD	SKILLS	N[a]	MEAN	SD
1. Washing face and hands	122	1.04	0.20	15. Blowing nose	122	1.18	0.41
2. Brushing teeth	121	1.09	0.31	16. Comprehending safety words	122	1.18	0.38
3. Urinating (female)	121	1.11	0.34	17. Telling authority you are sick	122	1.20	0.40
4. Urinating (male)	122	1.11	0.34	18. Taking a shower	122	1.21	0.43
5. Wiping mucous from face	122	1.12	0.40	19. Knowing objects to avoid	120	1.21	0.45
6. Defecating	122	1.12	0.35	20. Knowing objects harmful to eyes	121	1.21	0.40
7. Wiping food from face	122	1.15	0.44	21. Knowing objects harmful to ears	121	1.22	0.44
8. Knowing dangerous objects	120	1.15	0.40	22. Knowing objects harmful to nose	121	1.22	0.42
9. Knowing objects harmful if ingested	119	1.15	0.36	23. Drink from a glass	121	1.26	0.53
10. Wiping food from hands	122	1.16	0.43	24. Initiating own name and address (writing)	122	1.26	0.49
11. Picking up, chewing, swallowing, solid food	122	1.16	0.39	25. Naming flashcard safety words	122	1.26	0.56
12. Crossing intersection with light	120	1.17	0.40				
13. Menstrual care	122	1.17	0.38				
14. Crossing intersection without light	119	1.18	0.41				

[a]Some teachers did not rank all of the skills.

From W. L. Geiger, K. Brownsmith and C. Forgnone, "Differential importance of skills for TMR students as perceived by teachers," *Education and Training of the Mentally Retarded,* 1978, 13, 259–264. Reprinted by permission.

TABLE 11-5 25 Least Important Skills as Ranked by Teachers of TMR Students

SKILLS	N[a]	MEAN	SD	SKILLS	N[a]	MEAN	SD
526. Making a tile project	119	2.79	0.87	539. Applying eye make-up	121	2.99	0.93
527. Removing nail polish	115	2.83	0.88	540. Applying rouge	120	3.03	0.91
528. Applying face powder	121	2.83	0.89	541. Diving	121	3.04	0.90
529. Playing ping-pong	122	2.84	0.76	542. Using a duplicating machine	92	3.04	1.03
530. Weaving on upright loom	92	2.84	0.91	543. Doing needlepoint	92	3.04	0.94
531. Making decoupage project	118	2.86	0.82	544. Making a ring	91	3.05	0.88
532. Using typewriter	86	2.86	1.11	545. Knitting	92	3.05	0.94
533. Applying nail polish	120	2.92	0.86	546. Using a Xerox machine	91	3.11	1.07
534. Playing pool	122	2.92	0.80	547. Playing kazoo and xylophone	119	3.13	1.00
535. Embroidering	92	2.93	0.92	548. Making a macrame belt	91	3.13	0.89
536. Applying make-up base	121	2.96	0.86	549. Using a movie projector	92	3.14	1.00
537. Imprinting design on leather	92	2.98	0.92	550. Using a filmloop projector	92	3.15	0.99
538. Crocheting	92	2.98	0.91				

[a]Some teachers did not rank all of the skills.

From W. L. Geiger, K. Brownsmith and C. Forgnone, "Differential importance of skills for TMR students as perceived by teachers," *Education and Training of the Mentally Retarded*, 1978, 13, 259–264. Reprinted by permission.

TABLE 11-6 Skill Areas Listed in Order of Importance (most important to least important) by Teachers of TMR Students

SKILL AREAS	N[a]	MEAN	SD	SKILL AREAS	N[a]	MEAN	SD
Cleanliness	122	1.06	0.27	Counting and numeral identification	122	1.73	0.65
Safety skills	122	1.06	0.27	Maintenance	122	1.73	0.60
Eating	122	1.11	0.34	Recreation—individual	121	1.82	0.69
Health skills	122	1.13	0.34	Recreation—group	121	1.90	0.80
Dressing and undressing	122	1.24	0.46	Writing	122	2.02	0.81
Listening	122	1.31	0.46	Use of shop tools	122	2.02	0.83
Speaking	122	1.39	0.51	Measurement	122	2.10	0.77
Grooming	122	1.40	0.49	Reading	122	2.11	0.88
Sensory motor coordination	120	1.51	0.62	Recreational arts	122	2.13	0.85
Position of body in space	122	1.52	0.60	Personal public service skills	122	2.17	0.86
Housekeeping	122	1.63	0.59	Craft skills	122	2.24	0.86
Homemaking	120	1.66	0.56	Addition and subtraction	121	2.25	0.91
Money concepts	122	1.67	0.68	Clerical service skills	122	2.40	0.91

[a]Some teachers did not rank all of the skill areas.

From W. L. Geiger, K. Brownsmith and C. Forgnone, "Differential importance of skills for TMR students as perceived by teachers," *Education and Training of the Mentally Retarded*, 1978, 13, 259–264. Reprinted by permission.

ings. Reviewing these tables, it is apparent that teachers focus more on skills and skill areas that are critical for daily functioning.

The 550 skills specified by Geiger et al. is typical of more recent curriculum guides for trainable level students. Inspired by accountability and applied behavior analysis, program developers have given consumers many detailed guides that include extensive skill lists and task analyses of important behaviors (e.g., Fredericks, Baldwin, Grove, Riggs, Furey & Moore, 1977; Edgar, Sulzbacher, Swift, Harper, Baker & Alexander, 1975; Cohen, Gross & Haring, 1976; Snell, 1982; Wehman & McLaughlin, 1981). Some of these sequences (e.g., Cohen et al.) extend quite far down the developmental ladder and thus are helpful in planning programs for severely and profoundly retarded as well as moderately retarded students.

Academic and age-appropriate skills.   Recently some writers have suggested an expansion of curriculum for moderately retarded beyond its more traditional framework. Their position is that if we have the technical skills to effectively change behavior, why should there be a limit to the behavior we change? Accompanying this assumption of potential is the recent trend toward normalization and community integration. With these key elements, the stage was set for the creation of new learning plans. Two areas have clearly emerged. These include teaching more academic skills and teaching chronological age-appropriate skills. The ability of moderately retarded students to learn academic skills has traditionally been questioned (Kirk, 1972). Behavior analysis research during the past several years, however, has demonstrated that some of these students can learn to read if the teaching goals and strategies are carefully task analyzed (broken down into component parts) and sequenced (e.g., Brown & Perlmutter, 1971; Bijou, Birnbrauer, Kidder & Taugue, 1966; Hofmeister, 1969; Brown, Hermanson, Klemme, Haubrich & Ora, 1970; Domnie & Brown, 1977; Entriken, York & Brown, 1977; Vandever & Stubbs, 1977). Similar strategies have also been reported to be effective in teaching arithmetic skills (e.g., Brown, Bellamy & Gadberry, 1971; Bellamy & Buttars, 1975; Trace, Cuvo & Criswell, 1977; Borakove & Cuvo, 1976). Thus the academic learning potential for at least some moderately retarded students has been adequately documented.

Even with such encouraging results, however, a heavy emphasis on teaching academics to TMR students has been met with caution if not criticism (Burton, 1974; Hirshoren & Burton, 1979). Hirshoren and Burton (1979) felt that the strict teaching routine used in well-controlled studies would be difficult to implement in an actual classroom. They also noted the extensive amount of time required to teach the skills and questioned the usefulness of the skills by those who learned them. In their critique, they wrote: "the justification for teaching academics to these subjects cannot be based merely upon the fact that they can learn a few words or number facts . . . the price paid in terms of time and the usefulness of these skills by the subjects in their ultimate natural environment is yet to be resolved" (Hirshoren & Burton, 1979, pp. 178–179). Here we clearly see a concern for the questions raised earlier regarding adult needs and allotted learning time.

Teaching academic skills to moderately retarded students is intended to provide them with skills to allow more complete and normal life experiences. Teaching chronological age-appropriate skills has the same purpose. It also challenges many educational approaches used with moderately, severely, or profoundly retarded students. This is because often teachers teach those things that the student's mental age would indicate to be appropriate instead of those more congruent with his or her chronological age. According to Brown and his colleagues (Brown, Branston, Hamre-Nietupski, Pumpian, Certo & Gruenewald, 1979; Brown, Falvey, Vincent, Kaye, Johnson, Ferrara-Parrish & Gruenewald, 1980), this is referred to as a "bottom-up" curriculum. The student is placed in curriculum sequence that follows the normal continuum of development. He or she progresses through the sequence in the "natural" order, that is, going from the bottom up. This means that however long it takes to learn to complete a puzzle, that's how long puzzle-completion will remain an objective. While most children may learn this at the age of four or five years, the retarded person may not achieve it until thirteen or fourteen years of age. However, since such behavior is often considered prerequisite to more complex tasks, the retarded student stays with it until it's learned. Only after a skill on the sequence has been learned may he or she progress forward on the developmental curriculum.

According to Brown and his associates, the problem with the "bottom-up" curriculum is that putting a puzzle together is not normal or functional behavior for an adolescent, at least not the kind of puzzle enjoyed by a four-year-old child. Brown et al. (1979) stated that more CA appropriate functional skills should be taught. They wrote:

> Functional skills . . . refer to the variety of skills that are frequently demanded in natural domestic, vocational, and community environments. Functional skills are not limited to performances which affect the actual survival or physical well-being of an individual; they also include the variety of skills which influence a student's ability to perform as independently and productively as possible in home, school, and community. Nonfunctional skills, by contrast, are those that have an extremely low probability of being required in daily activities. (p. 83)

Examples of age-appropriate functional skills would include using coins to operate a vending machine, walking across bleachers, zipping jeans, and reading signs in public buildings. Parallel examples of nonfunctional skills would be placing pegs in a peg board, walking a balance beam, zipping a zipper board, and reading color words. Obviously the main concern of the age-appropriate philosophy is with adolescents and young adults. Brown, Pumpian, Baumgart, Vandeventer, Ford, Nisbet, Schroeder, and Gruenewald (1981) advocated that certain elements should characterize young retarded persons' curriculum. Besides being age-appropriate, it should be taught in nonschool as well as school environment; should not be based on "normal development" models; and should focus on skills needed for both the immediate and future environment of the individual.

Like academics, age-appropriate curricular suggestions have also been met with some criticism. Burton (1981) has warned that attempting to teach an individual some task for which he or she is not ready could result in frustration for both student and teacher. As you move further down the ladder of intelligence, a greater discrepancy appears between CA and MA. This discrepancy could present difficulties. Burton suggested that it is the teacher's responsibility to decide what is most appropriate for a student at a particular point in time. There is also some evidence that teaching skills in their normative sequence results in more learning than following a non-normative sequence with the students (Umbreit, 1980).

Other innovations. Besides academics and age-appropriate skills, other innovations have recently emerged in curricula for moderately retarded students. Some important trends include early intervention programs (Hayden, McGinness & Dmitriev, 1976; Hayden & Haring, 1976; Bricker, Bricker, Iacino & Dennison, 1976; Bricker & Bricker, 1976; Quick & Campbell, 1977), recreational and leisure skills programs (Schleien, Kierman & Wehman, 1981; Wehman, Schlein & Kierman, 1980); and community living and vocational skills programs (Wehman & J. Hill, 1980; Wehman & M. Hill, 1982; Gold, 1973, 1974, 1976; Katz, Goldberg & Shurka, 1977; Cuvo, Leaf & Borakove, 1978). Early intervention is common with children beginning public school programs when they are three years old. The goal is to foster the development of skills as rapidly as possible in order to inhibit the CA-MA gap.

At the other end of the educational period, greater emphasis is being placed on training for more complete adult living. Task analysis and direct teaching procedures have shown that moderately or even severely retarded persons can learn to complete complex assembly tasks (Gold, 1973, 1974, 1976). Similarly, skills required for at least semi-independent living have recently been taught and learned using operant techniques. Some have included laundry chores (Cuvo, Jacobi & Sipko, 1980); crossing the street (Page, Iwata & Neef, 1976); mending (Cuvo & Cronin, 1979); and driving (Zider & Gold, 1981).

Curriculum for Severely and Profoundly Mentally Retarded Persons

Having developed programs for moderately retarded students, parents, advocates, professionals, and lawmakers in the late '60s and '70s went on to secure educational rights for even the lowest functioning retarded individuals. Even more than for mildly and moderately retarded students, public school education was challenged to redefine its concept of education and once again to dig into its bag of innovations to provide an appropriate education for the severely and profoundly retarded (Luckey & Addison, 1974; Sontag, Burke & York, 1973). Roos (1971) stated a new definition of education:

> Education is the process whereby an individual is helped to develop new behavior or to apply existing behavior so as to equip him to cope more effectively with his total environment. It should be clear, therefore, that when we speak of education we do not limit ourselves to the so-called academics. We certainly include the development of basic self-help skills. Indeed, we include those very complex bits of behavior which help to define an individual as human. We include such skills as toilet training, dressing, communicating, and so on. (p. 2)

Because of the overall low level of functioning and deficient learning ability of these students, carefully planned learning goals and teaching methods were required to improve their behavioral repertoires. Curriculum guides were developed that itemized small learning targets and offered step-by-step approaches. Billingsley and Neafsey (1978) reviewed twenty-six of these guides. A common feature of most of them was the quantitative measurement of student learning across different training programs. The practice of directly measuring human behavior was a product of applied behavior analysis. Clearly, applied behavior analysis has been the backbone of most of the training efforts with severely and profoundly retarded persons. However, a number of researchers have also suggested Piagetian or sensory stimulation training as being useful (e.g., Kahn, 1979; Stephens, 1977).

Many of the curricular goals discussed in the previous section for moderate individuals are appropriate for persons who are severely or profoundly retarded. This is because some of these people are functioning adequately enough to work toward these goals. Other persons, however, are not developmentally at a level to perform even some rudimentary skills. Some are so extremely mentally, physically, and sensorily impaired that awareness of environmental stimuli is an important goal. For these individuals, education means improving their basic life-functioning systems so that person-person and person-environment interactions become possible. This must often precede even basic self-help skills or language development. Tawney, Knapp, O'Reilly, and Pratt (1979) targeted some of the behaviors that must be systematically taught to these individuals. Examples include:

Responding to social interaction
Attending to voice
Making sounds
Focusing attention
Attending to sounds
Reaching for objects
Grasping objects
Controlling head movements
Sitting
Chewing

Although legislation requiring public schools to teach profoundly retarded persons is now several years old, we still have much to learn about both the process and the outcome. Some professionals (e.g., Ellis, 1979; Bailey, 1981) have questioned the probability of successfully training many profoundly retarded persons to develop functional behaviors. Recently Stainback and Stainback (1983) reviewed the available literature on the educability of profoundly retarded individuals. Several studies were reported that supported the position that these persons were capable of learning. Still they were cautious in their conclusion:

Obviously, it would be inappropriate to interpret the findings of this research review as indicating that all profoundly retarded persons can learn every behavior taught to any individual or small group of profoundly retarded persons. (p. 97)

All of the answers and even many of the questions about teaching the severely and profoundly retarded have yet to surface. Teachers and other service personnel must deal with problems that were hardly considered fifteen or twenty years ago. Many of these students will have serious physical disabilities and will require extensive medication. The use of prosthetic devices is common. Support services of different sorts, such as physical and occupational therapy, special transportation, modified physical plants, manual or augmented communication are but a few of the extra ingredients necessary to comprise an educational program for many profoundly retarded persons. We should learn a great deal in the next several years about the most viable curricular goals and the best way to reach them.

CONCLUSION

Teaching mentally retarded persons is a complex task. In this chapter, we have touched on a few of the issues related to what to teach and how to teach. If little else, the reader should realize the intricacies of both domains. Deciding what to teach calls upon judgments about life potential and needs. Decisions must be made that require responsible thought and action. Deciding how to teach presents another kind of problem. Available methods and instructional devices call for an individual with technical sophistication adequate for the selection and implementation of the best set of tactics. The methods and the materials available to assist the teacher are overwhelming, but they are important and must be thoroughly studied. It is of necessity a life-long study.

STUDY QUESTIONS

1. Describe the similarities of the approaches used by Itard, Seguin, and Montessori to teach mentally retarded individuals.
2. How did the work of Decroly and Descoeudres differ significantly from Itard, Seguin, and Montessori?
3. What is the "units of instruction" approach?
4. What were the components of "occupational education"? In what way were academic skills incorporated into this curriculum?
5. What are the necessary components of individual educational plans? Who must be involved in its preparation?
6. What are some commonly used instructional materials in programs for mentally retarded students? What more recent advances have occurred?
7. What are the basic components of applied behavior analysis? In what areas of learning by retarded individuals has behavior analysis been used?
8. What factors must be considered in the development of curricula for mentally retarded students?
9. Outline the major elements of a curriculum for mildly mentally retarded students. How does career and vocational education fit within this framework?
10. Briefly describe the clinical teaching models used with mildly retarded individuals. Why have some criticized these models?
11. What are the major elements of a curriculum for moderately mentally retarded students?
12. What is meant by an age-appropriate curriculum? What has influenced some writers to suggest this approach?
13. What major problems currently exist in developing programs for severely retarded individuals?

12

Adult Abilities, Needs, and Services

THE DIFFICULTIES OF ADULTHOOD

When a child grows into adulthood, life changes. After years of the dependence that is more or less allowed for all children, the person enters a time of life when more independence is expected. For most nonretarded persons, this independence is cautiously welcomed. Proceeding through adolescence and into young adulthood, we seek the freedom to make our own choices and live our own lives. Still, we question some of our decisions, are concerned with many of our responsibilities, and occasionally look back to our elders for the guidance and advice that is no longer provided as a matter of course.

The mentally retarded adult is in many ways similar to other adults. Although reduced mental and behavioral abilities may decrease the opportunity for total independence, there is indeed a natural inclination toward a life style similar to nonretarded adults. Bostwick and Foss (1981) asked a group of mentally retarded adults (n = 58) to list their problems and a second group (n = 101) to rank order them. Table 12—1 presents these concerns under the areas of employment, community living, and social relations. As can be seen, these young adults (mean age, 20 years) had worries similar to many nonretarded persons their age. They worried about finding a job, how others treat them, and finding and keeping friends. In short, they worried about being considered adequate adults.

The purposes of this chapter are to discuss how retarded individuals succeed in attempting to fulfill the status of an adult and to examine variables related to their achievement. The chapter is divided into three major sections: adult adjustment of mildly retarded persons; adult adjustment of moderately and severely retarded persons; and sheltered workshops, activity centers, and competitive employment. The reader is referred to Chapters 7 and 10 for additional discussions on social characteristics and community living. Additionally, for the interested reader reviews of relevant literature have been written by Brolin (1976), Brolin and Kokaska (1979), Gold (1972), Goldstein (1964), Kokaska (1968), Kolstoe and Frey (1965), and Wolfensberger (1967).

ADJUSTMENT OF MILDLY RETARDED ADULTS

Over the years, different researchers have investigated the functioning of mentally retarded persons as adults. Most of the studies have focused on individuals classified as mildly mentally retarded. Goldstein (1964) reviewed several studies conducted in the early part of this century and continuing through World War II. Most of these investigated the status of previously institutionalized "high grade" (educable and borderline) re-

TABLE 12–1   Problems Encountered by Mentally Retarded Adults

DOMAIN	PROBLEM	RANK
Employment	Finding a job	1
	Getting to work on time	2
	Getting along with boss	3
	Remembering appointments	4
	Interviewing for a job	5
	Working fast enough	6
Community Living	Being treated differently	1
	Getting around to places	2
	Getting help from community	3
	Managing money	4
	Getting along with bad neighbor	5
	Making change with money	6
Social Relationships	Finding or keeping friends	1
	Talking in a group of people	2
	Getting parents to allow more freedom in making decisions	3
	Getting along with opposite sex	4
	Getting along as a family	5
	Getting along with police	6

From D. H. Bostwick and G. Foss "Obtaining consumer input: two strategies for identifying and ranking the problems of mentally retarded young adults," *Education and Training of the Mentally Retarded*, 1981, *16*, 207-212. Reprinted by permission.

tarded persons. The overall conclusion was that generally their adjustment was favorable. Goldstein (1964) summarized:

> Only one broad generalization may be derived . . . the probability is that the majority of high grade mentally retarded inmates of public institutions will make a relatively successful adjustment in their community when training, selection, placement, and supervision are all at an optimum. (p. 229)

Goldstein also found that among individuals at this level, no relationship existed between IQ or length of institutionalization and adult adjustment.

While some researchers were investigating previously institutionalized persons, others were analyzing the success of educable and borderline persons who had been enrolled in public school programs. Many of these studies compared mentally retarded adults to nonretarded adults. About the retarded adults, Goldstein (1964) drew the following conclusions:

1. Their overall adjustment is acceptable.
2. Their employability decreases during times of economic difficulty.

3. Their adjustment can be affected by the adequacy of community services.
4. Their employment is usually in semiskilled and unskilled jobs.

He also noted that various social and peripheral problems had deleterious effects on employment. Some of the more common difficulties were being punctual, dressing appropriately, getting to and from work, using a time clock, and giving immature responses. Even with such problems, Goldstein's conclusion was optimistic.

In a later review, Kokaska (1968) continued where Goldstein (1964) left off. He reviewed EMR adult adjustment studies written between 1948 and 1964. Eleven studies were thoroughly and systematically analyzed by Kokaska. His analysis indicated the following:

1. All subjects were former members of special classes with IQs ranging from 50 to 85.
2. Unemployment ranged from a low of 8.8% to a high of 23.3%. ("Employed" and "unemployed" were not consistently defined across studies.)
3. The percent of persons employed in different areas varied a great deal. From the studies reviewed the ranges were:

Skilled:	2.3% to 32.6%
Semiskilled:	8.3% to 54.9%
Unskilled:	2.2% to 75%
Service:	4.5% to 42.9%
Clerical:	4.3% to 30%

Overall, most were employed in unskilled areas although a number had moved up to semiskilled or skilled employment.

This last finding, that the mildly retarded adult could progress upward in job placement, was a favorable trend that had not been noted by Goldstein. Kokaska (1968) concluded:

The retarded individual has the capability to move through a number of work situations and in many instances increase his work skills when given the proper educational background and vocational training. (p. 376)

The early studies reviewed by Kokaska and Goldstein were generally interpreted as being positive. They indicated a favorable probability for employment and adjustment of most mildly retarded adults. Since these studies and reviews, a number of additional studies have appeared. In the following sections, some of the major findings of EMR adult adjustment studies reported since 1960 are presented.

Employment status

The reported percent of mildly retarded adults competitively employed or unemployed has varied greatly. Part of this variation is due to how "employment" had been defined by the researchers. For example, one of the lowest rates of unemployment (7.9%) was reported by Crain (1980). However, she based this figure on those adults considered to be in the "civilian labor force." (Membership in this group excludes those who are institutionalized, retired, work in their own homes, are in school, are ill, or who are voluntarily idle.) Thus the 7.9% unemployment rate she reported was based on only 68% of her sample (n = 130) who were considered to be in the civilian labor force. Similarly, Dinger (1961) reported that 83% of his follow-up sample (n = 333) were employed but his definition of employment included those who were in school and who were housewives along with those who had jobs. Actually, only 59% of the group fell in the latter group. Kidd, Cross, and Higginbotham (1967) also calculated a relatively high degree of employment (81%). Their definition of employment included those with full-time jobs along with housewives, those in the military, those with part-time jobs, and those in sheltered workshops.

Table 12—2 summarizes employment and/or unemployment levels reported in nine studies conducted between 1960 and 1980. The levels are reported according to the researchers' definitions of employment/unemployment. From the figures reported in Table 12—2, two points can be surmised. First, the majority of mildly retarded adults are able to secure employment although a large number of them are unemployed. Second, as earlier reviewers have noted, there is a lack of consistency in how figures are reported. Some researchers give specific figures, others do not. Some report levels of employment; some levels of unemployment. One conclusion is extremely clear. With the exception of Crain's (1980) analysis, all studies indicate much higher levels of unemployment for EMR adults than in society at large. An important question is: Why? What variables tend to affect the employability of these individuals?

Variables Related to Job Success of Mildly Retarded Adults

A few researchers have investigated different variables related to successful employment. Generally these variables fall into two categories: personalogical variables (those characterizing the individual) and treatment variables (those that characterize the education, training, or service provided to the individual).

One of the most thorough investigations of personalogical variables was conducted by Kolstoe (1961). He compared forty-one successfully employed mildly retarded adults and forty-one who were unemployed.

TABLE 12–2 Employment/Unemployment Levels Reported for Mildly Retarded Adults

SOURCE	TOTAL NUMBER	EMPLOYMENT/ UNEMPLOYMENT
Peterson & Smith (1960)	45	"Slightly over half" of the adults were employed.
Dinger (1961)	333	83% were employed; 12.9% were unemployed; 5% were deceased or could not be located
McFall (1966)	50	30% were employed at the time of the study; 26% had never been employed
Kidd et al. (1967)	209	81% were employed
Tobias (1970)	383	80% of the males were employed; 72% of the females were employed at the time of the study. Twenty percent had never been employed.
Chaffin et al. (1971)	30 from a work-study group; 23 from a comparison group	83% of the WS group was employed; 75% of the comparison group was employed
Brolin et al. (1975)	80	44% were unemployed
Redding (1979)	20 from a work-study group; 20 from a comparison group	More than 70% of both groups were employed
Crain (1980)	130	68% in the civilian labor force; 7.9% of this group unemployed

Thirty-six variables were compared. His most important findings indicated the following:

1. IQ scores in the mild to borderline range (50–90) made no difference in employability. This included Full Scale, Verbal, and Performance IQ's.
2. Chronological ages between eighteen and forty years made no difference in employability.
3. Academic ability levels were not related to employability.
4. Better physical appearance, general health, and motor coordination were most often associated with employment. Additionally, hearing aids and other visual signs of handicap reduced chances for employment.

5. Cheerfulness, cooperation, respect, minding one's own business, being on time, and showing initiative were related to employability.
6. The ability to do tasks involving assembly, sorting, manipulation, packaging, and using hand tools were positively related to employability.
7. Understanding work and producing quality work were related to employability.

Quite similar findings have been found by others. Brolin et al. (1975), Chaffin et al. (1971), Dinger (1961), and Kidd et al. (1967) all found no relationship between the mildly retarded adult's IQ and employment capability. Like Kolstoe, Brolin (1972) found that work habits, physical capacity, general health, and manual skills were related to achieving one's vocational potential.

In answer to our question, then, we can see that personal variables that are most characteristic of mild mental retardation (e.g., IQ, academic ability) are not necessarily interfering with their employment potential. On the other hand, what might be referred to as adaptive or social behaviors tend to bear on their success. And, of course, we cannot ignore the biases of society noted by Kolstoe (1961) when he found that more visibly handicapped persons were least often successful at being employed. In the years since Kolstoe's study, we may be hopeful that employers have become more accepting of differences.

While professionals may have little control over the thinking of society and employers, they have made various attempts to improve the prospect of employment by improving the skills and abilities of future employees. One effort has been to provide the mildly retarded individuals with work skills as a part of their public school experience. This is often done through work-study programs (Brolin, 1976; Kolstoe & Frey, 1965). Work-study programs are geared to prepare the individual for competitive employment. Students spend a significant portion of their school hours engaged in on-the-job training, generally in a community setting. This educational strategy can be contrasted with a more traditional academic approach in which the student remains in the classroom.

Chaffin et al. (1971), Brolin et al. (1975), and Redding (1979) followed up adults who had been enrolled in work-study programs and compared their later status to similar adults who had been in more traditional programs. Their findings were not entirely conclusive but were generally in favor of the work-study programs. Chaffin and his colleagues found that 83% of their work-study sample were employed at the time of follow-up as compared to 75% of the nonwork-study students. More dramatic, however, were the differences in salaries. While the work-study group earned over $90 per week, the nonwork-study group received an average of only $63 per week. Brolin et al. (1975) found similar results. Although 44% of their total sample were unemployed, the former work-study participants more often had an average or better level of adjustment (29%) than did those who had been in a traditional academic program (17%). Likewise, Redding (1979) reported his work-study group to be employed more often, in more skilled occupations, earning more money, and more often being totally self-supporting.

Another employment-oriented service often offered to handicapped persons, including the mentally retarded, is vocational rehabilation. Working with young adults who have difficulty securing jobs, this program provides a variety of services to help the person become successfully employed. These services may include counseling, various forms of therapy, or arranging for direct instructional activities. In addition, assistance may be provided in finding the right job for a person.

Brolin (1972) conducted a study to determine if "adequate" vocational rehabilitation services resulted in better vocational adjustment than "inadequate" services. Studying groups of EMR adults considered to differ in this regard, Brolin found that those who received more adequate services were more likely to reach their potential level of employment. Still he found many that had received adequate services but were not employed or not employed to their potential. Brolin concluded that vocational rehabilitation services can certainly improve the employability of individuals, but much remains to be done before the system will be totally successful.

It is apparent that training and rehabilitation services can improve the chance of successful employment for mildly retarded adults, although not always to the degree desirable. These treatment variables must certainly be considered when we judge the employment status of the mildly retarded. In the majority of the studies reviewed here and by Kokaska (1968) and Goldstein (1964), no mention was made of how well prepared the adults were for employment. If we are to do justice in judging the success of these individuals, we must also judge the preparation they received before entering the world of work. There seems to be little knowledge in this area.

Types of Jobs Held by Mildly Retarded Adults

Mildly retarded adults have been hired to do a number of different jobs. Most of these have been in the area of service work; domestic worker, hospital worker, dishwasher, janitor; or unskilled work; laborer, gardener, gas station attendant (Dinger, 1961; McFall, 1966; Tobias, 1970; Brolin ct al., 1975; Crain, 1980). Some researchers have found mildly retarded adults (albeit a fewer number) employed in more skilled jobs; clerical work or sales, heavy equipment operator, mechanics (McFall, 1966; Kidd et al., 1967; Tobias, 1970; Brolin et al., 1975; Crain, 1980). Brolin and his colleagues (1975) listed the various jobs held by the adults in their study. Eighty individuals had held 136 jobs since leaving high school. These are listed in Table 12–3. As can be seen, 50% of the jobs held were in the service occupations. Other areas employed considerably fewer individuals. The distribution is probably a fair indication of areas of employment of most mildly retarded adults.

Wages of Mildly Retarded Adults

Given the types of jobs held by mildly retarded adults, one might expect that their income would be below average. In fact, most studies indicate this to be true. After several years of inflation, it would be difficult to accurately interpret the relative amount of income reported in many of the studies, but of those that compared the wages of their retarded subjects with nonretarded workers', the former's were always lower (Peterson & Smith, 1960; Kidd et al., 1967). A major exception was reported by Crain (1980). She reported that her subjects had annual incomes ranging from $2,340 to $23,000 with a median income of $7,280. This median was noted to be $1,000 above the poverty level with only one subject having an annual income below the poverty level. She also noted that the median income compared rather favorably with the median income in the city of St. Louis, Missouri ($7,390) although it was considerably lower than the St. Louis County median income ($12,392).

Conclusion

The overall adjustment of mildly retarded adults in regard to employment status, types of jobs held, wages, and financial status is below the norm. Any optimism established in early studies should be tempered in light of the majority of recent findings. With the exception of some (e.g., Crain, Dinger), the general findings indicate higher unemployment than in the general population, a fairly restricted range of jobs, and lower wages. A major hope for the future seems to be the more widespread development of work-study programs. Some studies have reported important positive aspects of this approach. Special education for secondary-level mildly retarded persons must clearly have as its goal the functional preparation of individuals for competitive employment and successful living.

ADJUSTMENT OF MODERATELY AND SEVERELY RETARDED ADULTS

In comparison to studies of mildly retarded adults, there are relatively few that document the adult adjustment of moderately and severely mentally retarded adults. (There are virtually none on profoundly retarded

TABLE 12—3   Types of Jobs Held by Mildly Retarded Adults

CLASSIFICATION	JOB TITLE	N		PERCENT
Professional Managerial	Assistant manager (Take-out Restaurant)	1	1	1
Clerical and Sales	Inventory, Stock	4		
	Phone solicitor	3		
	Coupon sorting	3		
	Packaging	2		
	File clerk	2		
	Other	2	16	12
Service Occupations	Dishwasher, Kitchen help	20		
	Janitorial work	13		
	Busboy , Waitress	11		
	Nurse aide	8		
	Shoe repair	4		
	Laundry work	4		
	Maid	4		
	Nursery school aide	2		
	Presser	2		
	Other	2	70	50
Farming, Fishing & Related Occupations	Cemetery work	2		
	Greenhouse work	1	3	2
Processing	Rag cutter	3		
	Baker	1		
	Bottle washer	1		
	Laborer (cement industry)	1	6	4
Machine Trades Occupations	Mechanic's aide	3		
	Machine work	2		
	Bindery work	1	6	4
Bench work Occupations	Bag liner	2		
	Assembly line	2		
	Piece work–clothing	1		
	Bag trimmer	1	6	4
Structural Occupations	Shop work–assembly	4		
	Maintenance	4		
	Construction–Carpentry	3		
	Heavy equipment operator	1	12	9
Miscellaneous	Grocery carry-out	5		
	Gas station attendant	4		
	Car washer	4		
	Other	3	16	12
Total		136	136	100

From D. Brolin, R. Durand, K. Kromer and P. Muller "Post-school adjustment of educable retarded students," *Education and Training of the Mentally Retarded*, 1975, *10*, 144-149. Reprinted by permission.

adults. This is probably due to the recentness of these individuals being served in public school programs.)

The few studies that exist provide a great deal of information about how these persons fare in later years. Several of these studies examine how previously institutionalized individuals adapt to community living. A few of these are discussed in Chapter 10 and will not be reiterated in this section. Other studies (Delp and Lorenz, 1953; Saenger, 1957; Stanfield, 1973; and Tisdall, 1958) have reported follow-up results of individuals previously enrolled in public school classes for the trainable mentally retarded. These studies have looked at a number of marks of adjustment including family involvement, community mobility, social activity, and vocational activity.

Family Involvement

Follow-up of most moderately and severely retarded adults found them living with their parents and families. In their own home settings, their adjustment was judged favorably. They were often able to take care of their personal needs, had responsibilities for their own duties, and often contributed to the overall maintenance of the home. Saenger (1957), in his study of 520 adults who had been enrolled in special programs in New York City, reported that 75% of the parents interviewed felt their son or daughter was "easy to get along with." Twenty percent had a "major responsibility" around the house and 40% took care of their personal belongings, cleaned their rooms, made their beds, and so on. Stanfield, in a later study (1973), stated that 94% of his adult subjects (n = 120) could care for their personal needs and 90% had specific chores. Generally, parents felt that the public school training programs for their children had been beneficial in helping them attain some independence in the family structure.

While family relations between the retarded adult and other family members has usually been considered good, participation in family interactions has been restricted. Only 25% of Saenger's subjects played or talked much with family members. Stanfield's finding along this line was similar. Most of those living at home seem to spend much of their time engaged in solitary activity such as looking at magazines, listening to the radio, or watching TV.

The general picture of the adult moderately or severely retarded person living in the home is one that is both positive and negative. The ability to perform important daily living skills allows the individual some independence and thus reduces dependence on the parents. Clearly this is positive because it increases the probability that the retarded individual will be able to remain in the home. On the other hand, social interactions within the family are not always strong. While family relations are good, they are not ideal. Many parents fear leaving their adult children alone (Stanfield, 1973). Certainly a need for continuous responsibility would infringe upon more harmonious social relations. The fact that many of these adults lack self-confidence and personal independence (Saenger, 1957; Stanfield, 1973), does little to ease the problem. Given one goal, most parents would probably opt for more self-reliance.

Community Mobility

Most social activities of moderately and severely retarded adults tend to be limited to their home life or perhaps their immediate neighborhood (Delp and Lorenz, 1953; Saenger, 1957; Stanfield, 1973). Although 78% of the subjects researched by Saenger went out of their homes occasionally, the majority went out with family escorts. Only about one-third could leave the neighborhood or use public transportation. Stanfield's figures were similar. Sixty percent of his subjects were mobile in their own neighborhood but only 10% ventured into the broader community. Almost half (40%) never went unescorted beyond their front yard. When more distant excursions did occur, they often consisted of trips to the neighborhood supermarket or shopping center.

Several factors may account for the lack of greater community mobility. One may be fear by the parents on behalf of their dependent's safety. Another may be the lack of mobility experience on the adult's part. This could have a two-fold limiting effect. First, it could inhibit community travel because the person has not learned how to travel. Second, because of a lack of experience, the individual may never have been reinforced for traveling and thus not be motivated to do so.

This limitation may not be as great today as it was several years ago. Community mobility using public transportation is now considered to be an appropriate instructional goal for retarded students (Sowers, Rusch & Hudson, 1979). Given this important skill, movement through the larger community may become a greater possibility.

Social Activities[1]

Given a restricted degree of transportation, a restricted degree of social interaction (beyond the family) can be expected. Only about half of Saenger's subjects and two-thirds of Stanfield's subjects had friends. Most often these friends shared membership in the individual's sheltered workshop, activity center, or recreation program. Few retarded adults seem to have friends that they visited outside of these formally structured programs. Twenty-three percent of Stanfield's subjects did. However, as

[1]For more information on this topic, see Chapter 7.

he noted " . . . for the majority . . . there was virtually no social or recreational life apart from that with the immediate family" (p. 551).

Vocational Activity

For several reasons, vocational activity for moderately and severely retarded persons is an important goal. It is consistent with the values of our culture. Working persons are thought to be happier than those unemployed. Work provides an individual with adult status and society has more positive attitudes toward workers. The family of the adult retarded worker may be better adjusted because out-of-home activities are available. The worker may be able to earn some amount of income and thus be less of an economic burden. Additionally, the working retarded person may gain a degree of freedom through the attainment of personal material benefits. Work can also serve a therapeutic function by increasing positive social behavior and decreasing maladaptive behavior (Wolfensberger, 1967).

In follow-up studies of TMR adults, relatively few were engaged in competitive employment. Ten of the eighty-four adults in Delp and Lorenz's (1953) study had been gainfully employed. Twenty-seven percent of Saenger's 520 subjects were working for pay at the time of his study. In Tisdall's (1958) study, eight of forty-eight were employed, seven in a sheltered workshop. Stanfield (1973) reported forty-eight of his 120 subjects were employed in sheltered workshops with 80% of these earning less than $10 per week.

Retarded adults who were found to be engaged in competitive employment often had their jobs because of the assistance of parents, relatives, or friends. In Stanfield's study, two individuals were employed in family businesses, both working for their father. Most of Saenger's subjects who were employed either worked in a business owned by a parent or relative or worked where a parent or relative was employed. Noteworthy, however, was the fact that 42% of those working found their own jobs (Saenger, 1957).

Moderately retarded adults engaged in competitive employment are usually those who are higher functioning. Saenger's working subjects had better speech habits, could take care of their bodily needs, and had appropriate personal characteristics; that is, they were alert, responsive, and confident. In contrast, those who were lower functioning and had visibly apparent handicaps were more often unemployed.

During the time that these follow-up studies were conducted, competitive employment was not often a realized goal. While more recent studies have shown that this should not be accepted as an unmodifiable condition (Wehman & J Hill, 1981; Wehman, Hill, Goodall, Cleveland, Brooke & Pentecost, 1982), typical employment for moderately and severely retarded adults has been in sheltered workshops. These settings employ solely mentally retarded and/or other handicapped adults who are believed not to be capable of working on the "outside." Forty percent of Stanfield's graduates were employed in sheltered workshops. More recently, Whitehead (1979) estimated that over 200,000 severely handicapped adults were working in sheltered settings. This figure can expect to increase as more community living replaces institutional living.

Conclusion

In comparison to adult follow-up studies of mildly retarded persons, there are relatively few such studies for the moderately and severely retarded. The studies that have appeared tend to reveal certain life styles about a number of these individuals. They often live with their parents into their adult years, have restricted mobility and social interaction, and are employed in noncompetitive (sheltered workshop) settings. This should not lead one to conclude that these limits are universal. Certainly some moderately and severely retarded adults can fare much better. The variability in their success as adults may well be tied to the services they receive as much as to their cognitive ability. It is thus important that these services continue to be expanded and improved in all ways possible.

SHELTERED WORKSHOPS, ACTIVITY CENTERS, AND COMPETITIVE EMPLOYMENT

As stated earlier, vocational activity by mentally retarded adults is a desirable goal for several reasons. Perhaps the most important reason is because it is normally what adult people do. In our adherence to the normalization principle, our efforts lead us toward promoting normal lifestyles. It would therefore not be satisfactory for us to simply provide for the basic needs of the retarded adult. Instead, we should attempt whenever possible to assist the individual in achieving meaningful life experiences. Certainly one of the most important experiences is that of productive work activity.

Mentally retarded adults who work can be divided into two groups: those competitively employed and those employed in sheltered workshops. A third group includes those who do not work. They are sometimes provided services through adult activity centers. These are also referred to as developmental centers, day treatment programs, work activity centers, or adult day programs (Bellamy, Sheehan, Horner & Boles, 1980).

Traditionally, these three levels of engagement have roughly accommodated retarded individuals as a function of their intelligence level.

Most mildly retarded and fewer moderately or severely retarded persons were thought to be capable of competitive employment. Sheltered employment was designed for those not thought capable of performing regular employment duties. Adult activity centers were developed for adults not capable of even sheltered work. This would generally include some severely and most profoundly retarded persons residing in the community. Unfortunately, in several instances, these facilities would also include higher level adults who probably would have been able to perform some meaningful work.

In recent years, inspired by the normalization principle and armed with the skills of applied behavior analysis, many traditional assumptions and approaches have been challenged. Various experimental evidence has demonstrated that individuals with moderate, severe, or profound levels of retardation can learn the work skills necessary for jobs at relatively high levels (Bellamy et al., 1980; Bellamy, Peterson & Close, 1975; Gold, 1972; Pomerantz & Marholin, 1977; Wehman et al., 1982; Wehman & J. Hill, 1981; Wolfensberger, 1967). Some persons previously restricted to adult activity centers are functioning adequately in sheltered workshops. Others have been taken from sheltered workshops and become more gainfully employed in competitive jobs.

Progress such as this indicates that more work potential is available than has traditionally been thought. The nature of this progress is worthy of our attention. We will examine these recent trends and how they are affecting traditional practices. In order, we will look at adult activity centers, sheltered workshops, and competitive employment.

Adult Activity Centers

Adult activity centers are generally considered a primary community service for severely and profoundly retarded adults. Their main function is to provide day care for individuals not capable of even sheltered work skills. Often placement in an activity center is sought by parents after their children are too old for public school services. In other instances, persons who move into the community from public residential institutions are placed in activity centers for a portion of the day when they are not maintained in their community residential facility. Since the deinstitutionalization movement began, many new activity centers have appeared.

Bellamy and his colleagues (1980) conducted a national survey of adult centers, described the programs, and expressed some concerns about them. Based on responses from forty-nine states, the researchers found that approximately 2,000 centers were serving 105,500 individuals. Their self-described goals consisted of maximizing individual development, developing basic skills, providing respite care for parents and serving as a "first step" in a continuum of services. No paid work was included and only a minor emphasis was placed on the development of work skills.

Bellamy et al. (1980) concluded that the activity centers represented "indefinite placements for many severely handicapped individuals" (p. 312). They were concerned about the lack of true work opportunities and the funding system that tended to disallow these opportunities. Much of the funding for adult activity centers came from Title XIX (Medicaid) and Title XX (Social Services) funds and not from vocational rehabilitation agencies. Such funding practices tended to de-emphasize the need for productivity and, according to the authors, reflected a "welfare approach to services" (Bellamy et al., 1980).

Even though shortcomings such as these are undesirable, the need for basic service programs for many severely and profoundly retarded persons is apparent. This will become even more true as deinstitutionalization proceeds. Unfortunately, there may not be enough programs available; and of those that exist, many limit their clientele. Bellamy and his coworkers noted that many programs had restrictions on their number of admissions and sometimes were not able to serve all who had a need. In another study, Lynch and Gerber (1980) reported that in one large midwestern state, 68% of the activity centers surveyed would never accept individuals who were incontinent while most of the others would accept them only "some of the time."

Considering the need of many severely and profoundly retarded adults, limited access to activity centers must be reversed. Furthermore, consideration must be given to more work activities and moving capable individuals up the continuum to at least sheltered employment. A great deal of time in activity centers is devoted to arts and crafts as well as daily living skills (Lynch & Gerber, 1980). Wolfensberger (1967) suggested several years ago that if an individual is capable of arts and crafts and self-help skills, he or she is capable of at least sheltered employment.

Sheltered Workshops

Sheltered workshops (sometimes called rehabilitation workshops) generally have two goals. One, as we have already seen, is to provide employment for handicapped individuals. While most of these individuals are mentally retarded, persons with cerebral palsy, epilepsy, physical disabilities, psychiatric disorders, or other handicaps may also be employed in sheltered workshops. Many sheltered workshops will primarily serve only one disability area; for example, the mentally retarded.

The second goal of sheltered workshops is to provide vocational training in order to prepare persons for later competitive employment. Some sheltered workshops have this as their exclusive goal. Others do this and simultaneously provide permanent employment for some persons.

As we saw in the follow-up studies reviewed earlier, many moderately and some severely retarded special school graduates are employed in sheltered workshops. Previously institutionalized adults will also often be engaged in sheltered employment. Workshops are generally placed in communities although some will be operated by and in large institutions. The community placement is, of course, more desirable.

Sheltered workshops are essentially small, self-contained businesses operated by private organizations (such as Associations for Retarded Citizens) or state agencies. If private agencies operate them, they will generally receive supplementary funds from state or federal programs. The reason for this is that the workshops operate at a loss.

The workshop will usually employ a director or administrator, evaluators, work supervisors, counselors, a work procurement specialist, a job-placement specialist, and trainers (Brolin, 1976). The work performed often consists of subcontracts from community businesses or industry. These subcontracts are usually piecework jobs that the business does not want to be bothered with or can have more cheaply produced by the sheltered workshop. The nature of the work may range from painting soft drink cases to assembling electronic circuit boards, although they are usually quite simple tasks. Besides subcontracts, many sheltered workshops will have one or more ongoing vocational projects such as agricultural production. This will provide a steady source of work and income when subcontracts are not available. Ideally, subcontracts and other work should change often enough to provide the clients with new skills but should not change so dramatically as to preclude the use of learned skills (Pomerantz & Marholin, 1977; Wolfensberger, 1967).

The employees in sheltered workshops are paid for their work but the pay is usually only a fraction of the minimum wage. In most cases, paychecks are based on ability, with more productive workers receiving more money than slower or less productive individuals. Unfortunately, some retarded adults do not realize an association exists between their production rate and income. In one study, when this association was clarified by paying the workers immediately for their work, productivity increased substantially (Martin & Morris, 1980).

In recent years, many writers have voiced concerns about the traditional operation of sheltered workshops. In his analysis, Whitehead (1979) suggested procedures to increase productivity. His first suggestion was for sheltered workshops to seek better contracts. Gold (1972) noted that a gap exists between the potential of retarded workers and the tasks they are assigned. Whitehead agreed, stating that the subcontracts of the workshops are often too simple and earn low wages. He also called for more professionalism in the organization and operation of workshops, especially in such areas as job procurement, work organization, and operating efficiency. Additionally, Whitehead noted the need for better training of workshop staff, particularly those who provide direct training for the clients.

Sheltered workshops will probably remain the primary type of employment for many mentally retarded workers for several years. A key to increasing the adequacy of this service will be the realization that we have not yet achieved the potential working ability of many retarded persons. As stated above, a number of persons currently placed in activity centers could probably function quite well in sheltered workshops. The main reason for this is the improvement in training techniques that has occurred in the last several years. These techniques indicate that we can have greater expectations for lower functioning retarded persons and that it is possible to teach them more complex tasks. Severely and profoundly retarded persons (including some who were deaf and blind) have learned to assemble complex items such as bicycle brakes (Gold, 1974, 1976) and cam switch activators (Bellamy, Peterson & Close, 1975). Other research has shown that not only can some severely and profoundly retarded adults learn such skills, they can learn to perform at acceptably high rates of speed (Bates, Renzaglia & Clees, 1980; Martin & Morris, 1980).

Competitive Employment

For some people, work is a burden. For some, it is a pleasure. For most, it is probably a little bit of both but most definitely, it is a source of income. Competitive employment for the mentally retarded adult is this and more. It is an indication that adult status has been achieved. Competing for and getting a job in the community places a person squarely in the ranks of the mainstream of society. In other words, it is a chance to be like everyone else. Competitive employment is more desirable than sheltered work for other reasons as well. Better pay, fringe benefits (the latter is not often afforded in sheltered workshops), more of a chance to interact with nonretarded persons and thus improve socialization skills, a chance for promotion to a better or higher paying job, and a chance to contribute to the productivity of society instead of relying on it for support are clearly desirable outcomes.

Several types of jobs for mildly retarded adults have been discussed earlier (see Table 12–3). In addition, Becker (1973) reported the development of a vocational inventory approach that would be useful in helping retarded adolescents and adults decide on the types of jobs they would like. The inventory does not require reading. Individuals simply indicate their choices by pointing to pictures. Becker found that EMR adolescent males were interested in automotive mechanics, building trades, clerical work, animal care, food service, patient care, horticulture, janitorial work, personal service, laundry service, and materials handling. Females expressed interest in laundry service, light industrial work, personal service, food service, patient care, horticulture, and housekeeping. Other instruments of this nature were reviewed by Stodden, Ianacone, and Lazar (1979). They include the *VISA* (Vocational Interest and Sophistication Assessment) and the *WRIOT* (Wide Range Interest Opinion Test).

It will be important to train individuals to do jobs to which they will have access. Training for its own sake will not suffice. Planners must be able to determine that the jobs are available in the community for which the person is prepared. Some writers (e.g., Wolfensberger, 1967) have warned against the development of overspecialized skills. Others have noted that skills are not as important as attitudes and other personal characteristics (Kolstoe, 1961; Kolstoe & Frey, 1965). Still, it would be counterproductive to train agricultural skills to individuals residing in inner-city neighborhoods. This is not to say that skill training should be limited. It is simply to make the purpose of training more realistic.

Competitive employment opportunities for mildly retarded persons seems a realistic end for the process of education. But what about individuals in lower IQ ranges? Let us consider their potential for competitive employment.

Lack of employment, sheltered employment, and adult activity centers do not allow many people to achieve the work potential that they possess. Thus there is a movement underway in some areas to place moderately, severely, and profoundly retarded adults in competitive employment (Bellamy, Horner & Inman, 1979; Bellamy, Sheehan, Horner & Boles, 1980; Horner & Bellamy, 1979; Pomerantz & Marholin, 1977; Wehman & J. Hill, 1981; Wehman, Hill, Goodall, Cleveland, Brooke & Pentecost, 1982; Wehman & McLaughlin, 1980; Whitehead, 1979).

Traditionally, large numbers of handicapped persons have been employed in sheltered workshops or placed in adult activity centers. Often these programs intend to develop individuals for movement into higher levels; for example, activity centers to sheltered employment to competitive employment. According to some writers, however (Bellamy et al., 1980; Pomerantz & Marholin, 1977), the continuum does not always work and the large majority of individuals do not move up the ladder.

Part of the problem is that such facilities are funded based on the number of clients they serve instead of the number they place on jobs. This being the case, there is little motivation to move people into competitive employment. Another problem is that the Supplemental Security Income received by many mentally retarded workers, along with other social services, may cease if they earn too much money. Parents often fear this and are resistant to job placement for their adult children (Bellamy et al., 1980). Parents are also often under the impression that their children simply cannot work (sometimes having been told this for many years) and thus are not always fully cooperative. Finally, there is simply the problem of tradition and the belief that more severely retarded workers cannot perform jobs well enough to hold them in the open market. Several researchers have set out to disprove this latter notion and fight the tradition.

Mithaug, Hagmeier, and Haring (1977) suggested a model for relating training activities to job placement for severely handicapped persons. The procedures included the following:

1. Job assessment: Learn the requirements of jobs available in the community.
2. Client assessment: Determine the needs and available skills an individual has to perform in the available job.
3. Develop behavioral objectives to train the individual based on needs and job requirements.
4. Train the individual according to the behavioral objectives developed.

The important feature of this model is that specific jobs and their corresponding skills are determined before training begins. Structured training using the techniques of task analysis and applied behavior analysis is provided to develop the necessary skills.

Horner and Bellamy (1979) suggested a model of "structured employment." This plan calls for "extended employment that emphasizes high levels of individual productivity with ongoing training and support services not typically provided in industry" (p. 90). According to the plan, individuals with skills directly related to the production task and also indirectly related to it (e.g., grooming, hygiene, etc.) would be placed in competitive employment settings. Those without the indirect skills would remain in a sheltered setting until they had been learned. (Horner and Bellamy suggested that these indirect skills be learned during nonworking hours.) A candidate for competitive employment would be the person with direct and indirect skills. Regardless of whether the person was working in a sheltered workshop or in industry, Horner and Bellamy called for the work to be nontrivial and, following adequate training, provide a nontrivial wage. They also called for the work to be extended; that is, to be typical industrial vocational tasks as opposed to short-term simple contracts. On-the-job support and continued training opportunities would be provided for the employee.

One of the most persuasive presentations of the competitive employment abilities of sub-50 IQ individuals has been by Wehman and his colleagues working on "Project Employability." A number of publications over the last five years have documented the effectiveness of the project (c.f.: Wehman et al., 1982; Wehman & Hill, 1981; Wehman, Hill & Koehler, 1979; Wehman & McLauglin, 1980). The project has been in effect since 1978. It focuses on job placement, training, and follow-up of moderately and severely retarded and multiply-handicapped persons. The model followed is essentially that proposed by Mithaug et al. (1977) earlier. Jobs are located, employers are contacted, workers are placed and trained, and supervision is continued as long as it is needed. Attempts are made to match individuals with specific jobs based on variables such as dress, physical barriers, and work hours. During the training period, every effort is made to conduct on-the-job training. If this is not possible, training is conducted in public schools, activity centers, or sheltered workshops. Workers are drawn from all three settings as well as other agencies.

One of the most impressive aspects of the project is that the retarded individuals are contributing to the welfare of society instead of depending on it. Hill and Wehman (in press) reported that as of July, 1982, the total cost of the project to the taxpayer was $530,200. This figure included $470,639 in project costs plus $59,561 in tax credits to the employers for hiring handicapped persons. (Employers can receive a $3,000 per year person tax credit for hiring the handicapped.) In comparison, total public savings was $620,576. This figure included $186,190 *not paid* in Supplemental Security Income, $385,678 *not paid* for daily programming costs, and $48,708 *paid* in state and federal taxes by the retarded workers. Net savings to the public: $90,376. The annual income of the eighty workers placed on jobs as of July, 1982, averaged $4,600 per year. In comparison, the average annual income in sheltered workshops is $450 per year. Besides earning ten times the salary, the workers have been able to receive job benefits such as health insurance, life insurance, vacation with pay, sick leave, and perhaps intangible benefits that only they can perceive.

The ability of many moderately and severely retarded individuals to adequately participate in competitive employment is irrefutable. There are, of course, associated problems. Wehman et al. (1982) reported some difficulties and concerns of co-workers. These included a fear that they would have to absorb extra duties due to the client's slowness, unreasonable expectations, a lack of direct communication with the client, and existing prejudice. Such concerns are real and will have to be addressed. Part of the problem may be alleviated when it becomes apparent that the retarded workers can succeed on the job. Another part may simply have to wait for the passage of time.

If the concept of competitive employment for moderately and severely retarded adults is to become a successful practice, much work will have to be done. Structured training techniques will have to be carried out and these will have to be in the real world. As we know, generalization is a difficulty with retarded individuals. However, research is indicating that hard work and a willingness to try may compensate for this difficulty. The profession may be on the verge of opening a new world to these individuals.

CONCLUSION

It seems that historically much of our efforts on behalf of mentally retarded persons were directed toward the childhood years. This is probably as it should have been. However, slowly we have learned that mentally retarded children grow up. Sometimes they lose their "official" designation of "mental retardation" when they leave the public school system. This is particularly true of many mildly retarded persons whose difficulties were most readily apparent in the academic setting. Still, many of these and most all of the more severely retarded have difficulty in adapting to the adult world. The problem in adaption is no more evident than in the area of vocational success. This is a problem that cannot be ignored. It should provide a special significance for what we do with these individuals as children. If we are not adequately preparing them for adulthood; then what, indeed, is the purpose of our services?

Fortunately, we are in a better posture today than ever before to help these persons improve their adult status. We have developed a sound instructional technology and have come to realize that even very low IQ individuals can learn to perform complex jobs required in competitive employment. At this time two major tasks face the profession. The first is to take the technology out of the journals and put it to work where it is needed. The second is to let society know what we can do, and in turn, what mentally retarded individuals can do.

Wilcox and Bellamy (1982) called for development of transition plans. These individual plans would lay out the progression from the protective environs of the public school to the open world of the adult with necessary support provided along the way. The idea has much merit. After providing eighteen years of education, it seems such a waste not to help put the final touches on such an important and viable product.

STUDY QUESTIONS

1. What types of problems are encountered by mentally retarded adults?
2. What were the general findings in the early follow-up studies reviewed by Goldstein (1964) and Kokaska (1968)? What have more recent studies indicated?
3. What variables tend to affect the job success of mildly retarded adults?
4. What are work-study programs and how have they affected the employment of mildly retarded adults?

5. What kinds of jobs have most often been held by mildly retarded adults?
6. Describe the nature of the relationship of the moderately/severely retarded adult and his or her family.
7. How mobile are most moderately/severely retarded adults within their neighborhood and community?
8. What has been the general employment status of moderately, severely, and profoundly retarded adults?
9. What are adult activity centers, who are served by them, and what are their functions?
10. Describe the functioning of sheltered workshops.
11. Describe some of the recent models used to help moderately and severely retarded persons in the competitive job market.

13

Parents of Retarded Children

GENERAL CONSIDERATIONS

Having a child and experiencing the long process of parenthood could only be explained by using all of the words that describe the emotions, concerns, feelings, and attitudes of life. To be a parent exposes one to all of life's internal experiences. There is happiness and sorrow, pain and pleasure, joy and sadness, excitement and boredom, success and failure, satisfaction and frustration, and the many variations that lie within these opposites. They can change day to day or even minute to minute.

At best, a parent's lot is not an easy one. Performed correctly, the task is arduous. At the material level, the child's or children's basic needs must be provided and, for most, "basic" needs go beyond food, shelter, and clothing. Socially, the parent has the task of inculcating family and cultural values. The child will bear both the parents' name and the parents' beliefs.

Emotionally, parents and child will both give and receive. Love, understanding, discipline, and direction will flow on a two-way street. The parents will shape the child and the child will shape the parents.

Of course there are instances when being a parent is less than ideal. Many different factors can reduce the quality of parenthood. An unexpected child, an unemployed father, a troubled mother, a difficult pregnancy, problems with in-laws, or any number of other conditions can sharply affect what a child means to the parents and how the parents react to the child.

Undoubtedly one of the most difficult conditions is when the child is diagnosed as being mentally retarded. A baby born with obvious physical anomalies or who in the first few years of life fails to exhibit typical developmental successes can have a formidable effect on the parents as life continues. The emotional well-being of the parents and inordinate financial strains and the special needs of a retarded child cause problems within the family structure. In normal situations, parental responsibilities are awesome. When the child is mentally retarded, these responsibilities can be multiplied several times. The child will present difficulties that go well beyond those normally encountered during parenthood.

Given these difficulties, it might be easy to develop the notion that most parents of retarded children are voided of the positive experiences of being parents. Such a notion would be incorrect. As we have seen, mentally retarded individuals vary a great deal in their abilities and characteristics. The same is true of their parents. On the whole, it would probably be safe to say that the large majority of these parents love their special children dearly. There seems to be no evidence available to refute this conclusion.

Still their lives are more difficult than those of most parents. The mental and material strains they experience as they see their children fall behind, as they seek professional services, as they make critical decisions, and as they buffer their children from an uneducated society wear on them greatly.

The purpose of this chapter is to take a careful look at parents of mentally retarded children. We will consider what this role means and how it is managed. If our concern is with the general development and welfare of mentally retarded individuals, it would be shortsighted not to examine in some detail the most significant source of influence on their lives. During the last twenty or so years, parents of retarded children have come to be viewed in a different light by professionals in the field of mental retardation. Earlier, they were considered primarily from the point of view as needing services. Their reactions, concerns, and emotions were studied and analyzed. Like their retarded children, they were offered special services to better help them cope with their situation. While the analysis and services continue today (as they should), special parents are also now seen in another way. In this second fashion, they are being considered as important service providers for their children (Turnbull & Turnbull, 1982). In this role, they are required by law (PL 94–142) to be involved in the planning of special education services. They may also be educated to provide systematic training in the home, thereby extending the school's or service agency's efforts.

We will examine the parent from both angles. In the first section of this chapter, the general impact of a retarded child on parents will be studied. Attention will be given to the reactions, emotions, concerns, and needs of parents of mentally retarded children. In the second section, parent involvement in the education and training of their children will be considered.

THE IMPACT OF A RETARDED CHILD ON PARENTS

Having a mentally retarded child will cause parents to act and react in different ways at different points in time. Initially, a host of emotional reactions may permeate their daily lives, causing a great deal of stress. Usually, in time and sometimes with the aid of professional counseling, these difficult feelings will subside and life will become more emotionally bearable. Still, there will be problems that must be handled. Many of these will be like those of any parent. Others will be a result of the child's reduced level of development and solving them will require extraordinary effort. Throughout the process, parents may look for ways to help them cope. Parent organizations offer one such source of support; parent counseling offers another.

Finding the appropriate services for their child is another difficulty some parents may encounter. Because public schools are now providing special education for all handicapped children, there is less difficulty in this area today than in the past. Still, the best educational system cannot provide for all needs. There will be many that parents will have to seek out. At best this will often mean dealing with a complex bureaucratic network of agencies. At worst, it may mean doing without the services, traveling great distances to gain access to them, or institutionalizing the child because he or she cannot be adequately served in the community.

Beyond the school years, parents will be faced with the reality of their child as an adult and their own impending immortality. What will become of this person when the parents can no longer provide daily supervision? Again, appropriate services and facilities must be sought and difficult decisions must be made.

Throughout all of this, the retarded child will have an impact on the social structure of the family. Interactions of the parents and their nonretarded children may be affected. Relations between husbands and wives will almost certainly be modified by having a retarded child. Additionally, reactions from relatives and friends may hinder harmonious socialization. In turn, this may affect the functioning of the family unit.

All of these factors—emotional reactions, problems with the child, finding services, social difficulties within and outside of the family—interact considerably. Difficulties of one sort will have a bearing in another area. Amazingly, throughout this saga, most parents and families do remarkably well. They not only survive, but they experience a meaningful life.

Emotional Reactions

As mentioned earlier, parents of mentally retarded children are as different as are their children. No general description of emotional reaction will suffice or adequately describe how all parents react to the birth or diagnosis of a mentally retarded child. Years ago, Wolfensberger (1967) wrote:

> Almost an infinite variety of initial or early reactions have been described or mentioned in the literature, e.g., alarm, ambivalence, anger, anguish, anxiety, avoidance, bewilderment, bitterness, catastrophic reaction, confusion, death wishes, denial, depression, despair, disappointment, disbelief, disassociation, embarrassment, envy, fear, financial worries, frustration, grief, guilt, helplessness, hopelessness, identification, immobility, impulses to destroy the child, lethargy, mourning, over-identification, pain, projection, puzzlement, regret, rejection, remorse, self-blame, self-pity, shame, shock, sorrow, suicidal impulses, trauma, etc. The list is neither exhaustive of reactions that have been described nor of those conceivably possible. (p. 330)

Obviously, writers have interpreted reactions of parents in many different ways. One reason for this is that no single description fits all. It would be impossible to discuss all of these reactions. Still, there are some that should at least be briefly considered. Some discussed by Wolfensberger (1967) and/or Roos (1963) include the following:

Guilt.   Parents may feel guilty because they believe that in some way they caused their child's retardation. Often their belief is related to their sexual activity (premarital, extramarital) for which they believe God is punishing them. They may also feel guilty because of anger toward the child.

Ambivalence.   The parent is disappointed and frustrated yet feels a need to love and protect the child. The parent may also feel a need to place blame but cannot place it on the child.

Frustration.   There are many reasons why the parent may feel frustrated. There is a concern about social stigma, lack of services, financial demands, and delayed maturation. The parent may also feel frustrated because the family generation has not been successfully extended.

Loss of self-esteem.   Parents often view their children as extensions of themselves. Because their child is not their ideal, parents may feel they have failed and question their own worth.

Shame.   Retarded children are often pointed out as being different or sometimes even ridiculed. Parents may feel shame at such forms of rejection.

Depression.   Having a retarded child may result in deep disappointment and certainly concern for the future. Olshansky (1966) characterized many parents of retarded children as having "chronic sorrow."

Defensivenes.   Parents of retarded children often become sensitive to what they see as criticism about their children. They may become very resentful or even deny that the child is retarded.

Such emotional reactions as these are understandable. Again, however, it must be stressed that no two parents can be expected to react in the same way to the presence of a retarded child. It should also be kept in mind that we live in a different world today than existed twenty or twenty-five years ago. Individual rights and self-awareness, along with the recognition of handicapped persons as individuals, may lessen some of the emotional impact on parents that has existed in the past. In more recent writing, Roos (1978), who is both the parent of a retarded child and a well-known professional in the field, suggested that while some parents are overwhelmed, others not only cope but grow emotionally as the result of having a retarded child. He wrote: "It would be a serious mistake to assume that most parents of retarded children are emotionally disturbed" (Roos, 1978, p. 18). Another parent (Doolittle, 1978) wrote, "Fourteen years after the advent of retardation in our home, I see no signs of 'chronic sorrow' " (p. 9).

Giving some credence to this position, a recent study by Waisbren (1980) compared parents of handicapped children (mentally retarded, blind, cerebral palsied, and brain damaged) to parents of nonhandicapped children during the first eighteen months of the child's life. The coping abilities of the two groups were found to be "strikingly similar." There were no difference in their physical health, their social activity, their activities with their babies, their marital relations, or their future plans. Parents of the handicapped children did tend to feel more helpless and expressed more feelings of anger and rejection. Waisbren attributed some of the negative feelings to poor interactions with doctors and hospitals.

Some professionals have described parents as passing through stages of emotional adjustment or reaction. Wolfensberger (1967) suggested parents might experience three "crises." The first he called a "novelty shock crisis." This is likely to occur when the parents first discover their child is retarded. Usually it occurs at birth when there has been no forewarning of a problem. Wolfensberger states: "the crucial element here is not retardation at all; it is the demolition of expectancies" (p. 336).

The second crisis is the "value crisis." It occurs when the idea of the child being retarded is simply unacceptable to the parent. Different degrees of emotional rejection may occur and sometimes last throughout the parent's or child's life.

Finally, the "reality crisis" appears. At this stage, the day-to-day management of the child becomes the central issue. The parents' ability or inability to meet the child's needs may affect certain decisions, such as whether or not to place the child in an institution. Other influences, such as social pressure, are also examples of the reality crisis.

The hypothetical crises outlined by Wolfensberger (1967) can be understood in terms of the serious problems and decisions that parents must face. Their choices and actions are never easy and we should not hasten to pass judgment. We should, instead, make an attempt to understand these situations so future parents, retarded children, and society at large might benefit. Several dilemmas are discussed below.

Decisions about Institutionalization

For many parents a decision may have to ultimately be made as to whether the child should remain in the home or be placed out of the home in a public or community residential facility. As we saw in an earlier chapter, certain demographic data has been shown to affect the probability of this decision (see Chapter 10). Notwithstanding such data, the decision is a very personal one and certainly very trying.

While deinstitutionalization (and noninstitutionalization) is regarded as a positive move by many professionals and advocates for the mentally retarded, some parents have expressed concern and reservations about the practice. For some, deinstitutionalization has caused significant problems and additional emotional stress. For others it has been a source of confusion. One parent (Gorham, 1975) wrote:

> In the past we were made to feel guilty when we did not institutionalize our children; and now, under the new normalization principle, we are made to feel guilty if we do. (p. 522)

While many parents seem to endorse the *concepts* of deinstitutionalization and normalization, they have difficulty in applying them to their own children. In a study of 217 parents of institutionalized retarded persons, Ferrara (1979) found strong support toward normalization as long as it did not specifically apply to the parents' children. When the responses were child-specific, parents were not as supportive of normalization activities. Meyer (1980) questioned a similar group of parents (n = 273) and also found that most of them preferred that their child remain in the institution. Eighty-three percent felt that the institution was the best possible placement for their child. Their major concerns were the availability and quality of supervision, care, and resources outside of the institution.

One problem that must certainly face many of these parents is the emotional stress that might result if their child was to leave the institution. Willer, Intagliata, and Atkinson (1981) surveyed forty-three families of retarded individuals who had been released from an institution. Some of the former residents had returned to their natural homes (n = 15) while others had been placed in alternative community facilities (n = 28). Fifty percent of the families questioned expressed emotional problems related to deinstitutionalization. Many of the parents of the individuals replaced in their natural homes reported anxiety about the placement. They were concerned about the retarded person's disruptive behavior and their own ability to provide an appropriate environment. On the other hand, parents of persons placed in other settings often said they felt guilty because they could not allow the child to return to his or her original home.

Avis (1978), writing as both a professional and a parent, explained that many parents of institutionalized persons are experiencing "deinstitutionalization jet lag." They are being asked to accept a style of service for their mentally retarded child that is new and different. She described one elderly couple who told her they had heard on the evening news that many residents of a nearby institution would soon be coming home. They were worried about how they would explain the return of their daughter to their friends and relatives. Their daughter, it seems, had been born with Down's syndrome forty years ago. Their physician advised them that the baby would not live a year and so they authorized the child to be placed in the institution before they left the hospital. They then returned home without the child and sadly reported that their baby would not be coming home. When friends and relatives inferred the baby had died, the couple did not correct them. Now, forty years later, they felt in a bit of an awkward position when they considered the possibility of their daughter returning home. As Avis noted: " 'The baby will not live' is quite a distance from 'coming home to live' forty years later" (p. 172).

Many parents may elect to keep their child at home but ultimately realize that the child has become an adult and will probably out-live them. It is at this time that parents often start seeking alternative living arrangements for their adult-child. Often the choices are few. In the past, a large residential instituion might have been automatically selected. Today the parents might be directed toward a community facility if one is available and has room. Unfortunately, the placement may often disrupt the lives of the people involved and sometimes place great distances between parents and children.

As community support programs improve, we should be hopeful that more parents will opt to keep their children in their homes. The choice will never be an easy one. The physical and emotional strength required may simply not be present in many of the parents who need it the most. These are the ones who will have the greatest need for services. One thing is fairly certain: Once parents decide they need to remove their child from their home, the probability of a comfortable return seems low.

Problems at Home

While some parents will seek external placement, the large majority will keep their child at home at least until adulthood. In many such situations a pleasant life for the child, the parents, and other children will evolve. In the process of this evolution, however, it is realistic to expect that problems will arise. Some problems will be directly related to the child; others will be manifested in the adjustment of the family.

Skelton (1972) questioned 128 families about major concerns regarding their retarded children. Seven categories of problems were reported. In order of frequency, they were:

1. Concerns about the availability of educational programs
2. Inappropriate social behavior interfering with family life
3. Inability to care for the child because of other family concerns
4. Providing for the child's physical care and protection
5. Finding an appropriate living situation for later in life when parents can no longer care for the person
6. Finding appropriate recreational activities and companionship
7. Dealing with problems in the community

While the first problem hopefully is not as serious today as it was when Skelton conducted this study, the other problems may well be. As we know, deficits in social or adaptive behavior are one of the defining characteristics of mental retardation. While modification of behavior is possible, parents will always have to be able to expect some variation from the norm. This variation may be perceived as a problem. How it affects the parents and their interaction with the child will be different in each situation.

Parents of retarded children, like all parents, can expect different types of problems to occur depending on the age and/or developmental level of their child. Tavormina, Henggeler, and Gayton (1976) reported problems experienced by mothers of TMR children between two years and adolescence. Disobedience, stubbornness, and noncompliance were problems found in all age groups except adolescents. Parents of young children (2–4 years) were also concerned about developmental areas such as eating, talking, and walking. They described problems of impulsivity, sensitivity, and temperament. These tended to decrease as the child grew older. In the four- to six-year-old group, parents expressed concerns about aggression and personal hygiene. Temper tantrums and destructive behavior also appeared first at this age and continued to be reported at every stage thereafter. Many parents also stated that stereotyped behaviors were exhibited for the first time during the four- to six-year period.

Parents of older individuals, particularly adolescents, were most concerned about their children's social behavior. Apprehension was particularly noted in the area of social interactions. As the individual grows further away from childhood and closer to adulthood, parents are apt to be worried about the growing discrepancy between social age and chronological age. Appropriate training in social skills thus becomes more critical than ever as the child grows older.

Many parents will learn to deal effectively with these and other problems. Training parents in the use of behavior modification can help them help their children. Studies have shown quite conclusively that parents can be effective behavior managers (Berkowitz & Graziano, 1972; O'Dell, 1974). Yet there can be difficulties in communicating with parents and getting them to use the technology that has been developed (Baker, Heifetz & Murphy, 1980). Our efforts to reduce parents' problems with their children might well improve the relations between them. Simultaneously, however, we should remain mindful of the difficulties and realize that having a retarded child at home creates unique life problems for the parents.

Parent Adjustment

The parents and perhaps the entire family of the retarded child can experience extraordinary difficulties because of the child's presence. In turn, how the parents and family react to the child can affect his or her general welfare and development. For example, the parents out of necessity may devote a considerable amount of attention to the retarded child and less attention to a nonretarded sibling. As a result, the sibling may respond with aggression toward the retarded child. This may cause the retarded child to become more aggressive and thus require more attention. Such a sequence of interactions among family members could continue endlessly and, in fact, do. Some may be bad but others may be good.

The consensus in the research literature is that the presence of a retarded child can result in a variety of difficulties in family adjustment. If the child's presence is not a direct cause of problems, it may serve as a catalyst. In his review, Wolfensberger (1967) stated that most problems could be categorized as economic, social, or emotional. Economic or financial difficulties can result because of the extra cost involved in raising a handicapped child. Social and emotional difficulties can appear as parents interact with each other, their other children, or the rest of society.

In a study comparing thirty-four parents of handicapped children (physically handicapped and mentally retarded) with thirty-four parents of nonhandicapped children, Friedrich and Friedrich (1981) found several psychosocial differences. Families with handicapped children experienced a significantly greater amount of stress, less marital satisfaction, less psychosocial well-being, and less religiosity. Not all studies in this area, however, are as negative in their conclusions. Waisbren (1980) found many similarities between parents of handicapped and nonhandicapped children in a variety of areas including coping abilities, physical health, social activities, and marital relations. In a related but different type of study, Blackard and Barsh (1982) compared what professionals thought about parental problems with what the parents themselves thought. Generally, the professionals were much more pessimistic about the parents' prospects for adjustment than were the parents. The parents were more favorable in their judgments of family and marital relations, involvement in family activities, problems with siblings, financial impact, and their ability to find adequate services. Thus it may be that professionals perceive parents to have greater difficulties in adjustment than they actually do.

One problem not often realized but certainly of significance is the physical requirements placed on the parents. If their child is severely or profoundly retarded, parents may be required to provide for all of the child's daily care needs. This, of course, would require much physical activity. Even if the child is not severely handicapped, parents will have to "keep up" with him or her. This alone can produce fatigue. Often one of the greatest needs of parents is simply finding some relief. If they can locate a baby sitter or respite care service, this might provide them with the stamina needed to continue their child-rearing activities. Physical stress can compound the effects of emotional stress and vice versa. When dealing with parents of retarded children, professionals should keep in mind the 24-hours-a-day, 365-days-a-year job that these parents have.

Up to this point we have considered the impact of the retarded child on the family. It must also be realized that the family can have an impact on the child and that a variety of family conditions exist. Recently, Mink, Nihira, and Meyers (1983) conducted a study of 115 families with trainable level retarded children and found five distinctive types or "clusters" of families existed. They described the families as follows:

Cluster 1: Cohesive, harmonious (n = 35). In these families there was an absence of negative child influences and a low level of stressful life events. The majority of retarded children in these homes had Down's syndrome. The children earned high scores on personal-social responsibility, had high self-esteem, peer-acceptance, and self-concept.

Cluster 2: Control-oriented, somewhat nonharmonious (n = 34). These families had the highest socioeconomic level and a low level of stressful life events, but used physical punishment with their children. The children were low on all dimensions of the adaptive behavior scale and general social adjustment. Their self-sufficiency and self-esteem were also low.

Cluster 3: Low-disclosure, unharmonious (n = 7). Stressful life events and negative impact of the retarded child on the family were high in these families. The retarded children in this group had the highest IQs. These families had poor physical environments, social maturity, and also used physical punishment. Children were high on community self-sufficiency, personal-social responsibility, and adjustment at home. They also had high self-esteem and peer-acceptance.

Cluster 4: Child-oriented, expressive (n = 27). These families scored high on factors associated with the child's well being; for example, pride, affection, warmth, language stimulation, and the non-use of physical punishment. They scored low in the area of control. Few of the retarded children had a negative influence on these families. The children were rated high in personal self-sufficiency but average on most other measures.

Cluster 5: Disadvantaged with low morale (n = 12). These families scored extremely low in stimulation, expressiveness, intellectual-recreation, and residential area. The parents were often not well educated and there was a fairly high frequency of stressful life events. The impact of the retarded child on the family was poor. The children had very low IQs and were significantly low on personal self-sufficiency, community self-sufficiency, and self-esteem.

Mink et al. (1983) judged Clusters 1 and 4 as providing a good home environment for raising a retarded child. Cluster 5 was the worst; and Cluster 2 was in between while Cluster 3 was difficult to interpret. The one obvious conclusion that can be drawn is that families and their influences can vary. As Doolittle (1978), a parent, wrote:

> "The dynamics of each family, the religious and socioeconomic background, the availability of helpful services all effect the impact of the retarded child on the family." (p. 11)

Parent Support and Counseling

Because of their situation, parents—and sometimes entire families of retarded children—will seek support and guidance to help them cope. The assistance provided may take many forms but it is usually intended to help them make decisions, solve problems, and improve their personal adjustment.

One of the oldest forms of support offered to parents comes from other parents in the same situation. Because they have faced similar difficulties, parents feel comfortable in relying on each other for assistance. The largest organization for parents of retarded children is the National Association for Retarded Citizens (NARC, formerly the National Association for Retarded Children). Cain (1976) described the growth of this organization as it evolved from many smaller independent associations into a national organization in 1950.

The parents who formed the NARC were primarily concerned about securing educational and other services for their children and providing support for each other. They began by forming small private schools and then lobbying school boards and state legislatures for public school programs. As we saw earlier, they were ultimately successful in their efforts.

Of course, public school programs are not enough. Thus the NARC and its state and local affiliates provide support for community living facilities, sheltered workshops, preschool programs, diagnostic facilities, and parent education programs. In the past few years, NARC and various state ARCs have focused on advocacy for mentally retarded citizens. Much litigation on behalf of the mentally retarded has been supported by state ARCs.

The significance of parent organizations was recognized by Greer (1975), himself a parent, when he wrote:

> The best help can be found in interaction with parents who have experienced and solved such problems. Even though every family's situation is unique and what works for one family may not work for another, having someone with common problems with whom to interact is in itself therapeutic.
>
> Parents must realize also that only by banding together can they bring about the changes in society which are needed. Legislators and other government leaders listen to groups when they might not listen to individuals. Therefore, in order to exercise their "clout," parents of the handicapped must unite and seek common goals to alleviate society's barriers to their children's welfare. (p. 519)

Many times parents will seek professional counseling to help them with their special problems. The specific role of parental counseling will differ by situations. Sometimes it is to teach the parents how to better manage their children's behavior; other times it is to help them accept their child as is and/or to cope with emotional distress. Tavormina, Hampson, and Luscomb (1976) asked parents to evaluate the effectiveness of the particular type of counseling session they had attended. Parents who participated in adjustment sessions and talked about their problems with other parents felt they had learned to better accept their child and themselves. On the other hand, parents in a behavior management program were able to promote changes in their child's behavior and thus had greater satisfaction with their child. Both groups of parents agreed the counseling sessions were worthwhile. It may be that the specific content of the counseling session is not as important as the fact that there is someone to turn toward.

While this chapter is not intended to prepare parent counselors, some suggestions by Wolfensberger (1967) in this area may be insightful. It is hoped that most counselors or other professionals dealing with parents adhere to these suggestions. They are paraphrased below:

1. The counselor must be honest.
2. The counselor should be prepared with pertinent information for the parent.
3. Didactic counseling should be avoided until the facts have been presented.
4. Whenever possible, both parents should participate in counseling.

5. A diagnosis should be conveyed as a new beginning, not an end of professional involvement. Parents must know where to turn next.
6. The counselor must be extremely sensitive, especially when the diagnosis of retardation is being presented for the first time.
7. The parents should be provided a written report in order to avoid misunderstandings.
8. Agencies should try to maintain contact between the same counselor and parents in order to provide continuity.
9. Outdated, unclear, and offensive terminology should be avoided.
10. Care should be taken not to prognosticate or stereotype future abilities, particularly in cases of very young children.

Conclusion

In this section, we have seen that parents of retarded children are faced with dilemmas from the time of birth to adulthood. Throughout the process, the normal difficulties of parenting will be compounded by the problems of their special child. These problems in some cases may lead to emotional distress and may affect overall family adjustment. Fortunately, parent groups and support services exist to aid them. Without such services, their unique situations may be even more difficult, perhaps unbearable. We should not conclude that parents of retarded children do not love them or that they are not fully committed to their welfare. In most cases, this is simply not true. Still, we must realize the situation they are in. If for no other reason, we must understand their perspective when we deal with them as professionals or simply as members of society.

PARENTAL INVOLVEMENT IN THE EDUCATIONAL PROCESS

The way in which parents of retarded and other handicapped children are viewed by professionals has changed dramatically in the last several years. Today, parents are more likely to be looked upon as having a significant role in the education of their children. They are, in fact, considered to be a part of the educational team. Parent-professional partnerships are more and more becoming the desired strategy in special education programs (Simches, 1975; Turnbull, 1982).

This has not always been the case. Gorham (1975) expressed anger about some of the experiences she had as a parent trying to work with professionals in years past. She said parents had been "intimidated" by professionals and were "unreasonably awed" by them. Professionals were often criticized by parents for not sharing information about their children, for not providing the parents with useful management techniques, for providing only negative prognostic information, and for not helping parents face their dilemmas (Gorham, 1975; Roos, 1978; H. R. Turnbull, 1978).

As educational rights for handicapped individuals gained momentum, so did the right for their parents to be involved in the educational process. At a minimum, parents are now guaranteed the right to participate in the individual educational planning for their handicapped child. They also have the right to be provided all relevant information about their child's progress. As one parent of a retarded child, who also happens to be a professional, wrote:

> . . .access is not only invaluable to parents and professionals, it is imperative as a course of decent conduct between people and as a weapon against charlantry . . . (H. R. Turnbull, 1978, p. 119)

Rationale for Parent Involvement

There are several good reasons why parents of retarded children should be involved in their child's educational program. Perhaps the most basic reason is because they are usually interested in the child's welfare and they want to contribute to it. All parents are in a similar position. But parents of retarded children cannot assume that their child will learn or develop with the facility of normal children. Thus they tend to want to know more about what is going on in their child's educational program, what the child is being taught, and how well it is being learned.

Another reason for parental involvement is that parents know the child better than anyone else. They know the child's abilities and inabilities, what makes the child happy and sad, and often what the child needs to learn. Sometimes parents of mentally retarded children develop unreal expectations for their child and, of course, it is the professional's responsibility to gently direct them toward realistic goals. For the most part, however, parents are on target when it comes to determining what their children need to learn. Their input in this area should be given priority consideration.

Parents should also be included in the educational process because they can make it work more effectively. Research has shown that parents can be quite effective as teachers of their children and modifiers of their behavior (Berkowitz & Graziano, 1972; O'Dell, 1974). As such, they can continue training in the home where the school leaves off. Bricker and Bricker (1976) noted that not only can parents supplement the work of professionals but they can serve as an "ideal teacher" since they are apt to be very reinforcing to the child.

Finally, if parents are participants, they are more likely to be supportive of the educational system than antagonistic toward it. In the beginning (pre-1950s) parents' pleas for public school educational services were often rejected. When services were offered, parents had little choice in their nature, often being given a "take it or leave it" program (Simches, 1975). Strong animosity developed between some school systems and parent organizations.

By incorporating parents into the process today, schools can avoid such conflicts and even promote positive relations. It would be safe to surmise that parents of retarded children today are generally happier and more supportive of the school system than were parents twenty or maybe even ten years ago. In a recent study by Polifka (1981), it was found that the more parents were involved in planning their child's educational program, the more satisfied they were with it.

On the basis of the above reasons, it hardly seems logical not to involve parents in special education programs for their retarded children. It seems most fortunate that today there is opportunity for parental involvement. It might well be that the more participation by parents, the more development of their children will occur.

Degree of Parent Involvement

While involvement by parents is obviously desirable, we must realize that there are different degrees of involvement. From the preceding discussion, we might conclude that the more they are involved, the better. And we would probably be right. Yet we must remember that parents have other lives to live and other responsibilities to which they must attend. Some writers, including parents (MacMillan & Turnbull, 1983; Turnbull, 1982; Turnbull & Turnbull, 1982), have recently suggested that the degree of parent involvement in the child's educational program should be one of choice on the parents' part. Like the child's educational program, the amount of participation should probably be individually determined. We should not forget the difficulties of parents discussed in the earlier section of this chapter. To many parents, the school program offers a daily reprieve. Significant physical presence during the child's school activity may, for some, mean little chance to acquire needed rest. MacMillan and Turnbull (1983) suggested:

> . . .Special educators should be sensitive to the option that parents not be involved in the educational program at times in order that they be more effective in parenting (involvement with the child), or more effective in their involvement with other family members. Furthermore, when exercising this option for noninvolvement, the parent should not be made to feel guilty. (p. 5)

We might therefore expect a range of participation. Some parents will only be involved with the school program minimally; others may spend all of their free time working with their child (or other children) in the classroom or at home. The important thing is that they have the choice to do so. We can consider parental involvement as occurring on a continuum. On one end, there is no involvement at all or perhaps minimal involvement; for example, giving permission or uninformed consent (Yoshida & Gottlieb, 1977; Shevin, 1983). On the other end, the parent is as much involved in the program as is the teacher. In some programs for preschool age children, in fact, the parents have served as the primary instructors (c.f., Shearer & Shearer, 1976). The type of involvement by parents can be divided into two main parts: involvement in planning and involvement in teaching. In the following sections we will look at the role of parents in these activities.

Involvement in Planning

All parents of retarded children are expected, and required by law, to be involved in the planning of their child's IEP. How much a parent is involved, however, can vary a great deal. Yoshida and Gottlieb (1977) and Shevin (1983) presented descriptions of parent involvement in the planning process that ranged from quite insignificant to very extensive. During the input phase, Yoshida and Gottlieb noted that a parent could be a "permission giver" and an "information giver" or, in fact, state preferences for the type or nature of program their child should receive. The latter, of course, reflected more involvement. They also indicated that parents could be passive participants during planning; for example, they could attend the meeting but contribute little; or be active by suggesting placements and asking questions about the suitability of programs.

Shevin's (1983) analysis was similiar. Four levels of involvement were defined as follows:

> *Uninformed consent*: The parent signs the IEP form without consideration of implications or alternatives.
>
> *Uninformed participation*: The parent helps to identify goals and objectives but is not always knowledgeable about most realistic or immediate needs.
>
> *Informed consent*: Parents agree to the IEP after they are aware of the rationale, benefits, and possible alternatives.
>
> *Informed participation*: The parents become involved in goal and strategy development and continually monitor their child's progress. At this level, professionals and parents share the perception that parents should play an important role.

Shevin contended that too much emphasis has been placed on simply getting the parents to sign the IEP. Some parents accept this degree of involvement as satisfactory; while others would like the option to have more. Lusthaus, Lusthaus, and Gibbs (1981) surveyed parents and found they were most often cast in the role of giving and receiving information, a relatively basic position. In contrast, when asked what decisional control they desired, the three areas most often selected were types of records kept, types of medical services provided, and transference to another school. In a similar study of parents' opinions, Soffer (1982) found that parents were generally satisfied with their involvement in determining needs, goals, and objects. On the other hand, they desired greater participation in determining when the child's progress would be evaluated and how it would be evaluated.

From these two studies (Lusthaus et al., 1981; Soffer, 1982) we might conclude that generally parents' basic rights to participate in planning are being met. It seems, however, that they may want access to other areas of concern, particularly monitoring their child's progress.

There are two possible reasons why parental involvement in planning may be minimal. One is that this is all they desire and they trust the professionals to take care of the details. Turnbull and Turnbull (1982) expressed this sentiment when they wrote:

> Many parents do not believe that their child needs to be protected from the special education system. They consider the special education system their greatest ally. It follows that some will be reluctant to attack the system that helps them and their child. (p. 118)

If this is the position taken by a parent, it should be respected. On the other hand, it may be that professionals, as keepers of the gate, feel that parents are only capable of providing basic input. Some researchers have examined the opinions of professional staffing team members about the appropriate role for parents in planning. In a survey of 1,372 professional persons who were involved in staffing (planning) sessions, Yoshida, Fenton, Kaufman, and Maxwell (1978) found that the majority of them felt parents could only participate by gathering and presenting information to the committee. Yoshida and Gottlieb (1977) referred to this role as "information giving" and considered it rather minimal. Yoshida et al. (1978) found that less than 50% of their respondents felt that parents should be involved in others areas including reviewing educational progress (41%), reviewing the appropriateness of educational programs (37%), judging program alternatives (34%), and finalizing decisions (26%).

Additional research by Gilliam (1979) and Gilliam and Coleman (1981) is pertinent. In these studies, professionals were asked to rank order the status, importance, and contribution of different persons, including parents, made to IEP meetings. The subjects were asked to report their perceptions *prior* to the meetings and then *after* the meetings. On all variables, parents were perceived as being quite important before the meeting began. When it was over, however, the professionals' opinions changed and the ranking of parent significance and participation dropped significantly. Why did this happen? Perhaps because the parents actually contributed little to the staffing (Gilliam & Coleman, 1981). In comparison to the professionals, it may be that parents simply did not have the technical sophistication to make much of a contribution.

Involvement in Teaching

Parents of mentally retarded children are important teachers of their children. It can safely be assumed that many of the skills developed by retarded children can be directly attributed to the dedicated efforts of their mothers and fathers. It can also be assumed that parents of retarded children have more difficulty in teaching their children than do those of nonretarded children. This is simply because of the learning limitations inherent in mental retardation. It does not mean, however, that these parents' attempts are any less or that they are not meaningful for the child. It does mean that on some occasions, parents might seek help in developing their teaching skills and become more formalized and structured in their approaches. In these situations, parents will often attempt to learn from professionals how to better instruct their child and will usually try to coordinate their activities with the professionals.

One of the best examples of this type of coordination has been reported in some preschool programs for retarded children carried out at least partially in the home (Bricker & Bricker, 1976; Shearer & Shearer, 1976). Shearer and Shearer listed several advantages of this model. These could be applied to any home instructional program for mentally retarded children. They are as follows:

1. Since learning occurs in the natural environment, there is no problem in transferring learned skills.
2. Teaching at home allows the teacher (the parent) to have direct and constant access to behavior as it occurs. This means it can be more readily modified.
3. There is a better chance that learned behavior will be maintained and will generalize.
4. Home teaching means there is a greater chance for the entire family to participate in the teaching process.
5. There is no limit on the number or types of behavior that might occur, again improving chances for modifiability.
6. Parents with training experience will be able to deal with new behaviors as they occur.
7. Home training allows for the epitome of individualized instruction. (Shearer and Shearer, 1976)

If parents are to provide instruction in their home, it will be best for them and their children if they coordinate their efforts with school personnel. Sandler and Coren (1981) reported an integrated school and home training program in which parents participated in sessions and learned to model the teachers' instructional activities. The parents would observe the teachers, work with their child, and then receive feedback on their techniques. The large majority of parents felt the training program was extremely beneficial. In a later report, Sandler, Coren, and Thurman (1983) found that not only did mothers increase their knowledge of training techniques, but some improved their general interactions with their children. They also found a positive correlation to exist between the mother's attitudes and the gains made by the child as a result of the training.

Improving Parental Involvement

No doubt parents of retarded children in the large majority of instances have their child's interest in mind. We cannot expect all of them to be superparents, superteachers, and superpeople. We must keep in mind also, however, that the more and better their involvement with their children, the better the children will survive as individuals in a large society. Thus if anything can be done to improve parental involvement to whatever personal limits are possible, it should be done. Perhaps some affirmative action on the part of professionals would be helpful. Several suggestions have been made.

Strenecky, McLaughlin, and Edge (1979) advised schools to be clear in explaining problems and plans of action to parents. They suggested that parents should be made aware of not just test results, but the types of tests given and the reasons for the tests. They also suggested that structured learning activities be provided for parents who wish to implement formal teaching programs.

Goldstein and Turnbull (1982) advocated that efforts be made to increase the quantity and quality of parent involvement in IEP meetings. Their research revealed two strategies that were effective in improving participation. They included sending premeeting questions about the child to parents and having a counselor serve as a parent advocate during the meeting. Both strategies were reported to increase the parents' involvement.

Porcella (1980) described a program for severely and profoundly handicapped children that offered parents a "Request for Home Services" menu. From this menu, parents could select whatever service they needed: behavior management training, specific skill training, borrowing equipment or toys, books, legal rights information, and so on. According to Porcella, the most successful home training programs were those that were easy to conduct, could be worked into a routine, could be modeled for the parent, were suggested *by* the parent, and were reinforced by the school.

Regarding parent-teacher interactions, Mattson (1977) suggested that teachers collect as much information from the child's file as possible in order to be sensitive to possible parent or home problems. Any school meetings or home visits should be planned ahead and arranged at a time convenient for the parent or, preferably, both parents. He also suggested that time be spent establishing rapport and that technical jargon be avoided. Finally, teachers should always find something positive about the child to talk about with the parents. This may influence them to meet again.

Conclusion

We have reached a point in the history of services for mentally retarded individuals when the significance of what parents can contribute has been recognized. We have given the parents the right to participate in the planning of their child's educational needs albeit their participation is sometimes limited. Sometimes they choose limited involvement; sometimes it is all that is allowed. The former may be understandable; the latter should be challenged.

If we were to consider the needs and wants of parents of retarded persons to the same degree that we concern ourselves with the welfare of their children, both groups would probably benefit greatly. Sometimes the retarded child is but one difficulty in a host of problems faced by their parents. As Bricker and Casuso (1979) pointed out:

> ... other family needs must often be met before parents are able to learn to apply educational intervention strategies. (p. 109)

We have been teaching and working with retarded individuals for almost 200 years since Itard undertook his attempts. We have seriously involved their parents in our programs for only about ten of those years. Subsequent progress can certainly be improved if we continue to seek ways to facilitate parent involvement to whatever degree is possible.

STUDY QUESTIONS

1. How have professionals modified their view of parents of retarded children in recent years?
2. List and discuss some of the emotional reactions that may be initially experienced by parents of mentally retarded children. What "stages" of emotional development might a parent experience?
3. What concerns have parents expressed about deinstitutionalization?
4. What specific kinds of problems have parents expressed about raising a retarded child in the home? What can be done to help alleviate these problems?

5. Describe some of the elements that might characterize a "good" home for raising a retarded child.

6. Why is counseling important for some parents? What forms of counseling can be used? What are some of the guidelines that should be followed when counseling parents of retarded children?

7. Why should parents be included in their child's educational program?

8. In what ways can parents be involved in the educational program of their retarded child? What may influence their degree of involvement?

9. What are some possible tactics that might be used to increase parental involvement?

References

ABRAMOWICZ, H. & RICHARDSON, S. (1975). Epidemiology of severe mental retardation in children: Community studies. *American Journal of Mental Deficiency, 80*, 18–39.

ABRAMSON, S. F. & WUNDERLICH, R. A. (1972). Dental hygiene training for retardates: An application of behavioral techniques. *Mental Retardation, 10* (3), 6–8.

ABROMS, K. I. & BENNETT, J. W. (1980). Current genetic and demographic findings in Down's syndrome: How are they presented in college textbooks on exceptionality? *Mental Retardation, 18*, 101–107.

ABROMS, K. I. & BENNETT, J. W. (1983). Current findings in Down's syndrome. *Exceptional Children, 49*, 449–450.

ABT ASSOCIATES, (1974). *Assessment of selected resources for severely handicapped children and youth: Vol. 1: A state of the art paper.* Cambridge, Massachusetts: Abt Associates, Inc., (Eric Document Reproduction Service No. ED 134 614).

ACKERMAN, J. N. (1973). *Operant Conditioning Principles for the Classroom Teacher.* Glenview, IL: Scott-Foresman.

ADAMS, G. F. TALLON, R. J. & ALCORN, D. A. (1982). Attitudes toward the sexuality of mentally retarded and nonretarded persons. *Education and Training of the Mentally Retarded, 17*, 307–312.

AGRAN, M. & MARTIN, J. E. (1982). Use of psychotropic drugs by mentally retarded adults in community programs. *Journal of the Association for the Severely Handicapped, 7* (4), 54–59.

AIELLO, B. (1976). Especially for special educators—a sense of our own history. *Exceptional Children, 42*, 244–252.

ALGOZZINE, B., CHRISTIANSON, S. & YSSELDYKE, J. (1982). Probabilities associated with the referral and placement process. *Teacher Education and Special Education, 5* (3), 19–23.

ALLEN, G. (1958). Patterns of discovery in the genetics of mental deficiency. *American Journal of Mental Deficiency, 62*, 840–849.

ALLEY, G. & FOSTER, C. (1978). Nondiscriminatory testing of minority and exceptional children. *Focus on Exceptional Children, 9*(8), 1–14.

ALLINGTON, R. L. (1980). Word frequency and contextual richness on word identification of educable mentally retarded children. *Education and Training of the Mentally Retarded, 15*, 118–121.

ALOIA, G. F. (1975). Effects of physical stigmata and labels on judgments of subnormality by preservice teachers. *Mental Retardation, 13*(6), 17–21.

ALOIA, G. F., MAXWELL, J. A., & ALOIA, S. D. (1981). Influence of a child's race and the EMR label on initial impressions of regular classroom teachers. *American Journal of Mental Deficiency, 85,* 619–623.

ALPERN, G. D. & BOLL, T. J. (Eds.) (1971). *Education and care of moderately and severely retarded children.* Seattle, Washington: Special Child Publications.

AMERICAN PSYCHIATRIC ASSOCIATION. (1980). *Diagnostic and statistical manual of mental disorders* (3rd ed.) (DMS-III). Washington, D. C.: Author.

ANDERSON, E. M. & SPAIN, B. (1977). *The child with spina bifida.* London: Methuen.

ANDERSON, R. M., ZIA, B., SPRINGFIELD, H. L. & GREER, J. G. (1977). Educational media and materials for the handicapped. *Education and Training of the Mentally Retarded, 12,* 226–234.

APPEL, M. A. & TISDALL, W. J. (1968). Factors differentiating institutionalized from noninstitutionalized referred retardates. *American Journal of Mental Deficiency, 73,* 424–432.

ASHCROFT, S. C. (1977). Learning resources in special education: the quiet evolution. *Education and Training of the Mentally Retarded, 12,* 132–136.

AVIS, D. W. (1978). Deinstitutionalization jet lag. In A. P. Turnbull & H. R. Turnbull (Eds.). *Parents speak out: Views from the other side of the two-way mirror.* Columbus, Ohio: Charles E. Merrill.

AXELROD, S. (1977). *Behavior Modification for the Classroom Teacher.* New York: McGraw-Hill.

AYLLON, T., GARBER, S. & PISOR, K. (1976). Reducing time limits: A means to increase behavior of retardates. *Journal of Applied Behavior Analysis, 9,* 247–252.

AZRIN, N. H. & ARMSTRONG, P. M. (1973). The "mini-meal"—a method for teaching eating skills to the profoundly retarded. *Mental Retardation, 11*(1), 9–13.

AZRIN, N. H. & FOXX, R. M. (1971). A rapid method of toilet training the institutionalized retarded. *Journal of Applied Behavior Analysis, 4,* 89–99.

AZRIN, N. H., SCHAEFFER, R. M. & WESOLOWSKI, M. D. (1976). A rapid method for teaching profoundly retarded persons to dress by a reinforcement-guidance method. *Mental Retardation, 14*(6), 29–33.

AZRIN, N. H., SNEED, T. J. & FOXX, R. M. (1974). Dry bed training: Rapid elimination of childhood enuresis. *Behavior Research and Therapy, 12,* 147–156.

BAER, D. & GUESS, D. (1973). Teaching productive noun suffixes to severely retarded children. *American Journal of Mental Deficiency, 77,* 498–505.

BAILEY, J. S. (1981). Wanted: A rational search for the limiting conditions of habilitation in the retarded. *Analysis and Intervention in Developmental Disabilities, 1,* 45–52.

BAILEY, J. & MEYERSON, L. (1976). Vibration as a reinforcer with a profoundly retarded child. *Journal of Applied Behavior Analysis, 2,* 135–137.

BAKAN, R. (1970). Malnutrition and learning. *Phi Delta Kappan, 47,* 527–530.

BAKER, B. L., SELTZER, G. B. & SELTZER, M. M. (1974). *As close as possible.* Cambridge, Mass.: Harvard University, Behavioral Education Projects.

BAKER, B. L., HEIFETZ, L. J. & MURPHY, D. M. (1980). Behavioral training for parents of mentally retarded children: one-year follow-up. *American Journal of Mental Deficiency, 85,* 31–38.

BAKER, D. (1979). Severely handicapped: Toward an inclusive definition. *AAESPH Review, 4*(1), 52–65.

BALLA, D. (1976). Relationship of institutional size to quality of care: A review of the literature. *American Journal of Mental Deficiency, 81,* 117–124.

BALLA, D., BUTTERFIELD, E. C. & ZIGLER, E. (1974). Effects of institutionalization on retarded children: A longitudinal cross-institutional investigation. *American Journal of Mental Deficiency, 78,* 530–549.

BALLA, D. & ZIGLER, E. (1971). Luria's verbal deficiency theory of mental retardation and performance on sameness, symmetry, and opposition tasks: A critique. *American Journal of Mental Deficiency, 75,* 400–413.

BALLA, D. & ZIGLER, E. (1979). Personality development in retarded persons. In N. R. Ellis (Ed.). *Handbook of mental deficiency: psychological theory and research* (2nd ed.). Hillsdale, New Jersey: Lawrence Erlbaum Associates.

BALLARD, M., CORMAN, L., GOTTLIEB, J., & KAUFMAN, M. J. (1977). Improving the social status of mainstreamed retarded children. *Journal of Educational Psychology, 69,* 605–611.

BALTHAZAR, E. E. (1971). *Balthazar scales of adaptive behavior—I: Scales for functional independence.* Champaign, Illinois: Research Press.

BANDURA, A. (1971). Analysis of modeling processes. In A. Bandura (Ed.). *Psychological modeling: Conflicting theories.* Chicago: Aldine-Atherton.

BANK-MIKKELSON, N. E. (1969). A metropolitan area in Denmark: Copenhagen. In R. B. Kugel & W. Wolfensberger (Eds.), *Changing patterns in residential services for the mentally retarded.* Washington, D. C.: President's Committee on Mental Retardation.

BARLETT, R. H. (1977). Politics, litigation and mainstreaming: Special education's demise? *Mental Retardation, 15* (1), 24–26.

BARNES, L. & KRASNOFF, A. (1973). Medical and psychological factors pertinent to the rehabilitation of the epileptic. In A. B. Cobb (Ed.). *Medical and psychological aspects of disability.* Springfield, Illinois: Charles C Thomas.

BAROFF, G. S. (1982). Predicting the prevalence of mental retardation in individual catchment areas. *Mental Retardation, 20,* 133–135.

BARSCH, R. (1965). *A movigenic curriculum. Madison: Wisconsin State Department of Education.*

BATES, P. (1980). The effectiveness of interpersonal skills training on the social skill acquisition of moderately and mildly retarded adults. *Journal of Applied Behavior Analysis, 13,* 237–248.

BATES, P., RENZAGLIA, A. & CLEES, T. (1980). Improving the work performance of severely/profoundly retarded young adults: The use of a changing criterion procedural design. *Education and Training of the Mentally Retarded, 15,* 95–104.

BATSHAW, M. L. & PERRET, Y. M. (1981). *Children with handicaps: A medical primer.* Baltimore: Paul H. Brookes Publishing Co., Inc.

BAUMEISTER, A. A. (1970). The American residential institution: Its history and character. In A. A. Baumeister & E. Butterfield (Eds.). *Residential facilities for the mentally retarded.* Chicago: Aldine Publishing Company.

BAUMEISTER, A. A. (1981). The right to habilitation: What does it mean? *Analysis and Intervention in Developmental Disabilities, 1,* 61–74.

BAUMEISTER, A. A. & FOREHAND, R. (1973). Stereotyped acts. In N. R. Ellis (Ed.). *International review of research in mental retardation* (Vol. 6). New York: Academic Press.

BAUMEISTER, A. A. & MUMA, J. (1975). On defining mental retardation. *Journal of Special Education, 9*(3), 293–306.

BAUMEISTER, A. A. & ROLLINGS, J. P. (1976). Self-injurious behavior. In N. R. Ellis (Ed.). *International review of research in mental retardation* (Vol. 8). New York: Academic Press.

BAUMGART, D., BROWN, L., PUMPIAN, I., NISBET, J., FORD, A., SWEET, M., MESSINA, R. & SCHROEDER, J. (1982). Principle of partial participation and individualized adaptions in educational programs for severely handicapped students. *The Journal of the Association for the Severely Handicapped, 7*(2), 17–27.

BAUMGARTNER, B. B. (1960). *Helping the Trainable Mentally Retarded Child.* New York: Columbia University, Teachers College Press.

BAYLEY, N. (1969). *Bayley scales of infant development: Manual.* New York: The Psychological Corporation.

BECKER, R. L. (1973). Vocational choice: An inventory approach. *Education and Training of the Mentally Retarded, 8,* 128–136.

BECKER, W., ENGELMANN, S. & THOMAS, D. (1971). *Teaching: A course in applied psychology.* Chicago: Science Research Associates.

BECKMAN BRINDLEY, S. & TAVORMINA, J. B. (1978). Normalization: A new look. *Education and Training of the Mentally Retarded, 13,* 66–68.

BEIER, D. C. (1964). Behavioral disturbances in the mentally retarded. In H. A. Stevens & R. Heber (Eds.). *Mental retardation.* Chicago: University of Chicago Press.

BELLAMY, T. & BROWN, L. (1972). A sequential procedure for teaching addition skills to trainable retarded students. *Training School Bulletin, 69* (1), 31–44.

BELLAMY, T. & BUTTARS, K. (1975). Teaching trainable level retarded students to count money: toward personal independence through academic instruction. *Education and Training of the Mentally Retarded, 10,* 18–26.

BELLAMY, G. T., HORNER, R. H., INMAN, D. T. (1979). *Vocational habilitation of severely retarded adults.* Baltimore: University Park Press.

BELLAMY, G. T., PETERSON, L. & CLOSE, D. (1975). Habilitation of the severely and profoundly retarded: Illustrations of competence. *Education and Training of the Mentally Retarded, 10,* 174–186.

BELLAMY, G. T., SHEEHAN, M. R., HORNER, R. H. & BOLES, S. M. (1980). Community programs for severely handicapped adults: An analysis. *Journal of the Association for the Severely Handicapped, 5*(4), 307–324.

BELMONT, J. M. (1971). Medical-behavioral research in retardation. In N. R. Ellis (Ed.). *International review of research in mental retardation* (Vol. 5). New York: Academic Press.

BELMONT, J. M. & BUTTERFIELD, E. C. (1977). The instructional approach to developmental cognitive research. In R. V. Kail & J. W. Hagen (Eds.). *Perspectives on the development of memory and cognition.* Hillsdale, N. J.: Lawrence Erlbaum Associates.

BENSBERG, G. L. (Ed.). (1965). *Teaching the mentally retarded: A handbook for ward personnel.* Atlanta, GA: Southern Regional Education Board.

BEREITER, C. & ENGELMANN, S. (1966). *Teaching Disadvantaged Children in the Preschool.* Englewood Cliffs, New Jersey: Prentice-Hall.

BERKOWITZ, B. P., & GRAZIANO, A. M. (1972). Training parents as behavior therapists: A review. *Behavior Research and Therapy, 10,* 297–317.

BERKOWITZ, S., SHERRY, P. J. & DAVIS, B. A. (1971). Teaching self-feeding skills to retardates using reinforcement and fading procedures. *Behavior Therapy, 2,* 62–67.

BERKSON, G. (1963). Psychophysiological studies in mental deficiency. In N. R. Ellis (Ed.). *Handbook of mental deficiency: Psychological theory and research.* New York: McGraw-Hill.

BERNSTEIN, B. (1961). Social structure, language, and learning. *Educational Research, 3,* 163–176.

BEST-SIGFORD, B., BRUININKS, R. H., LAKIN, K. C., HILL, B. K. & HEAL, L. W. (1982). Resident release patterns in a national sample of public residential facilities. *American Journal of Mental Deficiency, 87,* 130–140.

BIALER, I. (1960). *Conceptualization of success and failure in mentally retarded and normal children.* Ann Arbor, Michigan: University Microfilms.

BIJOU, S. W. (1963). Theory and research in mental (developmental) retardation. *The Psychological Record, 13,* 95–110.

BIJOU, S. W., BIRNBRAUER, J. S., KIDDER, J. D. & TAGUE, C. (1966). Programmed instruction as an approach to the teaching of reading, writing, and arithmetic to retarded children. *Psychological Record, 16,* 505–522.

BILLINGSLEY, F. F. & NEAFSEY, S. S. (1978). Curriculum/training guides: A survey of content and evaluation procedures. *AAESPH Review, 3,* 42–57.

BINET, A. & SIMON, T. (1912). *A method for measuring the development of intelligence in young children.* Translated by C. H. Town. Lincoln, Illinois: The Courier Company.

BIRCH, H., RICHARDSON, S., BAIRD, D., HOROBIN, G., & ILLSLEY, R. (1970). *Mental subnormality in the community, a clinical and epidemiologic study.* Baltimore, Maryland: Williams & Wilkens.

BIRENBAUM, A. & RE, M. A. (1979). Resettling mentally retarded adults in the community—almost four years later. *American Journal of Mental Deficiency, 83,* 323–329.

BLACKARD, M. K. & BARSH, E. T. (1982). Parents' and professionals' perceptions of the handicapped child's impact on the family. *Journal of the Association of the Severely Handicapped, 7*(2), 62–70.

BLACKHURST, A. E. (1977). Competency-based special education personnel preparation. In R. D. Kneedler & S. G. Tarver (Eds.). *Changing perspectives in special education.* Columbus, Ohio: Chas. E. Merrill.

BLATT, B. (1979). A drastically different analysis. *Mental Retardation, 17,* 303–306.

BLATT, B. (1960). Some persistently recurring assumptions concerning the mentally subnormal. *Training School Bulletin, 57,* 48–59.

BLATT, B., BOGDAN, R., BIKLEN, D. & TAYLOR, S. (1977). From institution to community: A conversion model. In E. Sontag, J. Smith & N. Certo (Eds.). *Educational programming for the severely and profoundly handicapped.* Reston, Virginia: Division on Mental Retardation, The Council for Exceptional Children.

BLATT, B. & KAPLAN, F. (1966). *Christmas in purgatory.* Boston: Allyn & Bacon.

BLOOM, B. S. (1964). *Stability and chance in human characteristics.* New York: John Wiley & Sons.

BLOUNT, W. R. (1970). Retardates, normals, and U.S. moneys: Knowledge and preference. *American Journal of Mental Deficiency, 74,* 548–552.

BOGDAN, R. (1980). What does it mean when a person says "I am not retarded"? *Education and Training of the Mentally Retarded. 15*(1), 74–79.

BOGDAN, R. & TAYLOR, S. (1976). The judged, not the judges—An insider's view of mental retardation. *American Psychologist, 31*(1), 47–52.

BORAKOVE, L. S. & CUVO, A. J. (1976). Facilitative effects of coin displacement on teaching coin summation to mentally retarded adolescents. *American Journal of Mental Deficiency, 81,* 350–356.

BORING, E. (1950). *A history of experimental psychology.* New York: Appleton-Century-Crofts, Inc.

BOSTWICK, D. H. & FOSS, G. (1981). Obtaining consumer input: two strategies for identifying and ranking the problems of mentally retarded young adults. *Education and Training of the Mentally Retarded, 16,* 207–212.

BRADFIELD, H. R., BROWN, J., KAPLAN, P., RICKERT, E., & STANNARD, R. (1973). The special child in the regular classroom. *Exceptional Children, 39,* 384–390.

BREBNER, A., HALLWORTH, H. J. & BROWN, R. I. (1977). Computer-assisted instruction programs and terminals for the mentally retarded. In P. Mittler (Ed.). *Research to practice in mental retardation (Vol. II): Education and Training.* Baltimore: University Park Press.

BRICKER, D., BRICKER, W., IACINO, R. & DENNISON, L. (1976). Intervention strategies for the severely and profoundly handicapped child. In N. G. Haring & L. J. Brown (Eds.). *Teaching the severely handicapped* (Vol. I). New York: Grune & Stratton.

BRICKER, W. A. & BRICKER, D. D. (1976). The infant, toddler, and preschool research and intervention project. In T. D. Tjossein (Ed.). *Intervention Strategies for High Risk Infants and Young Children.* Baltimore: University Park Press.

BRICKER, D. & CASUSO, V. (1976). Family involvement: A critical component of early intervention. *Exceptional Children, 46,* 108–116.

BROLIN, D. E. (1977). Career development: A national priority. *Education and Training of the Mentally Retarded, 12,* 154–156.

BROLIN, D. E. (1973). Career education needs of secondary educable students. *Exceptional Children, 39,* 619–624.

BROLIN, D. (1972). Value of rehabilitation services and correlates of vocational success with the mentally retarded. *American Journal of Mental Deficiency, 76,* 644–651.

BROLIN, D. E. (1976). *Vocational Preparation of Retarded Citizens.* Columbus, Ohio: Charles E. Merrill.

BROLIN, D., CEGELKA, P., JACKSON, S. & WROBEL, C. (1977). *Official policy of the Council for Exceptional Children as legislated by the 1978 CEC Delegate Assembly.* Reston, Virginia: Council for Exceptional Children.

BROLIN, D. E. & D'ALONZO, B. J. (1979). Critical issues in career education for handicapped students. *Exceptional Children, 45,* 246–253.

BROLIN, D., DURAND, R., KROMER, K. & MULLER, P. (1975). Past-school adjustment of Educable Retarded Students. *Education and Training of the Mentally Retarded, 10*, 144–149.

BROLIN, D. E. & KOKASKA, C. J. (1979). *Career education for handicapped children and youth.* Columbus, Ohio: Chas. E. Merrill.

BROLIN, J. C. & BROLIN, D. E. (1979). Vocational education for special students. In D. Cullinan & M. Epstein (Eds.). *Special education for adolescents: Issues and perspectives.* Columbus, Ohio. Charles E. Merrill.

BRONFENBRENNER, U. (1976). Is early intervention effective? Facts and principles of early intervention: A summary. In A. M. Clarke and A. D. B. Clarke (Eds.). *Early experience: Myth and evidence.* New York: The Free Press.

BROOME, K. & WAMBOLD, C. L. (1977). Teaching basic math facts to EMR children through individual and small group instruction, pupil teaming, contingency contracting, and learning center activities. *Education and Training of the Mentally Retarded, 12*, 120–124.

BROWN, A. L. (1974). The role of strategic behavior in retardate memory. In N. R. Ellis (Ed.). *International review of research in mental retardation* (Vol. 7) New York: Academic Press.

BROWN, L. (1973). Instructional programs for trainable-level retarded students. In L. Mann & D. A. Sabatino (Eds.). *The first review of research of special education* (Vol. 2). Philadelphia: JSE Press.

BROWN, L., BELLAMY, T. & GADBERRY, E. (1971). A procedure for the development and measurement of rudimentary quantitative concepts in low functioning trainable students. *Training School Bulletin, 68*, 178–185.

BROWN, L., BRANSTON, M. B., HAMRE-NIETUPSKI, S., PUMPIAN, I., CERTO, N. & GRUENEWALD, L. (1979). A strategy for developing chronological age appropriate and functional curricular content for severely handicapped adolescents and young adults. *Journal of Special Education, 13*, 81–90.

BROWN, L., BRANSTON-McCLEAN, M., BAUMGART, D., VINCENT, L, FALVEY, M. & SCHROEDER, J. (1979). Utilizing the characteristics of current and subsequent least restrictive environments in the development of curricular content for severely handicapped students. *AAESPH Review, 4*(4), 407–424.

BROWN, L., FALVEY, M., VINCENT, L., KAYE, N., JOHNSON, F., FERRARA-PARISH, P. & GRUENEWALD, L. (1980). Strategies for generating comprehensive, longitudinal, and chronological-age-appropriate individualized educational programs for adolescent and young-adult severely handicapped students. *Journal of Special Education, 14*, 199–215.

BROWN, L., HERMANSON, J., KLEMME, H., HAUBRICH, P. & ORA, J. (1970). Using behavior modification principles to teach sight vocabulary. *Teaching Exceptional Children, 2*, 120–128.

BROWN, L., HUPPLER, B., PIERCE, L., YORK, B. & SONTAG, E. (1972). Teaching trainable level retarded students to read unconjugated action verbs. *Journal of Special Education, 6*, 237–246.

BROWN, L. & PERLMUTTER, L. (1971). Teaching functional reading to trainable level retarded students. *Education and Training of the Mentally Retarded, 6*, 74–84.

BROWN, L., PUMPIAN, I., BAUMGART, D., VANDEVENTER, P., FORD, A., NISBET, J., SCHROEDER, J. & GRUNEWALD, L. (1981). Longitudinal transition plans in programs for severely handicapped students. *Exceptional Children, 47*, 624–630.

BRUENING, S. E. & DAVIDSON, N. A. (1981). Effects of psychotropic drugs on intelligence test performance of institutionalized mentally retarded adults. *American Journal of Mental Deficiency, 85*, 575–579.

BRUININKS, R. H. (1974). Physical and motor development of retarded persons. In N. R. Ellis (Ed.). *International review of research in mental retardation* (Vol. 7). New York: Academic Press.

BRUININKS, R. H., HAUBER, F. A. & KUDLA, J. J. (1980). National Survey of community residential facilities: A profile of facilities and residents in 1977. *American Journal of Mental Deficiency, 84*, 470–478.

BRUININKS, R. H., RYNDERS, J. E., & GROSS, J. C. (1974). Social acceptance of mildly retarded pupils in resource rooms and regular classes. *American Journal of Mental Deficiency, 78*, 377–383.

BUDOFF, M. (1972). Providing special education without special classes. *Journal of School Psychology, 10*, 199–205.

BUDOFF, M., & GOTTLIEB, J. (1976). Special class students mainstreamed: A study of an aptitude (learning potential) X treatment interaction. *American Journal of Mental Deficiency, 81*, 1–11.

BUDOFF, M. & HUTTEN, L. (1982). Microcomputers in special education: Promises and pitfalls. *Exceptional Children, 49*, 123–128.

BUDOFF, M. & SIPERSTEIN, G. N. (1978). Low-income children's attitudes toward mentally retarded children. Effects of labeling and academic behavior. *American Journal of Mental Deficiency, 82*, 474–479.

BUDOFF, M., SIPERSTEIN, G. & CONANT, S. (1979). Children's knowledge of mental retardation. *Education and Training of the Mentally Retarded, 14*(4), 277–281.

BURTON, T. A. (1974). Education for trainables: An impossible dream? *Mental Retardation, 12*, 45–46.

BURTON, T. (1981). Deciding what to teach the severely/profoundly retarded student: A teacher responsibility. *Education and Training of the Mentally Retarded, 16*, 74–79.

BUTLER, E. W. & BJAANES, A. T. (1977). A typology of community care facilities and differential normalization outcomes. In P. Mittler (Ed.). *Research to practice in mental retardation* (Vol. I): *Care and Intervention.* Baltimore: University Park Press.

BUTTERFIELD, E. C. (1969). Basic facts about public residential facilities for the mentally retarded. In R. B. Kugel & W. Wolfensberger (Eds.). *Changing patterns in residential services for the mentally retarded.* Washington, D. C.: President's Committee on Mental Retardation.

BUTTERFIELD, E. C. & ZIGLER, E. (1965). The influence of differing institutional social climates on the effectiveness of social reinforcement in the mentally retarded. *American Journal of Mental Deficiency, 70,* 48–56.

BYRNES, M. M. & SPITZ, H. H. (1977). Performance of retarded adolescents and nonretarded children on the Tower of Hanoi problem. *American Journal of Mental Deficiency, 81,* 561–569.

CAIN, L. F. (1976). Parent groups: Their role in a better life for the handicapped. *Exceptional Children, 42,* 432–437.

CAIN, L. F., & LEVINE, S. (1963). Effects of community and institutional school programs on trainable mentally retarded children. *CEC Research Monograph,* No. B–1.

CALDWELL, B. (1970). The rationale for early intervention. *Exceptional Children, 36,* 717–727.

CAMPBELL, P. H., GREEN, K. M. & CARLSON, L. M. (1977). Approximating the norm through environmental and child-centered prosthetics and adaptive equipment. In E. Sontag, J. Smith & N. Certo (Eds.). *Educational programming for the severely and profoundly handicapped.* Reston, Virginia: Division on Mental Retardation, Council for Exceptional Children.

CAMPBELL, V., SMITH, R. & WOOL, R. (1982). Adaptive behavior scale differences in scores of mentally retarded individuals referred for institutionalization and those never referred. *American Journal of Mental Deficiency, 86,* 425–428.

CARPENTER, D. G. (1975a). Metabolic and transport anomalies. In C. H. Carter (Ed.). *Handbook of mental retardation syndromes* (3rd ed.). Springfield, Illinois: Charles C Thomas.

CARPENTER, D. G. (1975b). Teratogenesis. In C. H. Carter (Ed.) *Handbook of mental retardation syndromes* (3rd ed.), Springfield, Illinois: Charles C Thomas Publisher.

CARROLL, A. W. (1967). The effects of segregated and partially integrated school programs on self-concept and academic achievement of educable mentally retardates. *Exceptional Children, 34,* 93–99.

CARSRUD, A. L., CARSRUD, K. B., HENDERSON, O. P., ALISCH, C. J. & FOWLER, A. V. (1979). Effects of social and environmental change on institutionalized mentally retarded persons: The relocation syndrome reconsidered. *American Journal of Mental Deficiency, 84,* 266–272.

CARTER, C. H. (ED.) (1975). *Handbook of mental retardation syndromes* (3rd Ed.). Springfield, Illinois: Charles C Thomas.

CATTELL, P. (1972). *The Measurement of Intelligence in Infants and Young Children.* Revised 1960. New York: Johnston Reprint Corporation. (Revised from 1960 publication).

CAVALIER, A. R. & MCCARVER, R. B. (1981). *Wyatt v. Stickney* and mentally retarded individuals. *Mental Retardation, 19,* 209–214.

CEGELKA, W. J. (1978). Competencies of persons responsible for the classification of mentally retarded children. *Exceptional Children, 45,* 26–31.

CEGELKA, P. T. (1979). Career Education. In D. Cullinan & M. H. Epstein (Eds.). *Special education for adolescents: Issues and perspectives.* Columbus, Ohio: Charles E. Merrill.

CEGELKA, P. T. (1977). Exemplary projects and programs for the career development of retarded individuals. *Education and Training of the Mentally Retarded, 12,* 161–163.

CEGELKA, P. & CEGELKA, W. J. (1970). A review of the research: Reading and the educable mentally retarded. *Exceptional Children, 37,* 187–200.

CERTO, N., BROWN, L., BELMORE, K. & CROWNER, T. (1977). A review of secondary educational service delivery models for severely handicapped students in the Madison public schools. In E. Sontag, J. Smith, & N. Certo (Eds.). *Educational programming for the severely and profoundly handicapped.* Reston, Virginia: Division on Mental Retardation, The Council for Exceptional Children.

CHAFFIN, J. D., SPELLMAN, C. R., REGAN, C. E. & DAVISON, R. (1971). Two follow-up studies of former educable mentally retarded students from the Kansas work-study project. *Exceptional Children, 37,* 733–738.

CHAN, K. S. & RUEDA, R. (1979). Poverty and culture in education: Separate but equal. *Exceptional Children, 45,* 422–428.

CHILDS, R. E. (1979). A drastic change in curriculum for the educable mentally retarded child. *Mental Retardation, 17,* 299–301.

CHILDS, R. E. (1982). A study of the adaptive behavior of retarded children and the resultant effects of the use in the diagnosis of mental retardation. *Education and Training of the Mentally Retarded, 17,* 109–112.

CHRISTOPLOS, F. & RENZ, P. (1969). A critical examination of special education programs. *Journal of Special Education, 3,* 371–379.

CLARKE, A. D. B. & CLARKE, A. M. (1977). Prospects for prevention and amelioration of mental retardation. *American Journal of Mental Deficiency, 81,* 523–533.

CLARKE, A. M. & CLARKE, A. D. B. (Eds.). (1976). *Early experience: Myth and evidence.* New York. The Free Press.

CLAUSEN, J. (1962). Mental deficiency—development of a concept. *American Journal of Mental Deficiency, 71,* 727–745.

CLAUSEN, J. (1972). Quo vadis, AAMD? *Journal of Special Education, 6*(1). 51–61.

CLELAND, C. (1979). *The Profoundly Mentally Retarded.* Englewood Cliffs, N. J.: Prentice-Hall.

COCHRAN, W. E., SRAN, P. K. & VARANO, G. A. (1977). The relocation syndrome in mentally retarded individuals. *Mental Retardation, 15*(2), 10–12.

COHEN, H., CONROY, J. W., FRAZER, D. W., SNELBECKER, G. E. & SPREAT, S. (1977). Behavioral effects of interinstitutional relocation of mentally retarded residents. *American Journal of Mental Deficiency, 82,* 12–18.

COHEN, M., GROSS, P. & HARING, W. G. (1976). Developmental pinpoints. In N. G. Haring & L. J. Brown (Eds.). *Teaching the severely handicapped* (Vol. I). New York: Grune & Stratton.

COLE, M. & BRUNNER, J. S. (1971). Cultural differences and inferences about psychological processes. *American Psychologist, 26,* 867–876.

COLEMAN, A. E., AYOUB, M. M., & FRIEDRICH, D. W. (1976). Assessment of the physical work capacity of institutionalized mentally retarded males. *American Journal of Mental Deficiency, 80,* 629–635.

COLOMBATTO, J. J., ISETT, R. D., ROSZKOWSKI, M., SPREAT, S., D'ONOFRIO, A. & ALDERFER, R. (1982). Perspectives on deinstitutionalization: A survey of the members of the National Association of Superintendents of Public Residential Facilities for the Mentally Retarded. *Education and Training of the Mentally Retarded, 17,* 6–11.

CONNOLLY, J. M. (1975). The chromosome anomalies. In C. H. Carter (Ed.). *Handbook of mental retardation syndromes.* Springfield, Illinois: Charles C Thomas.

CORBETT, J. A., HARRIS, R. & ROBINSON, R. G. (1975). Epilepsy. In J. Wortis (Ed.). *Mental retardation and developmental disabilities*(Vol. VII). New York: Brunner/Mazel.

CORMAN, H. H. & ESCALONA, S. K. (1969). Stages of sensory-motor development: A replication study. *Merrill-Palmer Quarterly of Behavior and Development, 15,* 351–361.

CORMAN, L. & GOTTLIEB, J. (1978). Mainstreaming mentally retarded children: A review of research. In N. R. Ellis (Ed.). *International Review of Research in Mental Retardation* (Vol. 9). New York: Academic Press.

COUNCIL FOR EXCEPTIONAL CHILDREN. (1975). What is mainstreaming? *Exceptional Children, 42,* 174.

COURTNAGE, L. (1982). A survey of state policies on the use of medication in schools. *Exceptional Children, 49,* 75–77.

COVAL, T. E., GILHOOL, T. K. & LASKI, F. J. (1977). Rules and tactics in institutionalization proceedings for mentally retarded persons: The role of the courts in assuring access to service in the community. *Educational Training of the Mentally Retarded, 12,* 177–185.

CRAIN, E. J. (1980). Socioeconomic status of educable mentally retarded graduates of special education. *Education and Training of the Mentally Retarded, 15,* 90–94.

CRAWFORD, J. L., McMAHON, D. J., CONKLIN, G. S., GIORDANO, D., ALEXANDER, M. J. & KADYSZEWSKI, P. (1980). Assessing skilled functioning of mentally retarded persons. *Mental Retardation, 18,* 235–239.

CRAWLEY, S. B. & CHAN, K. S. (1982). Developmental changes in free-play behavior of mildly and moderately retarded preschool age children. *Education and Training of the Mentally Retarded, 17,* 234–239.

CROMWELL, R. L. (1963). A social learning approach to mental retardation. In N. R. Ellis (Ed.). *Handbook of mental deficiency: Psychological theory and research.* New York: McGraw-Hill.

CROMWELL, R. L. (1979). Personality evaluation. In A. A. Baumeister (Ed.), *Mental Retardation.* Chicago: Aldine.

CRONIS, T. G., SMITH, G. J. & FORGNONE, C. (1983). Mild mental retardation is not a mildly handicapping condition: Implications for a special curriculum. Manuscript submitted for publication.

CUVO, A. & CRONIN, K. (1979). Teaching mending skills to mentally retarded adolescents. *Journal of Applied Behavior Analysis, 12,* 401–406.

CUVO, A. J., JACOBI & SIPKO, R. (1981). Teaching laundry skills to mentally retarded students. *Education and Training of the Mentally Retarded, 16,* 54–64.

CUVO, A. J., LEAF, R. B. & BORAKOVE, L. S. (1978). Teaching janitorial skills to the mentally retarded: Acquisition, generalization, and maintenance. *Journal of Applied Behavior Analysis, 11,* 345–355.

D'AMELIO, D. (1971). *Severely retarded children: Wider horizons.* Columbus, Ohio: Charles E. Merrill Publishing Co.

DAS, J. P. (1973). Cultural deprivation and cognitive competence. In N. R. Ellis (Ed.). *International review of research in mental retardation* (Vol. 6). New York: Academic Press.

DAS, J. P. (1972). Patterns of cognitive ability in nonretarded and retarded children. *American Journal of Mental Deficiency, 77,* 6–12.

DAS, J. P. & CUMMINS, J. (1978). Academic performance and cognitive processes in EMR children. *American Journal of Mental Deficiency, 83,* 197–199.

DAS, J. P., KIRBY, J. & JARMAN, R. F. (1975). Simultaneous and successive synthesis: An alternative model for cognitive abilities. *Psychological Bulletin, 82,* 87–103.

DELP, H. A. & LORENZ, M. (1953). Follow-up study of 84 public school special class pupils with IQs below 50. *American Journal of Mental Deficiency, 58,* 175–182.

DEMAIN, G. C. & SILVERSTEIN, A. B. (1978). MA changes in institutionalized Down's syndrome persons: A semi-longitudinal approach. *American Journal of Mental Deficiency, 82,* 429–432.

DENHOFF, E. & ROBINAULT, I. P. (1960). *Cerebral palsy and related disorders—a developmental approach to dysfunction.* New York: McGraw-Hill.

DENNY, M. R. (1964). Research in learning and performance. In H. Stevens & R. Heber (Eds.). *Mental retardation: A review of research.* Chicago: University of Chicago Press.

DENNY, M. R. (1966). A theoretical analysis and its application to training the mentally retarded. In N. R. Ellis (Ed.). *International review of research in mental retardation* (Vol. 2). New York: Academic Press.

DENNY, M. R. & ADELMAN, H. M. (1955). Elicitation theory: I. An analysis of two typical learning situations. *Psychological Review, 62*, 290–296.

DENO, E. (1970). Special education as developmental capital. *Exceptional Children, 37*, 229–237.

DETTERMAN, D. K. (1979). Memory in the mentally retarded. In N. R. Ellis (Ed.), *Handbook of mental deficiency, Psychological theory and research* (2nd ed.). Hillsdale, New Jersey: Erlbaum.

DEUTSCH, C. P. (1964). Auditory discrimination and learning: Social factors. *Merrill-Palmer Quarterly, 10*, 177–296.

DEUTSCH, M. (1965). The role of social class in language development and cognition. *American Journal of Orthopsychiatry, 35*, 78–88.

DEVER, R. (1972). Linguistic aspects of the culturally disadvantaged child. In E. P. Trapp & P. Himelstein (Eds.). *Readings on the exceptional child* (2nd ed.) New York: Appleton-Century-Crofts.

DIBENEDETTO, T. A. (1976). Problems of the deaf-retarded: A review of the literature. *Education and Training of the Mentally Retarded, 11*, 164–171.

DINGER, J. C. (1961). Post-school adjustment of former educable retarded pupils. *Exceptional Children, 27*, 353–360.

DINGMAN, H. & TARJAN, G. (1960). Mental retardation and the normal distribution curve. *American Journal of Mental Deficiency, 64*, 991–994.

DOLL, E. A. (1936). *The Vineland social maturity scale: Revised condensed manual of directions.* Vineland, N. J.: The Training School.

DOLL, E. A. (1941). The essentials of an inclusive concept of mental deficiency. *American Journal of Mental Deficiency, 46*, 214–219.

DOLL, E. A. (1964). *Vineland Scale of Social Maturity.* Minneapolis: American Guidance Service.

DOLL, E. A. (1966). *Preschool Attainment Record.* Circle Pines, Minnesota: American Guidance Service.

DOMNIE, M. & BROWN, L. (1977). Teaching severely handicapped students reading skills requiring printed answers to who, what, and where questions. *Education and Training of the Mentally Retarded, 12*, 324–331.

DOOLITTLE, M. (1978). A mother probes impact of Down's child on her family. *Arise, 2*(3), 9–11.

DUFFEY, J. B. & FEDNER, M. L. (1978). Educational diagnosis with instructional use. *Exceptional Children, 44*, 246–251.

DUNLOP, K. H., STONEMAN, Z. & CANTRELL, M. L. (1980). Social interaction of exceptional and other children in a mainstreamed preschool class. *Exceptional Children, 47*, 132–141.

DUNN, L. M. (1956). A comparison of the reading processes of mentally retarded boys of the same mental age. In L. M. Dunn & R. J. Capobianco (Eds.). *Studies in the reading and arithmetic of mentally retarded boys.* Lafayette, Indiana: Child Development Publications.

DUNN, L. M. (1973). Children with mild general learning disabilities. In L. M. Dunn (Ed.). *Exceptional children in the schools: Special education in transition* (2nd ed.). New York: Holt, Rinehart & Winston.

DUNN, L. (1968). Special education for the mildly retarded—is much of it justifiable? *Exceptional Children, 35*(1), 5–24.

DUNN, L. M. (Ed.). (1973). *Exceptional children in the schools: Special education in transition* (2nd ed.). New York: Holt, Rinehart, and Winston.

DUPRAS, A. & TREMBLAY, R. (1976). Path analysis of parents conservatism toward sex education of their mentally retarded children. *American Journal of Mental Deficiency, 81*, 162–166.

DUSSAULT, H. H., COULOMBE, P., LABERGE, C., LETARTE, J., GUYDA, H. & KHOURY, K. (1975). Preliminary report on a mass screening program for neonatal hypothyroidism. *Journal of Pediatrics, 86*, 670–674.

DYBWAD, G. (1980). Avoiding misconceptions of mainstreaming, the least restrictive environment and normalization. *Exceptional Children, 47*, 85–88.

EDGAR, E., SULZBACHER, S., SWIFT, P. E., HARPER, C. T., BAKER, S. & ALEXANDER, B. (1975). An alternative to words and scores. The Washington State Cooperative Curriculum Project (WSCCP). *Education and Training of the Mentally Retarded, 10*, 259–261.

EDGERTON, R. B. (1967). *The cloak of competence: Stigma in the lives of the mentally retarded.* Berkeley: University of California Press.

EDGERTON, R. B. & BERCOVICI, S. M. (1976). The cloak of competence: Years later. *American Journal of Mental Deficiency, 80*, 485–497.

EDGERTON, R. B., EYMAN, R. K. & SILVERSTEIN, A. B. (1975). Mental retardation systems. In N. Hobbs (Ed.). *Issues in the classification of children* (Vol. 2). San Francisco: Jossey-Bass.

EDMONDSON, B., McCOMBS, K. & WISH, J. (1979). What retarded adults believe about sex. *American Journal of Mental Deficiency, 84*, 11–18.

EDMONDSON, B. & WISH, J. (1975). Sex knowledge and attitudes of moderately retarded males. *American Journal of Mental Deficiency, 80*, 172–179.

EDUCATION ADVOCATES COALITION. April 16, *Report by the Education Advocates Coalition on federal compliance activities to implement the Education for All Handicapped Children Act* (PL 94–142). April 16, 1980.

Education Daily, (1981 July). *14* (125).

Education of the Handicapped. (1981, May). Pennhurst ruling raises broader issues for handicapped law. 5–6.

ELLIS, D. (1979). Visual handicaps of mentally handicapped persons. *American Journal of Mental Deficiency, 83,* 497–511.

ELLIS, J. W. (1982). The Supreme Court and institutions: A comment on *Youngberg v. Romeo. Mental Retardation, 20,* 197–200.

ELLIS, N. R. (1969). A behavioral research strategy in mental retardation: Defense and critique. *American Journal of Mental Deficiency, 73,* 557–566.

ELLIS, N. R. (1970). Memory processes in retardates and normals. In N. R. Ellis (Ed.). *International review of research in mental retardation* (Vol. 4). New York: Academic Press.

ELLIS, N. R. (1981). On training the mentally retarded. *Analysis and Intervention in Developmental Disabilities, 1,* 99–108.

ELLIS, N. R. (1979). The Partlow case: A reply to Dr. Roos. *Law and Psychology Review, 5,* 15–49.

ELLIS, N. R. (1963). The stimulus trace and behavioral inadequacy. In N. R. Ellis (Ed.). *Handbook of mental deficiency: Psychological theory and research.* New York: McGraw-Hill.

ELLIS, N. R., BALLA, D., ESTES, O., WARREN, S. A., MEYERS, C. E., HOLLIS, J., ISAACSON, R. L., PALK, B. E. & SIEGEL, P. S. (1981). Common sense in the habilitation of mentally retarded persons: A reply to Menolascino and McGee. *Mental Retardation, 5,* 221–225.

ENTRIKIN, D., YORK, R. & BROWN, L. (1977). Teaching trainable level multiply handicapped students to use picture cues, context cues, and initial consonant sounds to determine the labels of unknown words. *AAESPH review, 2,* 169–190.

ERLENMEYER-KIMLING, L. & JARVIK, L. F. (1963). Genetics and intelligence: A review. *Science, 142,* 1477–1479.

EYMAN, R. K. & ARNDT, S. (1982). Life-span development of institutionalized and community-based mentally retarded residents. *American Journal of Mental Deficiency, 86,* 342–350.

EYMAN, R. K., BORTHWICK, S. A. & MILLER, C. (1981). Trends in maladaptive behavior of mentally retarded persons placed in community and institutional settings. *American Journal of Mental Deficiency, 85,* 473–477.

EYMAN, R. K., DEMAINE, G. C. & LEI, T. (1979). Relationship between community environments and resident changes in adaptive behavior: A path model. *American Journal of Mental Deficiency, 83,* 330–338.

EYMAN, R., DINGMAN, H. & SABACH, G. (1966). Association of characteristics of retarded patients and their families with speed of institutionalization. *American Journal of Mental Deficiency, 71,* 93–99.

EYMAN, R. K., O'CONNOR, G. O., TARJAN, G. & JUSTICE, R. S. (1972). Factors determining residential placement of mentally retarded children. *American Journal of Mental Deficiency, 76,* 692–698.

EYMAN, R. K., SILVERSTEIN, A. B., MCLAIN, R. & MILLER, C. (1977). Effects of residential settings on development. In P. Mittler (Ed.). *Research to practice in mental retardation (Vol. I): Care and intervention.* Baltimore: University Park Press.

FALBE-HANSEN, I. (1968). Congenital ocular anomalies in 800 mentally deficient patients. *Acta Ophthalmologica, 46,* 391–397.

FANCHER, R. (1979). *Pioneers in psychology.* New York: W. W. Norton & Co.

FARBER, B. (1959). Effects of a severely mentally retarded child on family integration. *Monographs of the Society for Research in Child Development, 24.*

FARBER, B. (1968). *Mental retardation: Its social context and social consequences.* Boston: Houghton-Mifflin.

FARBER, B. (1959). *Prevalence of exceptional children in Illinois in 1958.* Springfield, Illinois: Illinois Superintendent of Public Instruction.

FARBER, B., JENNE, W. & TOIGO, R. (1960). Family crisis and the decision to institutionalize the retarded child. *Monograph, Council for Exceptional Children.*

FEINGOLD, B. (1974). *Why Your Child is Hyperactive.* New York: Random House.

FERRARA, D. M. (1979). Attitudes of parents of mentally retarded children toward normalization activities. *American Journal of Mental Deficiency, 84,* 145–151.

FINKELSTEIN, N. W. & RAMEY, C. T. (1980). Information from birth certificates as a risk index for educational handicap. *American Journal of Mental Deficiency, 84,* 546–552.

FIORELLI, J. C. (1982). Community residential services during the 1980s. Challenges and future trends. *Journal of the Association of the Severely Handicapped, 7(4),* 14–18.

FISHER, M. A. & ZEAMAN, D. (1973). An attention-retention theory of retardate discrimination learning. In W. R. Ellis (Ed.). *International review of research in mental retardation* (Vol. 6). New York: Academic Press.

FISHER, M. A. & ZEAMAN, D. (1970). Growth and decline of retardate intelligence. In N. R. Ellis (Ed.). *International review of research in mental retardation* (Vol. 4). New York: Academic Press.

FLAVELL, J. (1963). *The developmental psychology of Jean Piaget.* Princeton, N. J.: Van Nostrand.

FOLEY, J. M. (1979). Effects of labeling and teacher behavior on children's attitudes. *American Journal of Mental Deficiency, 83,* 380–384.

FOLK, M. C. & CAMPBELL, J. (1978). Teaching functional reading to the TMR. *Education and Training of the Mentally Retarded, 13,* 322–326.

FOSTER, G. & KEECH, V. (1977). Teacher reactions to the label of educable mentally retarded. *Education and Training of the Mentally Retarded, 12,* 307–311.

FOTHERINGHAM, J. B., SKELTON, M. & HODDINOLT, B. A. (1971). *The retarded child and his family: The effects of home and institution.* Toronto, Ontario: Institute for Studies in Education.

FOX, R. & ROTATORI, A. F. (1982). Prevalence of obesity among mentally retarded adults. *American Journal of Mental Deficiency, 87,* 228–230.

FOX, R., SWITZKY, H., ROTATORI, A. F. & VITKUS, P. (1982). Successful weight loss techniques with mentally retarded children and youth. *Exceptional Children, 49,* 238–244.

FRANKEL, F. & SIMMONS, J. Q. (1976). Self-injurious behavior in schizophrenic and retarded children. *American Journal of Mental Deficiency, 80,* 512–522.

FRANKEL, M. G., HAPP, E. W. & SMITH, M. P. (1966). *Functional teaching of the mentally retarded.* Springfield, Illinois: Charles C Thomas.

FRANKENBURG, W. K. (1977). Early detection of children with handicapping conditions: Implications for educators. In B. M. Caldwell & D. J. Stedman (Eds.). *Infant education: A guide for helping handicapped children in the first three years.* New York: Walker & Co.

FRANKENBURG, W. K. & DODD, J. B. (1969). *Denver developmental screening test.* Denver: University of Colorado Medical Center.

FRANZINI, L. R., LITROWNIK, A. J. & MAGY, M. A. (1978). Immediate and delayed reward preferences of TMR adolescents. *American Journal of Mental Deficiency, 82,* 406–409.

FRANZINI, L. R., LITROWNIK, A. J. & MAGY, M. A. (1980). Training trainable mentally retarded adolescents in delay behavior. *Mental Retardation, 18,* 45–47.

FREDERICKS, H. D., BALDWIN, V. L., GROVE, D., RIGGS, C., FUREY, V. & MOORE, W. (1977). Curriculum for the severely handicapped. *Education and Training of the Mentally Retarded, 12,* 316–324.

FREEMAN, S. & ALGOZZINE, B. (1980). Social acceptability as a function of labels and assigned attributes. *American Journal of Mental Deficiency, 84,* 589–595.

FRIEDRICH, W. W. & FRIEDRICH, W. L. (1981). Psychosocial assets of parents of handicapped and nonhandicapped children. *American Journal of Mental Deficiency, 85,* 551–553.

GABLE, R. A., HENDRICKSON, J. M. & STRAIN, P. S. (1978). Assessment, modification, and generalization of social interaction among severely retarded, multihandicapped children. *Education and Training of the Mentally Retarded, 13,* 279–286.

GADOW, K. D. (1980). *Children on medication: A primer for school personnel.* Reston, Virginia: The Council for Exceptional Children.

GADOW, K. D. (1982). Problems with students on medication. *Exceptional Children, 49,* 20–27.

GADOW, K. D. & KALACHNIK, J. (1981). Prevalence and pattern of drug treatment for behavior and seizure disorders of TMR students. *American Journal of Mental Deficiency, 85,* 588–595.

GAMPEL, D. H., GOTTLIEB, J. & HARRISON, R. H. (1974). A comparison of the classroom behaviors of special class EMR, integrated EMR, low IQ and nonretarded children. *American Journal of Mental Deficiency, 79,* 16–21.

GARBER, H. & HEBER, R. (1973). *The Milwaukee Project: Early intervention as a technique to prevent mental retardation.* Storrs: University of Connecticut, Technical Paper.

GARBER, H. & HEBER, R. (1977). The Milwaukee Project: Indications of the effectiveness of early intervention in preventing mental retardation. In P. Mittler (Ed.). *Research to practice in mental retardation* (Vol. 1). *Care and Intervention.* Baltimore: University Park Press.

GARCIA, E., GUESS, D. & BYRNES, J. (1973). Development of syntax in a retarded girl using procedures of imitation, reinforcement, and modeling. *Journal of Applied Behavior Analysis, 6,* 299–310.

GARDNER, W. I. (1974). *Children with learning and behavior problems: A behavior management approach.* Boston: Allyn & Bacon.

GARFIELD, S. L. (1963). Abnormal behavior and mental deficiency. In N. R. Ellis (Ed.). *Handbook of mental deficiency: Psychological theory and research.* New York: McGraw-Hill.

GARFIELD, S. L. & WITTSON, C. (1960). Some reactions to the revised "Manual on Terminology and Classification in Mental Retardation." *American Journal of Mental Deficiency, 64,* 951–953.

GEIGER, W. L., BROWNSMITH, K. & FORGNONE, C. (1978). Differential importance of skills for TMR students as perceived by teachers. *Education and Training of the Mentally Retarded, 13,* 259–264.

GELOF, M. (1963). Comparison of systems of classification relating degree of retardation to measured intelligence. *American Journal of Mental Deficiency, 68,* 299–301.

GESSELL, A. & AMATRUDE, C. S. (1952). *Developmental diagnosis.* London: Cassell & Co., Ltd.

GICKLING, E. E. & THEOBALD, J. T. (1975). Mainstreaming: Affect or effect. *Journal of Special Education, 9,* 317–328.

GILLIAM, J. E. (1979). Contributions and status rankings of educational planning committee participants. *Exceptional Children, 45,* 466–468.

GILLIAM, J. E. & COLEMAN, M. C. (1981). Who influences IEP committee decisions? *Exceptional Children, 47,* 642–644.

GILLUNG, T. B. & RUCKER, C. N. (1977). Labels and teacher expectations. *Exceptional Children, 43,* 404–405.

GINSBURG, B. E. & LAUGHLIN, W. S. (1971). Race and intelligence, what do we really know? In R. Cancro (Ed.). *Intelligence: Genetic and environmental influences.* New York: Grune & Stratton.

GINSBURG, H. & OPPER, S. (1969). *Piaget's theory of intellectual development: An introduction.* Englewood Cliffs, N. J.: Prentice-Hall.

GIRARDEAU, F. L. (1971). Cultural-familial retardation. In N. R. Ellis (Ed.). *International review of research in mental retardation* (Vol. 5). New York: Academic Press.

GOLD, M. W. (1973). Research on the vocational habilitation of the retarded: The present, the future. In N. R. Ellis (Ed.). *International Review of Research in Mental Retardation* (Vol. 6). New York: Academic Press.

GOLD, M. W. (1974). Redundant cue removal in skill training for the retarded. *Education and Training of the Mentally Retarded, 9,* 5–8.

GOLD, M. W. (1976). Task analysis of a complex assembly task by the retarded blind. *Exceptional Children, 43,* 78–84.

GOLDBERG, I. & CRUICKSHANK, W. (1958). The trainable but noneducable: Whose responsibility? *National Education Association Journal, 47,* 622–623.

GOLDSTEIN, H. (1956). *Report number two on study projects for trainable mentally handicapped children.* Springfield, Illinois: Superintendent of Public Instruction.

GOLDSTEIN, H. (1964). Social and occupational adjustment. In H. A. Stevens & R. Heber (Eds.). *Mental retardation: A review of research.* Chicago: University of Chicago Press.

GOLDSTEIN, S., STRICKLAND, B., TURNBULL, A. P. & CURRY, L. (1980). An observational analysis of the IEP conference. *Exceptional Children, 46,* 278–286.

GOLDSTEIN, S. & TURNBULL, A. P. (1982). Strategies to increase parent participation in IEP conferences. *Exceptional Children, 48,* 360–361.

GOLLAY, E. (1977). Deinstitutionalized mentally retarded people: A closer look. *Education and Training of the Mentally Retarded, 12,* 137–144.

GONZALEZ, G. (1974). Language, culture, and exceptional children. *Exceptional Children, 40,* 565–570.

GOODMAN, H., GOTTLIEB, J. & HARRISON, H. (1972). Social acceptance of EMRs integrated into a nongraded elementary school. *American Journal of Mental Deficiency, 76,* 412–417.

GORHAM, K. A. (1975). A lost generation of parents. *Exceptional Children, 41,* 521–525.

GOTTLIEB, J. (1980). Improving attitudes toward retarded children by using group discussion. *Exceptional Children, 47,* 106–111.

GOTTLIEB, J. (1981). Mainstreaming: Fulfilling the promise? *American Journal of Mental Deficiency, 86,* 115–126.

GOTTLIEB, J. (1982). Mainstreaming. *Education and Training of the Mentally Retarded, 17,* 79–82.

GOTTLIEB, J. & BUDOFF, M. (1973). Social acceptability of retarded children in nongraded schools differing in architecture. *American Journal of Mental Deficiency, 78,* 15–19.

GOTTLIEB, J., COHEN, L. & GOLDSTEIN, L. (1974). Social contact and personal adjustment as variables relating to attitudes toward EMR children. *Training School Bulletin, 71,* 9–16.

GOTTLIEB, J. & CORMAN, L. (1975). Public attitudes toward mentally retarded children. *American Journal of Mental Deficiency, 80*(1), 72–80.

GOTTWALD, H. (1970). Public awareness about mental retardation. CEC Research Monograph. Reston, Virginia: Council for Exceptional Children.

GRALIKER, B. V., KOCH, R. & HENDERSON, R. A. (1965). A study of factors influencing placement of retarded children in a state residential institution. *American Journal of Mental Deficiency, 69,* 553–559.

GREENSPAN, S. (1979). Social intelligence in the retarded. In N. R. Ellis (Ed.). *Handbook of mental deficiency: Psychological theory and research* (2nd ed.) Hillsdale, New Jersey: Lawrence Erlbaum Associates.

GREENWALD, C. A. & LEONARD, L. B. (1979). Communication and sensorimotor development in Down's syndrome children. *American Journal of Mental Deficiency, 84,* 296–303.

GREER, B. G. (1975). On being the parent of a handicapped child. *Exceptional Children, 41,* 519.

GRESHAM, F. M. (1982). Misguided mainstreaming: The case for social skills training with handicapped children. *Exceptional Children, 48,* 422–433.

GROSSMAN, H. (1983). *Classification in mental retardation.* Washington, D.C.: American Association on Mental Deficiency.

GROSSMAN, H. J. (Ed.). (1973). *Manual on terminology and classification in mental retardation.* Washington, D. C.: American Association on Mental Deficiency.

GROSSMAN, H. J. (Ed.). (1977). *Manual on terminology and classification in mental retardation.* Washington, D. C.: American Association on Mental Deficiency.

GUILFORD, J. P. (1967). *The Nature of Human Intelligence.* New York: McGraw-Hill.

GULLY, K. J. & HOSCH, H. M. (1979). Adaptive behavior scale: Development as a diagnostic tool via discriminant analysis. *American Journal of Mental Deficiency, 83,* 518–523.

GUSKIN, S. (1963). Social psychologies of mental deficiencies. In N. R. Ellis (Ed.). *Handbook of mental deficiency: Psychological theory and research.* New York: McGraw-Hill.

GUSKIN, S. L. & SPICKER, H. H. (1968). Educational research in mental retardation. In N. R. Ellis (Ed.). *International Review of Research in Mental Retardation* (Vol. 3). New York: Academic Press.

GUTHRIE, G. M., BUTLER, A. & GORLOW, L. (1962). Patterns of self-attitudes of retardates. *American Journal of Mental Deficiency, 66,* 222–239.

GUTHRIE, R. (1972). Mass screening for genetic disease. *Hospital Practice, 7,* 93.

HALL, K. (1967). Allergy of the nervous system. *Annals of Allergy, 36*, 49–64.

HALL, J. E. & MORRIS, H. L. (1976). Sexual knowledge and attitudes of institutionalized and noninstitutionalized retarded persons. *American Journal of Mental Deficiency, 80*, 382–387.

HALL, R. V. (1975). *Managing behavior, Part 2. Behavior modification: Basic principles* (rev. ed.). Lawrence, Kansas: H & H Enterprises.

HALPERN, A., RAFFIELD, P., IRVIN, L. K. & LINK, R. (1975). *Test book for the social and prevocational information battery.* Montery, California: CTB/McGraw-Hill.

HAMILTON, J., ALLEN, P., STEPHENS, L. & DAVALL, E. (1969). Training mentally retarded females to use sanitary napkins. *Mental Retardation, 7*(1), 40–43.

HAMMILL, D. & WIEDERHOLT, J. L. (1972). *The resource room: Rationale and implementation.* Philadelphia: Buttonwood Farms.

HAMRE-NIETUPSKI, S., NIETUPSKI, J., BATES, P. & MAURER, S. (1982). Implementing a community-based educational model for moderately/severely handicapped students: Common problems and suggested solutions. *The Journal of the Association of the Severely Handicapped, 7*(4), 38–43.

HARDMAN, M. J. & DREW, C. J. (1975). Incidental learning in the mentally retarded: A review. *Education and training of the mentally retarded, 10*, 3–9.

HARDMAN, M. & DREW, C. (1977). The physically handicapped retarded individual: A review. *Mental Retardation, 15*(5), 43–48.

HATCHER, R. P. (1976). The predictability of infant intelligence scales: A critical review and evaluation. *Mental Retardation, 14*(4), 16–19.

HAYDEN, A. H. & HARING, N. G. (1976). Programs for Down's syndrome children at the University of Washington. In T. D. Tjossem (Ed.). *Intervention strategies for high risk infants and young children.* Baltimore: University Park Press.

HAYDEN, A. H., McGINNESS, G. & DMITRIEV, V. (1976). Early and continuous intervention strategies for severely handicapped infants and very young children. In N. G. Haring & L. J. Brown (Eds.). *Teaching the Severely Handicapped* (Vol. I). New York: Grune & Stratton.

HAYES, J. & HIGGINS, S. T. (1978). Issues regarding the IEP: Teachers on the front line. *Exceptional Children, 44*, 267–273.

HAYWOOD, H. C. & TAPP, J. T. (1966). Experience and the development of adaptive behavior. In N. R. Ellis (Ed.). *International review of research in mental retardation* (Vol. 1). New York: Academic Press.

HEAL, L. W., SIGELMAN, C. K. & SWITZKY, H. N. (1978). Research on community alternatives for the mentally retarded. In N. R. Ellis (Ed.). *International Review of Research in Mental Retardation* (Vol. 9). New York: Academic Press.

HEBB, D. O. (1949). *The organization of behavior.* New York: John Wiley & Sons.

HEBER, R. (1970). *Epidemiology of mental retardation.* Springfield, Illinois: Charles C Thomas.

HEBER, R. (1959). A manual on terminology and classification in mental retardation. *Monograph Supplement of the American Journal of Mental Deficiency* (No. 64).

HEBER, R. (1961). A manual on terminology and classification in mental retardation. *Monograph Supplement of the American Journal of Mental Deficiency* (2nd ed.).

HEBER, R. (1961). Modifications in the manual on terminology and classification in mental retardation. *American Journal of Mental Deficiency, 65*(4), 499–500.

HEBER, R. (1964). Personality. In H. A. Stevens & R. Heber (Eds.). *Mental Retardation.* Chicago: University of Chicago Press.

HEBER, R. & DEVER, R. B. (1970). Research on education and habilitation of the mentally retarded. In H. C. Haywood (Ed.). *Social-cultural aspects of mental retardation.* New York: Appleton-Century-Crofts.

HEBER, R., DEVER, R. B. & CONRY, J. (1968). The influence of environmental and genetic variables on intellectual development. In H. J. Prehm, L. A. Hamerlynck, & J. E. Crosson (Eds.). *Behavioral research in mental retardation.* Eugene, Oregon: University of Oregon.

HEBER, R. & GARBER, H. (1975). The Milwaukee Project: A study of the use of family intervention to prevent cultural-familial mental retardation. In B. Z. Friedlauder, G. M. Sterrit, & G. E. Kirk (Eds.). *Exceptional infant (Vol. 3): Assessment and intervention.* New York: Brunner/Mazel.

HELLER, H. W. (1979). A suggested approach for the establishment of realistic goals of achievement for educable mentally retarded. *Education and Training of the Mentally Retarded, 14*, 156–158.

HERRNSTEIN, R. & BORING, E. (1965). *A source book in the history of psychology.* Cambridge: Harvard University Press.

HESHUSIUS, F. (1982). Sexuality, intimacy, and persons we label mentally retarded: What they think—what we think. *Mental Retardation, 20*, 164–168.

HESS, R. D. & SHIPMAN, V. C. (1965). Early experience and the socialization of cognitive modes in children. *Child Development, 36*, 869–886.

HILL, J. (1980). Use of an automated recreational device to facilitate independent leisure and motor behavior in a profoundly retarded male. In P. Wehman & J. Hill (Eds.). *Instructional Programming for Severely Handicapped Youth.* Richmond: Virginia Commonwealth University.

HILL, M. & WEHMAN, P. (In Press). Cost benefit analysis of placing moderately and severely handicapped individuals into competitive employment. *Journal of the Association for the Severely Handicapped.*

HIRSHOREN, A. & BURTON, T. A. (1979). Teaching academic skills to trainable mentally retarded children: A study in tautology. *Mental Retardation, 17*, 177–179.

HOBBS, M. A. (1964). A comparison of institutionalized and noninstitutionalized mentally retarded. *American Journal of Mental Deficiency, 69*, 206–210.

HOBBS, N. (1975). *The Futures of Children.* San Francisco: Jossey-Bass.

HOBSON, P. A. & DUNCAN, P. (1979). Sign learning and profoundly retarded people. *Mental Retardation, 17*(1), 33–37.

HOFMEISTER, A. M. (1969). An investigation of academic skills in trainable mentally retarded adolescents and young adults. *Dissertation Abstracts, 3786–A.*

HOFMEISTER, A. M. (1982). Microcomputers in perspective. *Exceptional Children, 49,* 115–121.

HOLLAND, R. P. (1980). An analysis of the decision-making processes in special education. *Exceptional Children, 46,* 551–554.

HOMME, L. (1969). *Contingency contracting in the classroom.* Champaign, Illinois: Research Press.

HORNER, D. & KEILITZ, I. (1975). Training mentally retarded adolescents to brush their teeth. *Journal of Applied Behavior Analysis, 8,* 301–309.

HORNER, R. H. & BELLAMY, G. T. (1979). Structured employment: Productivity and productive capacity. In G. T. Bellamy, G. O'Connor & P. C. Karan (Eds.). *Vocational rehabilitation of severely handicapped persons.* Baltimore: University Park Press.

HOROWITZ, F. D. & PADEN, L. Y. (1973). The effectiveness of environmental intervention programs. In B. M. Caldwell & H. N. Riccinti (Eds.). *Review of child development and research* (Vol. 3). Chicago: University of Chicago Press.

HOTTEL, J. (1958). *An evaluation of Tennessee's day class program for severely mentally retarded trainable children.* Nashville, Tennessee: State Department of Education.

HOUSE, B. J., HANLEY, M. J. & MAGID, D. F. (1980). Logographic reading by TMR adults. *American Journal of Mental Deficiency, 85,* 161–170.

HOWELL, K. W., KAPLAN, J. S. & O'CONNELL, C. Y. (1979). *Evaluating exceptional children: A task analysis approach.* Columbus, Ohio: Charles E. Merrill.

HUBERTY, T., KOLLER, J. & TEN BRINK, T. (1980). Adaptive behavior in the definition of mental retardation. *Exceptional Children, 46*(4), 256–261.

HUDSON, F., REISBERG, T. E. & WOLF, R. (1983). Changing teachers' perceptions of mainstreaming. *Teacher Education and Special Education, 6,* 18–24.

HULL, J. T. & THOMPSON, J. C. (1980). Predicting adaptive functioning of mentally retarded persons in community settings. *American Journal of Mental Deficiency, 85,* 253–261.

HUMPHREYS, L. G. & PARSONS, C. K. (1979). Piagetian tasks measure intelligence and intelligence tests assess cognitive development: A reanalysis. *Intelligence, 3,* 369–382.

HUNT, J. McV. (1961). *Intelligence and Experience.* New York: The Ronald Press.

HUNT, J. McV. & KIRK, G. E. (1971). Social aspects of intelligence. In R. Cancro (Ed.) *Intelligence: Genetic and environmental influences.* New York: Grune & Stratton.

HUNT, J. McV. (1969). *The challenge of incompetence and poverty.* Urbana: University of Illinois Press.

HURLEY, D. L. (1975). Reading comprehension skills *vis à vis* the mentally retarded. *Education and Training of the Mentally Retarded, 10,* 10–14.

IANO, R. P. (1972). Shall we disband special classes? *The Journal of Special Education.*

IANO, R. P., AYRES, D., HELLER, H. B., McGETTIGAN, J. F. & WALKER, V. S. (1974). Sociometric status of retarded children in an integrative program. *Exceptional Children, 40,* 267–271.

ISAACSON, R. L. & VAN HARTESVELDT, C. (1978). The biological basis of an ethic for mental retardation. In N. R. Ellis (Ed.). *International review of research in mental retardation* (Vol. 9). New York: Academic Press.

IRVIN, L. K. & HALPERN, A. S. (1977). Reliability and validity of the social and prevocational information battery for mildly retarded individuals. *American Journal of Mental Deficiency, 81,* 603–605.

JANICKI, M. P., MAYEDA, T. & EPPLE, W. A. (1983). Availability of group homes for persons with mental retardation in the United States. *Mental Retardation, 21,* 45–51.

JARMAN, R. F. (1978). Patterns of cognitive ability in retarded children: A reexamination. *American Journal of Mental Deficiency, 82,* 344–348.

JENKINS, J. R. & MAYHALL, W. F. (1973). Discribing resource teacher programs. *Exceptional Children, 35–36.*

JENSEN, A. R. (1969). How much can we boost IQ and scholastic achievement? *Harvard Educational Review, 39,* 1–123.

JENSEN, A. R. (1970). A theory of primary and secondary familial mental retardation. In N. R. Ellis (Ed.). *International review of research in mental retardation* (Vol. 4). New York: Academic Press.

JOHNSON, G. O. (1962). Special education for the mentally retarded—a paradox. *Exceptional Children, 29,* 62–69.

JOHNSON, G. O. & CAPOBIANCO, R. J. (1957). *Research project on severely retarded children.* New York: Interdepartmental Health Resources Board.

JOHNSON, G. O., CAPOBIANCO, R. J. & BLAKE, K. (1960). An evaluation of behavior changes in trainable mentally deficient children. *American Journal of Mental Deficiency, 64,* 881–893.

JONES, A. & ROBSON, C. (1979). Language training and the severely mentally handicapped. In N. R. Ellis (Ed.). *Handbook of mental deficiency, psychological theory, and research* (2nd ed.). Hillsdale, New Jersey: Erlbaum.

JONES, R. L. (1973). Accountability in special education: Some problems. *Exceptional Children, 39,* 631–642.

JUSTEN, J. E. III. (1976). Who are the severely handicapped? A problem in definition. *AAESPH Review, 1*(5), 1–11.

KABACK, M. M., BECKER, M. H. & RUTH, M. V. (1974). Compliance factors in a voluntary heterozygote screening program. *Birth Defects, 10,* 145–163.

KAHN, J. V. (1979). Applications of the Piagetian literature to severely and profoundly mentally retarded persons. *Mental Retardation, 17,* 273–280.

KAHN, J. (1976). Utility of the Uzgiris and Hunt scales of sensorimotor development with severely and profoundly retarded children. *American Journal of Mental Deficiency, 80,* 663–665.

KAMHI, A. G. (1981). Developmental vs. difference theories of mental retardation: A new look. *American Journal of Mental Deficiency, 86,* 1–7.

KANNER, L. (1964). *A History of the Care and Study of the Mentally Retarded.* Springfield, Illinois: Charles C Thomas.

KATZ, S., GOLDBERG, J. & SHURKA, E. (1977). The use of operant techniques in teaching severely retarded clients work habits. *Education and Training of the Mentally Retarded, 12,* 14–20.

KAUFMAN, K. R. & KATZ-GARRIS, L. (1979). Epilepsy, mental retardation, and anticonvulsant therapy. *American Journal of Mental Deficiency, 84,* 256–259.

KAUFMAN, M. E. & ALBERTO, P. A. (1976). Research on efficacy of special education for the mentally retarded. In N. R. Ellis (Ed.). *International Review of Research in Mental Retardation* (Vol. 8). New York: Academic Press.

KAUFMAN, M. J., GOTTLIEB, J., AGARD, J. A. & KUKIC, M. B. (1975). Mainstreaming: Toward an explanation of a construct. *Focus on Exceptional Children, 7*(3), 1–12.

KAZDIN, A. E. (1975). *Behavior Modification in Applied Settings.* Homewood, Illinois: Dorsey Press.

KEITH, K. D. (1979). Behavior analysis and the principle of normalization. *AAESPH Review, 4,* 148–151.

KELLER, S. (1963). The social world of the urban slum child: Some early findings. *American Journal of Orthopsychiatry, 33,* 823–831.

KEPHART, N. C. (1960). *The Slow Learner in the Classroom.* Columbus, Ohio: Charles E. Merrill.

KERN, W. H. & PFAEFFLE, H. A. (1962). A comparison of social adjustment of mentally retarded children in various educational settings. *American Journal of Mental Deficiency, 67,* 407–413.

KERSHNER, J. R. (1970). Intellectual and social development in relation to family functioning: A longitudinal comparison of home vs. institutional effects. *American Journal of Mental Deficiency, 75,* 276–284.

KIDD, J. (1977). Comments from the executive director. *Education and Training of the Mentally Retarded, 12*(3), 303–304.

KIDD, J. W. (1970). Pro—the efficacy of special class placement for educable mental retardates. Paper presented at the 48th Annual Convention, *Council for Exceptional Children.*

KIDD, J., BARTLETT, R., FORGNONE, C., GOLDSTEIN, H., GORTON, C., MORENO-MILNE, N., ROSEBORO, D. & WHITE, R. (1979). An open letter to the Committee on Terminology and Classification of AAMD from the Committee on Definition and Terminology of CEC-MR. *Education and Training of the Mentally Retarded, 14*(2), 74–76.

KIDD, J. W., CROSS, T. J. & HIGGINBOTHAM, J. L. (1967). The world of work for the educable mentally retarded. *Exceptional Children, 33,* 648–649.

KIRK, S. A. (1972). *Educating exceptional children* (2nd ed.). Boston: Houghton-Mifflin.

KIRK, S. A. (1970). The effects of early intervention. In H. C. Haywood (Ed.). *Social-cultural aspects of mental retardation.* New York: Appleton-Century-Croft.

KIRK, S. A. (1964). Research in education. In H. A. Stevens & R. Heber (Eds.). *Mental Retardation.* Chicago: University of Chicago Press.

KIRK, S. A. & JOHNSON, G. O. (1951). *Educating the retarded child.* Boston: Houghton-Mifflin.

KIRK, S. & WEINER, B. (1959). The Anondaga census—fact or artifact. *Exceptional Children, 25,* 226–228, 230–231.

KLAUS, R. A. & GRAY, S. W. (1968). The early training project for disadvantaged children: A report after five years. *Monographs of the Society for Research in Child Development, 33.*

KLINE V. ARMSTRONG.(1979). 476 Supp. 583 (E.D. Pa.).

KNAPCZYK, D. R. (1979). The presence of allergies among severely handicapped persons. *AAESPH Review, 4,* 354–363.

KNOFF, H. M. (1983). Effect of diagnostic information on special education placement decisions. *Exceptional Children, 49,* 440–444.

KOEGEL, P. & EDGERTON, R. B. (1982). Labeling and the perception of handicap among black mildly mentally retarded adults. *American Journal of Mental Deficiency, 87,* 266–276.

KOKASKA, C. J. (1968). The occupational status of the educable mentally retarded: A review of follow-up studies. *Journal of Special Education, 2,* 369–377.

KOKASKA, C. J. (1968). *The vocational preparation of the educable mentally retarded.* Ypsilanti: Eastern Michigan University Press.

KOLSTOE, B. (1972). *Mental retardation: An educational viewpoint.* New York: Holt, Rinehart & Winston.

KOLSTOE, O. P. (1961). An examination of some characteristics which discriminate between employed and not employed mentally retarded males. *American Journal of Mental Deficiency, 66,* 472–482.

KOLSTOE, O. P. (1972). Programs for the mildly retarded: A reply to the critics. *Exceptional Children, 39,* 51–56.

KOLSTOE, O. P. (1976). *Teaching Educable Mentally Retarded Children* (2nd ed.). New York: Holt, Rinehart & Winston.

KOLSTOE, O. P. & FREY, R. M. (1965). *A high school work-study program for mentally subnormal students.* Carbondale: Southern Illinois University Press.

KOORLAND, M. A. & MARTIN, M. B. (1975). *Elementary principles and procedures of the standard behavior chart* (3rd ed.). Gainesville, Florida: Odyssey Learning Center.

KOUNIN, J. (1941a). Experimental studies of rigidity: I. The measurement of rigidity in normal and feeble-minded persons. *Character and Personality, 9,* 251–272.

KOUNIN, J. (1941b). Experimental studies of rigidity: II. The explanatory power of the concept of rigidity as applied to feeble-mindedness. *Character and Personality, 9,* 273–282.

KRAGER, J. M., SAFER, D. J. & EARHARDT, J. (1977). Medication used to treat hyperactive children: Follow-up survey results. Unpublished manuscript.

KURTZ, P. D.& NEISWORTH, J. T. (1976). Self-control possibilities for exceptional children. *Exceptional Children, 42,* 212–217.

LABOV, W. (1969). The logic of nonstandard English. *Monograph Series on Language and Linguistics, 2,* 1–43.

LABOV, W. (1970). The logic of nonstandard English. In F. Williams (Ed.). *Language and Poverty.* Chicago: Markham.

LAIDLER, J. (1976). Nutritional assessment of common problems found among the developmentally disabled. *Mental Retardation, 14*(4), 24–28.

LAKIN, K. C., KRANTZ, G. C., BRUININKS, R. H., CLUMPER, J. L. & HILL, B. K. (1982). One hundred years of data on populations of public residential facilities for mentally retarded people. *American Journal of Mental Deficiency, 87,* 1–8.

LALLY, M. (1981). Computer-assisted teaching of sight word recognition for mentally retarded school children. *American Journal of Mental Deficiency, 85,* 383–388.

LANCE, W. D. (1977). Technology and media for exceptional learners: Looking ahead. *Exceptional Children, 44,* 92–97.

LANDESMAN-DWYER, S. (1981). Living in the community. *American Journal of Mental Deficiency, 86,* 223–234.

LANDESMAN-DWYER, S., BERKSON, G. & ROMER, D. (1979). Affiliation and friendship of mentally retarded residents in group homes. *American Journal of Mental Deficiency, 83,* 571–580.

Larry P. v. Riles, (1979, October). No. C-71-2270 RFP (W.D. Cal.).

LARSEN, L., GOODMAN, L. & GLEAN, R. (1981). Issues in the implementation of extended school year programs for handicapped students. *Exceptional Children, 47,* 256–263.

LAWRENCE, E. A. & WINSCHEL, J. F. (1973). Self-concept and the retarded: Research and issues, *Exceptional Children, 39,* 310–319.

LAWRENCE, E. A. & WINSCHEL, J. F. (1975). Locus of control: Implications for special education. *Exceptional Children, 41,* 483–490.

LEJEUNE, J., GAUTIER, M. & TURPIN, R. (1963). Study of the somatic chromosomes of nine mongoloid idiot children. In S. H. Boyer (Ed.). *Papers on human genetics.* Englewood Cliffs, New Jersey: Prentice-Hall.

LEMKAU, P. & IMRE, P. (1969). Results of a field epidemiologic study. *American Journal of Mental Deficiency, 73,* 858–863.

LENNEBERG, E. H. (1967). *Biological foundations of language.* New York: Wiley.

LEONARD, J. (1981). 180 day barrier: Issues and concerns. *Exceptional Children, 47,* 246–253.

LEVINSON, E. (1962). *Retarded Children in Maine: A Survey and Analysis.* Orono, Maine: University of Maine Press.

LEWIS, E. D. (1933). Types of mental deficiency and their social significance. *Journal of Mental Science, 79,* 298–304.

LEWIS, E. O. (1929). *Report on an investigation into the incidence of mental deficiency in six areas, 1925–1927.* London: H. M. Stationary Office.

LEWIN, K. (1936). *A Dynamic Theory of Personality.* New York: McGraw-Hill.

LEYSER, Y. & GOTTLIEB, J. (1980). Improving the social status of rejected pupils. *Exceptional Children, 46,* 459–461.

LI, A. K. F. (1981). Play and the mentally retarded child, *Mental Retardation, 19,* 121–126.

LILLY, M. S. (1971). A training based model for special education. *Exceptional Children, 37,* 745–749.

LIPMAN, R. S. (1970). The use of psychopharmacological agents in residential facilities for the retarded. In F. J. Menolascino (Ed.). *Psychiatric approaches to mental retardation.* New York: Basic Books.

LITROWNIK, A. J., CLEARY, C. P., LECKLITER, G. L. & FRANZINI, L. R. (1978). Self-regulation in retarded persons: Acquisition of standards for performance. *American Journal of Mental Deficiency, 83,* 86–89.

LITROWNIK, A. J., FRANZINI, L. R., GELLER, S. & GELLER, M. (1977). Delay of gratification: Decisional self-control and experience with delay intervals. *American Journal of Mental Deficiency, 82,* 149–154.

LITROWNIK, A. J., FRIETAS, J. L. & FRANZINI, L. R. (1978). Self regulation in mentally retarded children: Assessment and training of self-monitoring skills. *American Journal of Mental Deficiency, 82,* 499–506.

LITTON, F. W. (1978). *The education of the trainable mentally retarded: Curriculum, methods, materials.* St. Louis: C. V. Mosby.

LIVINGSTON, S. (1972). *Comprehensive management of epilepsy in infancy, childhood, and adolescence.* Springfield, Illinois: Charles C Thomas.

LLOYD, L. L. (1970). Audiologic aspects of mental retardation. In N. R. Ellis (Ed.). *International review of research in mental retardation* (Vol. 4). New York: Academic Press.

LUCKEY, R. E. & ADDISON, M. R. (1974). The profoundly retarded: A new challenge for public education. *Education and Training of the Mentally Retarded, 9,* 123–130.

LUCKEY, R. & NEMAN, R. (1976). Practices in estimating mental retardation prevalence. *Mental Retardation, 14,* 16–18.

LUSTHAUS, C. S., LUSTHAUS, E. W. & GIBBS, H. (1981). Parents' role in the decision process. *Exceptional Children, 48* 256–257.

LYNCH, K. P. & GERBER, P. J. (1980). A survey of community sheltered facilities: Implications for mandated school programs. *Education and Training of the Mentally Retarded, 15,* 264–269.

MACDONALD, D. (1965). Our invisible poor. In L. A. Ferman, J. L. Kornbluh & A. Haber (Eds.). *Poverty in America.* Ann Arbor, Michigan: University of Michigan Press.

MACEACHRON, A. E. (1979). Mentally retarded offenders: Prevalence and characteristics. *American Journal of Mental Deficiency, 84,* 165–176.

MACMILLAN, D. L. (1971). Special education for the mildly retarded: Servant or savant. *Focus on Exceptional Children, 2*(9), 1–11.

MACMILLAN, D. L. & BORTHWICK, S. (1980). The new educable mentally retarded population: Can they be mainstreamed? *Mental Retardation, 18,* 155–158.

MACMILLAN, D. L., JONES, R. L. & ALOIA, G. F. (1974). The mentally retarded label: A theoretical analysis and review of research. *American Journal of Mental Deficiency, 79,* 241–261.

MACMILLAN, D. L., JONES, R. L. & MEYERS, C. E. (1976). Mainstreaming the mildly retarded: Some questions, cautions, and guidelines. *Mental Retardation, 14*(1), 3–10.

MACMILLAN, D. L., MEYERS, C. E. & MORRISON, G. M. (1980). System-identification of mildly mentally retarded children: Implications for interpreting and conducting research. *American Journal of Mental Deficiency, 85,* 108–115.

MACMILLAN, D. L. & SEMMEL, M. I. (1977). Evaluation of mainstreaming programs. *Focus on Exceptional Children, 9*(4), 1–14.

MACMILLAN, D. L. & TURNBULL, A. D. (1983). Parent involvement in special education: Respecting individual preferences. *Education and Training of the Mentally Retarded, 18,* 5–9.

MAHONEY, G., GLOVER, A. & FINGER, I. (1981). Relationship between language and sensorimotor development of Down's syndrome and nonretarded children. *American Journal of Mental Deficiency, 86,* 21–27.

MAHONEY, K., VAN WAGENEN, R. K. & MEYERSON, L. (1971). Toilet training of normal and retarded children. *Journal of Applied Behavior Analysis, 4,* 173–181.

MALPASS, L. F. (1963). Motor skills in mental deficiency. In N. R. Ellis (Ed.). *Handbook of mental deficiency: Psychological theory and research.* New York: McGraw-Hill.

MANEY, A. C., PACE, R. & MORRISON, D. F. (1964). A factor analytic study of the need for institutionalization: Problems and populations for institutional development. *American Journal of Mental Deficiency, 69,* 372–384.

MARGOLIS, J. & CHARITONIDIS, T. (1981). Public reactions to housing for the mentally retarded. *Exceptional Children, 48,* 68–70.

MARHOLIN, D., TOUCHETTE, P. E. & STEWART, M. R. (1979). Withdrawal of chronic chlorpromazine medication: An experimental analysis. *Journal of Applied Behavior Analysis, 12,* 159–171.

MAROZAS, D., MAY, D. & LEHMAN, L. (1980). Incidence and prevalence: Confusion in need of clarification. *Mental Retardation, 18,* 229–230.

MARTIN, A. S. & MORRIS, J. L. (1980). Training a work ethic in severely mentally retarded workers, providing a context for the maintenance of skill performance. *Mental Retardation, 18,* 67–71.

MARTIN, G. L., KEHOE, B., BIRD, E., JENSEN, V. & DARBYSHIRE, M. (1971). Operant conditioning in the dressing behavior of severely retarded girls. *Mental Retardation, 9*(3), 27–30.

Maryland Association for Retarded Citizens v. The State of Maryland. Equity No. 100/182/77676 (Circuit Court, Baltimore City, April 9, 1974).

MASCARI, B. G. & FORGNONE, C. (1982). A follow-up study of EMR students four years after dismissal from the program. *Education and Training of the Mentally Retarded, 17,* 288–292.

MASON, J. M. (1978). Role of strategy in reading by mentally retarded persons. *American Journal of Mental Deficiency, 82,* 110–118.

MATARAZZO, J. (1972). *Wechsler's measurement and appraisal of adult intelligence* (5th ed.). Baltimore: The Williams & Wilkins Co.

Mattie T. v. *Holladay,* No. DC-75-31-S (N.D. Miss., July 28, 1977).

McCLELLAND, D. C. (1973). Testing for competence rather than for "intelligence." *American Psychologist, 1–14.*

MATTSON, B. D. (1977). Involving parents in special education: Did you really reach them? *Education and Training of the Mentally Retarded, 12,* 358–360.

McCANDLESS, B. R. (1964). Relation of environmental factors to intellectual functioning. In H. A. Stevens & R. Heber (Eds.). *Mental Retardation.* Chicago: The University of Chicago Press.

McCANDLESS, B. R. (1970). Modeling and power in cognitive development. In H. C. Haywood (Ed.). *Social-cultural aspects of mental retardation.* New York: Appleton-Century-Crofts.

McCARTHY, J. H. (1968). An overview of the IMC network. *Exceptional Children, 35,* 263–266.

McCARVER, R. B. & CRAIG, E. M. (1974). Placement of the retarded in the community: Prognosis and outcome. In N. R. Ellis (Ed.). *International review of research in mental retardation* (Vol. 7). New York: Academic Press.

McCORMICK, M., BALLA, D. & ZIGLER, E. (1975). Resident care practices in institutions for retarded persons: A cross-institutional cross-cultural study. *American Journal of Mental Deficiency, 80,* 1–17.

McDEVITT, S. C., SMITH, P. M., SCHMIDT, D. W. & ROSEN, M. (1978). The deinstitutionalized citizen: Adjustment and quality of life. *Mental Retardation, 16*(1), 22–24.

McDOWELL, E. B. (1964). *Teaching the Severely Subnormal.* London: Edward Arnold.

McFALL, T. M. (1966). Postschool adjustment: A survey of fifty former students of classes for the educable mentally retarded. *Exceptional Children, 32,* 633–634.

McGREW, J. B. (1977). Establishing a public school program for the severely handicapped. In E. Sontag, J. Smith & N. Certo (Eds.). *Educational programming for the severely and profoundly handicapped.* Reston, VA: Division on Mental Retardation, The Council for Exceptional Children.

McMAHON, J. (1983). Extended school year programs. *Exceptional Children, 49,* 457–460.

MENOLASCINO, F. J. & McGEE, J. J. (1981). The new institutions: Last ditch arguments. *Mental Retardation, 19,* 215–220.

MENOLASCINO, F. J., McGEE, J. J. & CASEY, K. (1982). Affirmation of the rights of institutionalized retarded citizens (Implications of *Youngberg* v. *Romeo*). *Journal of the Association of the Severely Handicapped, 7*(3), 63–72.

MERCER, C. D. & ALGOZZINE, B. (1977). Observational learning and the retarded: Teaching implications. *Education and Training of the Mentally Retarded, 12,* 345–353.

MERCER, C. D. & SNELL, M. E. (1977). *Learning theory research in mental retardation: Implications for teaching.* Columbus, Ohio: Charles E. Merrill.

MERCER, C. R. (1966). Patterns of family crisis related to reacceptance of the retardate. *American Journal of Mental Deficiency, 71,* 19–32.

MERCER, J. (1971). The meaning of mental retardation. In R. Koch and J. Dobson (Eds.). *The mentally retarded child and his family.* New York: Brunner-Mazel.

MERCER, J. (1973a). *Labeling the mentally retarded.* Berkeley: University of California Press.

MERCER, J. (1973b). The myth of 3% prevalence. In R. Lyman, C. Meyers & G. Tarjan (Eds.). *Sociobehavioral studies in mental retardation.* Washington, D. C.: American Association on Mental Deficiency.

MERCER, J. (1975). Psychological assessment and the rights of children. In N. Hobbs (Ed.). *Issues in the classification of children* (Vol. I). San Francisco: Jossey-Bass.

MERCER, J. (1970). Sociological perspectives on mild mental retardation. In H. C. Haywood (Ed.). *Social-cultural aspects of mental retardation.* New York: Appleton-Century-Crofts.

MERCER, J. R. & LEWIS, J. F. (1978). *System of multicultural pluralistic assessment.* New York: Psychological Corporation.

MESIBOV, G. B. (1976a). Alternatives to the principle of normalization. *Mental Retardation, 14*(5), 30–32.

MESIBOV, G. B. (1976b). Mentally retarded people: 200 years in America. *Journal of Clinical Child Psychology, 5.*

MEYER, R. J. (1980). Attitudes of parents of institutionalized mentally retarded individuals toward deinstitutionalization. *American Journal of Mental Deficiency, 85,* 184–187.

MEYERS, C. E., MacMILLAN, D. I., & YOSHIDA, R. K. (1975) Correlates of success in transition of MR to regular classes (Final Report, Grant No. OEG-0-73-5263). Pomona, California: U. S. Department of Health, Education & Welfare.

MEYERS, C. E., NIHIRA, K. & ZETLIN, A. (1979). The measurement of adaptive behavior. In N. R. Ellis (Ed.). *Handbook of mental deficiency, psychological theory, and research* (2nd ed.). Hillsdale, New Jersey: Lawrence Erlbaum Publishers.

MEYERSON, L. A. (1971). Somatopsychology of physical disability. In W. Cruickshank (Ed.). *Psychology of exceptional children and youth* (3rd ed). Englewood Cliffs, N. J.: Prentice-Hall.

MILGRAM, N. A. (1971). Cognition and language in mental retardation: A reply to Balla and Zigler. *American Journal of Mental Deficiency, 76,* 33–41.

MILLER, C. R. (1976). Subtypes of the PMR: Implications for placement and progress. In C. C. Cleland,

J. Schwartz, & L. W. Talkington (Eds.). *The Profoundly Mentally Retarded*. Austin, Texas: Western Research Conference and the Hogg Foundation.

MILLER, J. O. (1970). Cultural deprivation and its modification: Effects of intervention. In H. C. Haywood (Ed.). *Social-cultural aspects of mental retardation*. New York: Appleton-Century-Crofts.

MILLHAM, J., ATKINSON, B. L. & NATHAN, M. (1980). Mentally retarded individuals as informants on the AAMD adaptive behavior scale. *Mental Retardation, 18*, 82–84.

MILUNSKY, A. (1976). A prenatal diagnosis of genetic disorders. *New England Journal of Medicine, 295*, 377–380.

MINK, I. T., NIHIRA, K. & MEYERS, C. E. (1983). Taxonomy of family life-styles: I. Homes with TMR Children. *American Journal of Mental Deficiency, 87*, 484–497.

MITCHELL, L., DOCTOR, R. M. & BUTLER, D. C. (1978). Attitudes of caretakers toward the sexual behavior of retarded persons. *American Journal of Mental Deficiency, 83*, 289–296.

MITHAUG, D. E., HAGMEIER, L. D. & HARING, N. G. (1977). The relationship between training activities and job placement in vocational education of the severely and profoundly handicapped. *AAESPH Review, 2*(2), 25–45.

MITHAUG, D. E. & HANAWALT, D. A. (1978). The validation of procedures to assess prevocational task preferences in retarded adults. *Journal of Applied Behavior Analysis, 11*, 153–162.

MOLLOY, J. S. (1972). *Trainable Children: Curriculum and Procedure* (rev. ed.). New York: John Day.

MOLNAR, G. E. (1978). Analysis of motor disorder in retarded infants and young children. *American Journal of Mental Deficiency, 83*, 213–222.

MOREHEAD, D. M. & MOREHEAD, A. (1974). From signal to sign: A Piagetian view of thought and language during the first two years. In R. L. Schrifelbusch & L. L. Lloyd (Eds.). *Language perspectives—acquisition, retardation, and intervention*. Baltimore: University Park Press.

MOSIER, H. D., GROSSMAN, J. H. & DINGHAM, H. F. (1965). Physical growth in mental defectives. *Pediatrics, 36* (Part II), 465–519.

MURPHY, R. & DOUGHTY, N. (1977). Establishment of controlled arm movement in profoundly retarded students using response contingent vibratory stimulation. *American Journal of Mental Deficiency, 82*, 212–216.

NAGLER, B. (1972). A change in terms or concepts? A small step forward or a giant step backward? *Journal of Special Education, 6*(1), 61–64.

NAZZARO, J. N. (1977). *Exceptional timetables: Historic events affecting the handicapped and the gifted*. Reston, Va.: The Council for Exceptional Children.

NEISWORTH, J. & GREER, J. (1975). Functional similarity of learning disability and mild retardation. *Exceptional Children, 42*, 17–21.

NEISWORTH, J. T., JONES, R. T. & SMITH, R. M. (1978). Body-behavior problems: A conceptualization. *Education and Training of the Mentally Retarded, 13*, 265–271.

NEISWORTH, J. T. & SMITH, R. M. (1973). *Modifying retarded behavior*. Boston: Houghton-Mifflin.

NELSON, R., PEOPLES, A., HAY, L., JOHNSON, T. & HAY, W. (1976). The effectiveness of speech training techniques based on operant conditioning: A comparison of two methods. *Mental Retardation, 14*(3), 34–38.

New York ARC v. Rockefeller, No. 72 356, 72/357, E. D. New York (1975).

New York State Association for Retarded Citizens v. Rockefeller. U.S. Dist. Court, E.D., N.Y., (1972).

NIHIRA, K., FOSTER, R., SHELLHAAS, M. & LELAND, H. (1974). *AAMD adaptive behavior scale*. Washington, D. C.: American Association on Mental Deficiency.

NIHIRA, K., MINK, I. T. & MEYERS, C. E. (1981). Relationship between home environment and social adjustment of TMR children. *American Journal of Mental Deficiency, 86*, 8–15.

NIRJE, B. (1969). The normalization principle and its human management implications. In R. B. Kugel & W. Wolfensberger (Eds.). *Changing patterns in residential services for the mentally retarded*. Washington, D. C.: President's Committee on Mental Retardation.

O'BRIEN, F., AZRIN, N. & BUGLE, C. (1972). Training profoundly retarded children to stop crawling. *Journal of Applied Behavior Analysis, 5*, 131–137.

O'BRIEN, F., BUGLE, C. & AZRIN, N. H. (1972). Training and maintaining a retarded child's proper eating. *Journal of Applied Behavior Analysis, 5*, 67–72.

O'CONNOR, G. (1976). *Home is a good place: A national perspective of community residential facilities for developmentally disabled persons* (Monograph No. 2). Washington, D. C.: American Association on Mental Deficiency.

O'DELL, S. (1974). Training parents in behavior modification: A review. *Psychological Bulletin, 81*, 418–433.

ODOM, S. L. (1981). The relationship of play to developmental level in mentally retarded children. *Education and Training of the Mentally Retarded, 16*, 136–141.

OLSHANSKY, S. (1966). Parent responses to a mentally defective child. *Mental Retardation, 4*(4), 21–23.

OPTON, E. (1979). A psychologist takes a closer look at the recent landmark *Larry P.* opinion. *APA Monitor, 12*(10), 1, 4–5.

ORELOVE, F. P. (1982). Acquisition of incidental learning in moderately and severely handicapped adults. *Education and Training of the Mentally Retarded, 17*, 131–136.

ORLANDO, C. P. (1973). Review of reading research in special education. In L. Mann & D. A. Sabatina (Eds.). *The first review of special education*. Philadelphia, PA: JSE Press.

PALMER, D. J. (1980). The effect of educable mental retardation descriptive information on regular classroom teachers' attributions and instructional prescriptions. *Mental Retardation, 18*, 171–175.

PALMER, D. J. (1983). An attributional perspective on labeling. *Exceptional Children, 49*, 423–429.

PAGE, E. B. (1975). Miracle in Milwaukee: Raising the IQ. In B. Z. Friedlander, G. M. Sterrit, & G. E. Kirk (Eds.). *Exceptional infant (Vol. 3): assessment and intervention*. New York: Brunner/Mazel.

PAGE, T., IWATA, B. & NEEF, N. (1976). Teaching pedestrian skills to retarded persons: generalization from the classroom to the natural environment. *Journal of Applied Behavior Analysis, 9*, 433–444.

Parents in Action on Special Education (PASE) v. Hannon, No. 74-C-3586 (E.D. Ill., 1974).

PATRICK, J. L., & RESCHLY, D. J. (1982). Relationship of state educational criteria and demographic variables to school-system prevalence of mental retardation. *American Journal of Mental Deficiency, 86*, 351–360.

PAVENSTEDT, E. (1965). A comparison of child-rearing environment of upper–lower and very low–lower class families. *American Journal of Orthopsychiatry, 35*, 89–98.

PAYNE, D., JOHNSON, R. C. & ABELSON, J. A. (1969). *A comprehensive description of institutionalized retardates in the western United States*. Boulder, Colorado: Western Interstate Commission for Higher Education.

PAYNE, J. E. (1976). The deinstitutionalization backlash. *Mental Retardation, 14*(3), 43–45.

PAYNE, J., MERCER, C. & EPSTEIN, M. (1974). *Education and rehabilitation techniques*. New York: Behavioral Publications.

PECK, C. A. & SEMMEL, M. I. (1982). Identifying the least restrictive environment (LRE) for children with severe handicaps: Toward an empirical analysis. *The Journal of the Association for the Severely Handicapped, 7*(1), 56–63.

PECK, J. R. (1960). A comparative investigation of the learning and social adjustment of trainable children in public school facilities, segregated community centers, and state residential centers. USOE Project No. 6430. U. S. Office of Education.

PECK, J. R. & SEXTON, C. L. (1961). Effects of various settings on trainable children's progress. *American Journal of Mental Deficiency, 66*, 62–68.

Pennsylvania Association for Retarded Citizens (PARC) v. The Commonwealth of Pennsylvania. 343 F. Supp. 279 (E.D., Pa.), 1972.

PENNYPACKER, H. S., KOENIG, C. H. & LINDSLEY, O. R. (1972). *Handbook of the standard behavior chart*. Kansas City: Precision Media.

PENROSE, L. Mental deficiency. (1972). *Journal of Special Education, 6*(1), 65–66.

PERKINS, S. A. (1977). Malnutrition and mental development. *Exceptional Children, 43*, 214–219.

PERRY, N. (1960). *Teaching the Mentally Retarded Child*. New York: Columbia University Press.

PETERSON, L & SMITH, L. L. (1960). A comparison of the post-school adjustment of educable mentally retarded adults—with that of adults of normal intelligence. *Exceptional Children, 26*, 404–408.

PFEIFFER, S. J. (1982). The superiority of team decision making. *Exceptional Children, 49*, 68–69.

PHILLIPS, J. L. & BALTHAZAR, E. E. (1979). Some correlates of language deterioration in severely and profoundly retarded long-term institutionalized residents. *American Journal of Mental Deficiency, 83*, 402–408.

PIPER, T. J. & MACKINNON, R. C. (1969). Operant conditioning of a profoundly retarded individual reinforced via a stomach fistule. *American Journal of Mental Deficiency, 73*, 627–630.

POLIFKA, J. C. (1981). Compliance with Public Law 94–142 and consumer satisfaction. *Exceptional Children, 48*, 250–253.

POMERANTZ, D. J. & MARHOLIN, D. (1977). Vocational habilitation: A time for change. In E. Sontag, J. Smith, & W. Certo (Eds.). *Educational programming for the severely and profoundly handicapped*. Reston, Virginia: Division on Mental Retardation, The Council for Exceptional Children.

PORCELLA, A. (1980). Increasing parent involvement. *Education and Training of the Mentally Retarded, 15*, 155–157.

PORTER, R. B. & MILAZZO, T. C. (1958). A comparison of mentally retarded adults who attended a special class with those who attended regular school classes. *Exceptional Children, 24*, 410–412, 420.

President's Committee on Mental Retardation. (1970). *The six-hour retarded child*. Washington, D. C.: Author.

PRICE, M. & GOODMAN, L. (1980). Individualized education programs: A cost study. *Exceptional Children, 46*, 446–454.

QUAY, L. C. (1963). Academic skills. In N. R. Ellis (Ed.), *Handbook of mental deficiency: Psychological theory and research*. New York: McGraw-Hill.

QUICK, A. D. & CAMPBELL, A. A. (1977). A model for preschool curriculum. *Mental Retardation, 15*(2), 42–46.

RAMEY, C. T. & BROWNLEE, J. R. (1981). Improving the identification of high risk infants. *American Journal of Mental Deficiency, 85*, 504–511.

RAMEY, C. T., STEDMAN, D. J., BORDERS-PATTERSON, A. & MENGEL, W. (1978). Predicting school failure from information available at birth. *American Journal of Mental Deficiency, 82*, 525–534.

RASCHKE, D. & YOUNG, A. (1976). A comparative analysis of the diagnostic-prescriptive and behavioral analysis models in preparation for the development of a dialectic pedagogical system. *Education and Training of the Mentally Retarded, 11,* 135–145.

REDDING, S. F. (1979). Life adjustment patterns of retarded and nonretarded low functioning students. *Exceptional Children, 45,* 367–368.

REED, E. W. & REED, S. C. (1965). *Mental Retardation: A Family Study.* Philadelphia: Saunders.

REESE-DUKES, J. L. & STOKES, E. H. (1978). Social acceptance of elementary educable mentally retarded pupils in the regular classroom. *Education and Training of the Mentally Retarded, 13,* 356–361.

REGER, R. (1973). What is a resource room program? *Journal of Learning Disabilities, 6,* 609–614.

REGER, R. & KOPPMANN, M. (1971). The child oriented resource room program. *Exceptional Children, 37,* 460–462.

REID, D. H. & HURLBUT, B. (1977). Teaching nonvocal communication skills to multihandicapped retarded adults. *Journal of Applied Behavior Analysis, 10,* 591–603.

REITER, S. & LEVI, A. M. (1981). Leisure activities of mentally retarded adults. *American Journal of Mental Deficiency, 86,* 201–203.

REMINGTON, R. E., FOXEN, T. & HOGG, J. (1977). Auditory reinforcement in profoundly retarded multiply handicapped children. *American Journal of Mental Deficiency, 82,* 145–148.

RESCHLY, D. & JIPSON, F. (1976). Ethnicity, geographic locale, sex, and urban-rural residence as variables in the prevalence of mild retardation. *American Journal of Mental Deficiency, 81,* 154–161.

REYNOLDS, G. S. (1975). *A Primer of Operant Conditioning* (rev. ed.). Glenview, Ill.: Scott, Foresman.

REYNOLDS, M. C. (1962). A framework for considering some issues in special education. *Exceptional Children, 28,* 367–370.

REYNOLDS, M. C. & BALOW, B. (1972). Categories and variables in special education. *Exceptional Children, 38,* 357–366.

REYNOLDS, M.. C., ELLIS, R. & KILAND, V. R. (1953). *A study of public school children with severe mental retardation.* St. Paul, Minn.: Minnesota State Department of Education.

REYNOLDS, M. C. & ROSEN, S. W. (1976). Special education: Past, present, and future. *Education Forum,* May.

REYNOLDS, W. M. & REYNOLDS, S. (1979). Prevalence of speech and hearing impairments of noninstitutionalized mentally retarded adults. *American Journal of Mental Deficiency, 84,* 62–66.

RICHARDSON, S. A., KOLLER, H., KATZ, M. & McLERAN, J. (1981). A functional classification of seizures and its distribution in a mentally retarded population. *American Journal of Mental Deficiency, 85,* 457–466.

ROBINAULT, I. P. (Ed.). (1973). *Functional aids for the multiply handicapped.* New York: Harper & Row.

ROBINAULT, I. P. & DENHOFF, E. (1973). The multiple dysfunctions called cerebral palsy. In A. B. Cobb (Ed.) *Medical and psychological aspects of disability.* Springfield, Illinois: Charles C Thomas.

ROBINSON, N. (1980). Editors note: terminology, classification, and description in mental retardation research. *American Journal of Mental Deficiency, 85,* 107.

ROBINSON, N. M. & ROBINSON, H. B. (1976). *The Mentally Retarded Child* (2nd ed.). New York: McGraw-Hill.

ROGERS, C. (1947). Some observations on the organization of personality. *American Psychologist, 2,* 358–368.

ROMER, D. & BERKSON, G. (1981). Social ecology of supervised communal facilities for mentally disabled adults: IV. Characteristics of social behavior. *American Journal of Mental Deficiency, 86,* 28–38.

ROOS, P. (1979). Custodial care for the "subtrainable"—revisiting an old myth. *Law & Psychology Review, 5,* 1–14.

ROOS, P. (1971). Current issues in the education of mentally retarded persons. In W. J. Cegelka (Ed.). *Proceedings: Conference on the education of mentally retarded persons.* Arlington, Texas: National Association for Retarded Citizens.

ROOS, P. (1963). Psychological counseling with parents of retarded children. *Mental Retardation, 1,* 345–350.

ROOS, P. (1978). Parents of mentally retarded children—misunderstood and mistreated. In A. P. Turnbull & H. R. Turnbull (Eds.). *Parents speak out: Views from the other side of the two-way mirror.* Columbus, Ohio: Chas. E. Merrill.

ROSENBERG, S. (1970). Problems of language development in the retarded. In H. C. Haywood (Ed.). *Sociocultural aspects of mental retardation.* New York: Appleton-Century-Crofts.

ROSENZWIEG, L. E. & LONG, J. (1960). *Understanding and Teaching the Dependent Retarded Child* (2nd ed.). Darien, Connecticut: Educational Publishing Corporation.

ROTTER, J. B. (1954). *Social learning and clinical psychology.* Englewood Cliffs, New Jersey: Prentice-Hall.

RYNDERS, J. E. & FRIEDLANDER, B. Z. (1972). Preferences in institutionalized severely retarded children for selected visual stimulus material presented as operant reinforcement. *American Journal of Mental Deficiency, 76,* 568–573.

RYNDERS, J. & HORROBIN, J. (1975). Project EDGE: The University of Minnesota's communication stimulation program for Down's syndrome infants. In B. Friedlander, G. Sterritt, & G. Kirk (Eds.). *Exceptional infant: Assessment and intervention* (Vol. 3). New York: Brunner/Mazel.

RYNDERS, J. E., SPIKER, D. & HORROBIN, J. M. (1978). Underestimating the educability of Down's syndrome children: Examination of methodological problems in recent literature. *American Journal of Mental Deficiency, 82,* 440–448.

SABAGH, G., LEI, T. & EYMAN, R. (1972). The speed of hospitalization revisited: A replication of a preadmission waiting list cohort in a hospital for the retarded. *Social Problems, 19,* 373–382.

SABATINO, D. A. (1972). Resource rooms: The Renaissance in special education. *The Journal of Special Education, 6,* 335–347.

SAENGER, G. (1957). *The adjustment of severely retarded adults living in the community.* Albany, N. Y.: New York State Interdepartmental Health Resources Board.

SAENGER, G. (1960). *Factors influencing the institutionalization of mentally retarded individuals in New York City: A study of the effects of services, personnel characteristics, and family background on the decision to instutionalize.* Albany: New York State Department of Health Resources Board.

SAILOR, W. & HARING, N. (1977). Some current directions in education of the severely/multiply handicapped. *AAESPH Review, 2*(2), 67–86.

SALISBURY, C., WAMBOLD, C. & WALTER, G. (1978). Manual communication for the severely handicapped: An assessment and instructional strategy. *Education and Training of the Mentally Retarded, 13,* 393–397.

SALVIA, J. & YSSELDYKE, J. E. (1978). *Assessment in special and remedial education.* Boston: Houghton-Mifflin Co.

SANDLER, A. & COREN, A. (1981). Integrated instruction at home and school: Parents' perspective. *Education and Training of the Mentally Retarded, 16,* 183–187.

SANDLER, A., COREN, A. & THURMAN, S. K. (1983). A training program for parents of handicapped preschool children: Effects upon mother, father, and child. *Exceptional Children, 49,* 355–358.

SANDLER, A. & ROBINSON, R. (1981). Public attitudes and community acceptance of mentally retarded persons: A review. *Education and Training of the Mentally Retarded, 16,* 97–103.

SANDLER, A. & THURMON, S. K. (1981). Status of community placement research: Effects on retarded citizens. *Education and Training of the Mentally Retarded, 16,* 245–251.

SARASON, S. B. (1953). *Psychological problems in mental deficiency* (2nd ed.). New York: Harper & Row.

SATTLER, J. M. (1974). *Assessment of children's intelligence* (Rev. reprint). Philadelphia: W. B. Saunders Company.

SATTLER, J. (1982). *Assessment of children's intelligence* (2nd Ed.). Philadelphia: W. B. Saunders Co.

Scanlon v. Battle, 66 L. Ed. 2d, 837, (1981).

SCHEERENBERGER, R. C. (1983). *A history of mental retardation.* Baltimore: Brookes Publishing Co.

SCHEERENBERGER, R. C. (1982). Public residential services, 1981: Status and trends. *Mental Retardation, 20,* 210–215.

SCHEERENBERGER, R. C. (1976). A study of public residential facilities. *Mental Retardation, 14*(1), 32–35.

SCHEERENBERGER, R. C. (1978). Public residential services for the mentally retarded. In N. R. Ellis (Ed.). *International review of research in mental retardation* (Vol. 9). New York: Academic Press.

SCHEERENBERGER, R. C. & FELSENTHAL, D. (1977). Community settings for MR persons: Satisfaction and activities. *Mental Retardation, 15*(4), 3–7.

SCHIEFELBUSCH, R. L. & LLOYD, L. L. (EDS.). (1974). *Language perspectives—acquisition, retardation, and intervention.* Baltimore: University Park Press.

SCHILIT, J. & CALDWELL, M. L. (1980). A word list of essential career/vocational words for mentally retarded students. *Education and Training of the Mentally Retarded, 15,* 113–117.

SCHLEIEN, S. J., KIERNAN, J. & WEHMAN, P. (1981). Evolution of an age-appropriate leisure skills program for moderately retarded adults. *Education and Training of the Mentally Retarded, 16,* 13–19.

SCHROEDER, G. L. & BAER, D. M. (1972). Effects of concurrent and serial training on generalized vocal imitation in retarded children. *Developmental Psychology, 6,* 293–301.

SCHROEDER, S. R., MULICK, J. A. & SCHROEDER, C. S. (1979). Management of severe behavior problems of the retarded. In N. R. Ellis (Ed.). *Handbook of mental deficiency: Psychological theory and research* (2nd ed.). Hillsdale, New Jersey: Lawrence Erlbaum Associates.

SCHWARTZ, C. (1977). Normalization and idealism. *Mental Retardation, 15*(6), 38–39.

SCHWARTZ, L. & OSEROFF, A. (1975). *The clinical teacher for special education, Final report* (Vol. 1). Tallahassee, Florida: The Florida State University.

SCOTT, K. G. (1978). Learning theory, intelligence, and mental development. *American Journal of Mental Deficiency, 82,* 325–336.

SCRIMSHAW, N. (1968). Infant malnutrition and adult learning. *Saturday Review, 16,* 64–84.

SEGUIN, E. (1866). *Idiocy: And its treatment by the physiological method.* New York: William Wood.

SEITZ, S. & GESKE, D. (1976). Mothers' and graduate trainees' judgments of children: Some effects of labeling. *American Journal of Mental Deficiency, 81,* 362–370.

SELLS, C. J. & BENNETT, F. C. (1977). Prevention of mental retardation: The role of medicine. *American Journal of Mental Deficiency, 82,* 117–129.

SEMMEL, M. I., GOTTLIEB, J. & ROBINSON, N. M. (1979). Mainstreaming: Perspectives on educating handicapped children in the public schools. In D. Berliner (Ed.). *Review of research in education* (Vol. 7). Washington, D. C.: American Educational Research Association.

SEVERANCE, L. J. & GASSTROM, L. L. (1977). Effects of the label "mentally retarded" on causal explanations for success and failure outcomes. *American Journal of Mental Deficiency, 81,* 547–555.

SHALOCK, R. L. & HARPER, R. S. (1978). Placement from community-based mental retardation programs: How well do clients do? *American Journal of Mental Deficiency, 83,* 240–247.

SHALOCK, R. L., HARPER, R. S. & CARVER, G. (1981). Independent living placement: Five years later. *American Journal of Mental Deficiency, 86,* 170–177.

SHALOCK, R. L., HARPER, R. S. & GENUNG, T. (1981). Community integration of mentally retarded adults: Community placement and program success. *American Journal of Mental Deficiency, 85,* 478–488.

SHEARE, J. B. (1974). Social acceptance of EMR adolescents in integrated programs. *American Journal of Mental Deficiency, 78,* 678–682.

SHEARER, D. E. & SHEARER, M. S. (1976). The Portage Project: A model for early childhood intervention. In T. D. Tjossem (Ed.). *Intervention strategies for high risk infants and young children.* Baltimore: University Park Press.

SHELLHAAS, M. D. & NIHIRA, K. (1969). Factor analysis of reasons retardates are referred to an institution. *American Journal of Mental Deficiency, 74,* 171–179.

SHEPERD, G. (1967). Selected factors in the reading ability of educable mentally retarded boys. *American Journal of Mental Deficiency, 71,* 536–570.

SHEVIN, M. (1983). Meaningful parent involvement in long-range educational planning for disabled children. *Education and Training of the Mentally Retarded, 18,* 17–21.

SHOTEL, J. R., IANO, R. P. & McGETTIGAN, J. F. (1972). Teacher attitudes associated with integration of handicapped children. *Exceptional Children, 38,* 677–683.

SILVA, D. A. (1979). The use of medication in a residential institution for mentally retarded persons. *Mental Retardation, 17,* 285–288.

SILVERSTEIN, A. B., AGUILAR, B. F., JACOBS, L. J., LEVY, J. & RUBENSTEIN, D. M. (1979). Imitative behavior by Down's syndrome persons. *American Journal of Mental Deficiency, 83,* 409–411.

SILVERSTEIN, A. B., PEARSON, L. B., COLBERT, B. A., CORDEIRO, W. J., MARWIN, J. L. & NAKAJI, M. J. (1982). Cognitive development of severely and profoundly mentally retarded individuals. *American Journal of Mental Deficiency, 87,* 347–350.

SIMCHES, R. F. (1975). The parent-professional partnership. *Exceptional Children, 41,* 565–566.

SIMEONSSON, R. J. (1977). Infant assessment and developmental handicaps. In B. M. Caldwell, D. J. Stedman (Eds.). *Infant education: A guide for helping handicapped children in the first three years.* New York: Walker & Co.

SIMPSON, G. G. & BECK, W. S. (1965). *Life: An Introduction to Biology.* New York: Harcourt, Brace & World.

SINGH, N. W. & AMAN, M. G. (1981). Effects of thioridozine dosage on the behavior of severely mentally retarded persons. *American Journal of Mental Deficiency, 85,* 580–587.

SITKO, M. C. & SEMMEL, M. I. (1973). Language and language behavior of the mentally retarded. In L. Mann & D. A. Sabatino (Eds.). *The first review of special education* (Vol. 1). Philadelphia: JSE Press.

SITLINGTON, P. L. (1981). Vocational and special education in career programming for the mildly handicapped adolescent. *Exceptional Children, 47,* 592–598.

SKEELS, H. M. (1966). Adult status of children with contrasting early life experiences. *Monographs of the Society for Research in Child Development, 31* (No. 3, Serial No. 105).

SKEELS, H. M. & DYE, H. B. (1939). A study of the effects of differential stimulation on mentally retarded children. *Proceedings and Addresses of the American Association on Mental Deficiency, 44,* 114–136.

SKELTON, M. (1972). Areas of parental concern about retarded children. *Mental Retardation, 10*(1), 38–41.

SKINNER, B. F. (1938). *The Behavior of Organisms: An Experimental Analysis.* New York: Appleton-Century-Crofts.

SKINNER, B. F. (1953). *Science and Human Behavior.* New York: Macmillan.

SMITH, C. A. (1947). Effects of maternal undernutrition upon the newborn infant in Holland. *Journal of Pediatrics, 30,* 229.

SMITH, D. W. & WILSON, A. A. (1973). *The child with Down's syndrome (Mongolism).* Philadelphia: Saunders.

SMITH, I. L. & GREENBERG, S. (1975). Teacher attitudes and the labeling process. *Exceptional Children, 41,* 319–324.

SMITH, R. M. & NEISWORTH, J. T. (1975). *The Exceptional Child: A Functional Approach.* New York: McGraw-Hill.

SNELL, M. E. (Ed.). (1982). *Systematic instruction of the moderately and severely handicapped* (2nd ed.). Columbus, Ohio: Charles E. Merrill.

SOFFER, R. M. (1982). IEP decisions in which parents desire greater participation. *Education and Training of the Mentally Retarded, 17,* 67–70.

SONTAG, E., BURKE, B. J. & YORK, R. (1973). Considerations for serving the severely handicapped in the public schools. *Education and Training of the Mentally Retarded, 8,* 20–26.

SONTAG, E., SMITH, J. & SAILOR, W. (1977). The severely/profoundly handicapped: Who are they? Where are we? *Journal of Special Education, 11*(1), 5–11.

SOWERS, J., RUSCH, F. F., CONNIS, R. T. & CUMMINGS, L. T. (1980). Teaching mentally retarded adults to time-manage in a vocational setting. *Journal of Applied Behavior Analysis, 13,* 119–128.

SOWERS, J., RUSCH, F. R. & HUDSON, C. (1979). Training a severely retarded young adult to ride the city bus to and from work. *AAESPH Review, 4*(1), 15–23.

SPITZ, H. H. (1979). Beyond field theory in the study of mental deficiency. In N. R. Ellis (Ed.). *Handbook of mental deficiency: Psychological theory and research* (2nd ed.). Hillsdale, New Jersey: Erlbaum.

SPITZ, H. H. (1973). Consolidating facts into the schematized learning and memory system of educable retardates. In N. R. Ellis (Ed.). *International Review of Research in Mental Retardation* (Vol. 6). New York: Academic Press.

SPITZ, H. H. (1963). Field theory in mental deficiency. In N. R. Ellis (Ed.). *Handbook of mental deficiency: Psychological theory and research.* New York: McGraw-Hill.

SPITZ, H. H. (1966). The role of input organization in the learning and memory of mental retardates. In N. R. Ellis (Ed.), *International review of research in mental retardation* (Vol. 2). New York: Academic Press.

SPITZ, H. H. (1976). Toward a relative psychology of mental retardation, with special emphasis on evolution. In N. R. Ellis (Ed.). *International review of research in mental retardation* (Vol. 8). New York: Academic Press.

SPITZ, H. H. & BORYS, S. V. (1977). Performance of retarded adolescents and non-retarded children on one- and two-bit logical problems. *Journal of Experimental Child Psychology, 23,* 415–429.

SPITZ, H. H. & WINTERS, E. A. (1977). Tic-tac-toe performance as a function of maturational level of retarded adolescents and non-retarded children. *Intelligence, 1,* 108–117.

SPOONER, F. & DYKES, M. K. (1982). Epilepsy: Impact upon severely and profoundly handicapped persons. *Journal of the Association for the Severely Handicapped, 7*(3), 87–96.

SPRADLIN, J. E. (1963). Language and communication of mental defectives. In N. R. Ellis (Ed.), *Handbook of mental deficiency: Psychological theory and research.* New York: McGraw-Hill.

SPRAGUE, R. L. (1977). Overview of psychopharmocology for the retarded in the United States. In P. Mittler (Ed.). *Research to practice in mental retardation (Vol. III): Biomedical aspects.* Baltimore: University Park Press.

STAINBACK, S. B. & STAINBACK, W. C. (1975). A defense of the concept of the special class. *Education and Training of the Mentally Retarded, 10,* 91–93.

STAINBACK, W. & STAINBACK, S. (1983). A review of research on the educability of profoundly retarded persons. *Education and Training of the Mentally Retarded, 18,* 90–100.

STALLARD, C. K. (1982). Computers and education for exceptional children: Emerging practices. *Exceptional Children, 49,* 102–104.

STANFIELD, J. S. (1973). Graduation: What happens to the retarded child when he grows up? *Exceptional Children, 39,* 548–552.

STEDMAN, D. J. (1977). Early childhood intervention programs. In B. M. Caldwell & D. V. Stedman (Eds.) *Infant education: A guide for helping handicapped children in the first three years.* New York: Walker and Company.

STEIN, Z., SUSSER, M., SAENGER, G. & MAROLLA, F. (1975). *Famine and human development: The Dutch hunger winter of 1944–1945.* New York: Oxford University Press.

STEPHENS, B. (Ed.). (1971). *Training the Developmentally Young.* New York: John Day.

STEPHENS, B. (1977). A Piagetian approach to curriculum development. In E. Sontag, J. Smith & N. Certo (Eds.). *Educational programming for the severely and profoundly handicapped.* Reston, Virginia: Division on Mental Retardation, Council for Exceptional Children.

STEPHENS, B. & McLAUGHLIN, J. A. (1974). Two year gains in reasoning by retarded and nonretarded persons. *American Journal of Mental Deficiency, 79,* 116–126.

STEPHENS, B., McLAUGHLIN, J. A., MILLER, C. K. & GLASS, G. V. (1972). Factorial structure of selected psychoeducational measures and Piagetian reasoning assessments. *Developmental Psychology, 6,* 343–348.

STERICK, G. (1979). A follow-up study of ten children who learned to read in a class for trainable students. *Education and Training of the Mentally Retarded, 14,* 170–176.

STERN, W. (1914). Über die psychologishen methoden der intelligenzprufüng. *Ber. V. Kongress Exp. Psychol., 1912, 16,* 1–160. American translation by G. M. Whippelo, the psychological methods of testing intelligence. *Educational Psychology Monographs,* No. 13, Baltimore: Warwich & York.

STODDEN, R. A., IANACONE, R. N. & LAZAR, A. L. (1979). Occupational interests and mentally retarded people: Review and recommendations. *Mental Retardation, 17,* 294–298.

STOKES, T. F., BAER, D. M. & JACKSON, R. L. (1974). Programming the generalization of a greeting response in four retarded children. *Journal of Applied Behavior Analysis, 7,* 599–610.

STRAIN, P. S. & SHORES, R. E. (1977). Social reciprocity: A review of research and educational implications. *Exceptional Children, 43,* 526–530.

STRAUSS, A. A. & LEHTINEN, L. E. (1947). *Psychopathology and education of the brain injured child.* New York: Grune & Stratton.

STRENECKY, B. J., McLAUGHLIN, J. A. & EDGE, D. (1979). Parent involvement: A consumer perspective—In the schools. *Education and Training of the Mentally Retarded, 14,* 54–56.

SULZER-AZAROFF, B. & MAYER, G. R. (1977). *Applying behavior analysis procedures with children and youth.* New York: Holt, Rinehart, and Winston.

SUTTER P., TADASHI, M., CALL, T., YANAGI, G. & YEE, S. (1980). Comparison of successful and unsuccessful community placed mentally retarded persons. *American Journal of Mental Deficiency, 85,* 262–267.

SWITZKY, H. N., HAYWOOD, H. C. & ROTATORI, A. F. (1982). Who are the severely and profoundly mentally retarded. *Education and Training of the Mentally Retarded, 17,* 268–272.

TABA, H. (1964). Cultural deprivation as a factor in school learning. *Merrill-Palmer Quarterly, 10,* 147–159.

TARJAN, G. (1973). Sex: A tri-polar conflict in mental retardation. In R. K. Eyman, C. E. Meyers & G. Tarjan (Eds.). *Socio-behavioral studies in mental retardation.* Washington, D. C.: American Association on Mental Deficiency.

TARJAN, G., WRIGHT, S., EYMAN, R. & KEERAN, C. (1973). Natural history of mental retardation: Some aspects of epidemiology. *American Journal of Mental Deficiency, 77,* 369–379.

TAVORMINA, J. B., HAMPSON, R. B. & LUSCOMB, R. L. (1976). Participants' evaluations of the effectiveness of their parent counseling groups. *Mental Retardation, 14*(6), 8–9.

TAVORMINA, J. B., HENGGELER, S. W. & GAYTON, W. F. (1976). Age trends in parental assessments of the behavior problems of their retarded children. *Mental Retardation, 14*(1), 38–39.

TAWNEY, J. W., KNAPP, D. S., O'REILLY, C. D. & PRATT, S. S. (1979). *Programmed environments curriculum.* Columbus, Ohio: Charles E. Merrill.

TAYLOR, R. (1980). Use of the AAMD classification system: A review of recent research. *American Journal of Mental Deficiency, 85,* 116–119.

TAYLOR, R. L., SMILEY, L. R. & ZIEGLER, E. W. (1983). The effect of labels and assigned attributes on teacher perceptions of academic and social behavior. *Education and Training of the Mentally Retarded, 18,* 45–51.

TEFFREY, D., MARTIN, G. L., SAMELS, J. L. & WATSON, C. (1970). Operant conditioning of grooming behavior in severely retarded girls. *Mental Retardation, 8*(4), 29–33.

TERMAN, L. M. (1916). *The Measurement of Intelligence.* Boston: Houghton & Mifflin.

TERMAN, L. & MERRILL, M. (1973). *Stanford-Binet Intelligence Scale, 1972 norms edition.* Boston: Houghton-Mifflin Co.

TERRELL, G., JR., DURKIN, K. & WIESLEY, M. (1957). Social class and the nature of the incentive in discrimination learning. *Journal of Abnormal and Social Psychology, 59,* 270–272.

TETZLAFF, D. M. & SEDLAK, R. A. (1978). Organizational structures of TMH classes in Illinois. *Education and Training of the Mentally Retarded, 13,* 287–293.

THIEL, G. W. (1981). Relationship of IQ, adaptive behavior, age, and environmental demand to community placement success of mentally retarded adults. *American Journal of Mental Deficiency, 86,* 208–211.

THEONE, J., HIGGINS, J., KRIEGER, I., SCHMICKEL, R. & WEISS, L. (1981). Genetic screening for mental retardation in Michigan. *American Journal of Mental Deficiency, 85,* 335–340.

THOMAS, M. A. (1979). Adapt the program to fit the needs: A conversation with Kenneth E. Wyatt about the least restrictive environment for mentally retarded students. *Education and Training of the Mentally Retarded, 14,* 191–197.

THOMAS, M. A. (1981). Educating handicapped students via microcomputer/videodisc technology: A conversation with Ron Thorkildsen. *Education and Training of the Mentally Retarded, 16,* 264–269.

THOMASON, J. & ARKELL, C. (1980). Educating the severely/profoundly handicapped in the public schools: A side by side approach. *Exceptional Children, 47,* 114–122.

THOMPSON, T. & CAREY, A. (1980). Structured normalization: Intellectual and adaptive behavior changes in a residential setting. *Mental Retardation, 18,* 193–197.

THOMPSON, W. R. & GRUSEC, J. (1970). Studies in early experience. In P. H. Mussen (Ed.). *Carmichael's manual of child psychology* (Vol. I). New York: John Wiley & Sons.

THRONE, J. M. (1975). Normalization through the normalization principle: Right ends, wrong means. *Mental Retardation, 13*(5), 23–25.

THRONE, J. M. (1979). Deinstitutionalization: Too wide a swath. *Mental Retardation, 17,* 171–175.

THURMAN, S. K. (1981). Least restrictive environments: Another side of the coin. *Education and Training of the Mentally Retarded, 16,* 68–70.

TIZARD, J. & GRAD, J. C. (1961). *The mentally handicapped and their families* (Maudsley Monograph No. 7). London: Oxford University Press.

TISDALL, W. J. (1958). A follow-up of trainable mentally handicapped children in Illinois. Unpublished Masters thesis, University of Illinois.

TJOSSEM, T. D. (Ed.). (1976). *Intervention strategies for high risk infants and young children.* Baltimore: University Park Press.

TOBIAS, J. (1970). Vocational adjustment of young retarded adults. *Mental Retardation, 3*(8), 13–16.

TOLLIVER, B. (1975). Discrimination against minority students in special education. *Education and Training of the Mentally Retarded, 10,* 188–192.

TRACE, M. W., CUVO, A. J. & CRISWELL, J. L. (1977). Teaching coin equivalence to the mentally retarded. *Journal of Applied Behavior Analysis, 10,* 85–92.

TREDGOLD, A. F. (1908). *Mental Deficiency.* London: Bailliera, Tindall & Fox.

TREDGOLD, A. (1937). *A Textbook of Mental Deficiency* (6th ed.). Baltimore: Wood.

TURNBULL, A. P. (1982). Parent-professional interactions. In M. E. Snell (Ed.), *Systematic instruction of the moderately and severely handicapped* (2nd ed.). Columbus, Ohio: Chas. E. Merrill.

TURNBULL, A. P., STRICKLAND, B. B. & BRANTLEY, J. C. (1978). *Developing and implementing individualized education programs.* Columbus, Ohio: Chas. E. Merrill.

TURNBULL, A. P., STRICKLAND, B. & GOLDSTEIN, S. (1978). Training professionals and parents in developing and implementing the IEP. *Education and Training of the Mentally Retarded, 13,* 414–423.

TURNBULL, A. P. & TURNBULL, H. R. (1982). Parent involvement in the education of handicapped children: A critique. *Mental Retardation, 20,* 115–122.

TURNBULL, H. R. (1978). Jay's story. In A. P. Turnbull & H. R. Turnbull (Eds.). *Parents speak out: Views from the other side of the two-way mirror.* Columbus, Ohio: Chas. E. Merrill.

TURNBULL, H. R. (1982). Youngberg v. Romeo: An essay. *Journal of the Association of the Severely Handicapped, 7*(3), 3–6.

TURNURE, J. E. & ZIGLER, E. (1964). Outerdirectedness in the problem-solving of normal and retarded children. *Journal of Abnormal and Social Psychology, 69,* 427–436.

UMBREIT, J. (1980). Effects of developmentally sequenced instruction on the rate of skill acquisition by severely handicapped students. *Journal of the Association for the Severely Handicapped, 5*(2), 121–129.

U. S. Department of Education. (1980). *Second annual report to Congress on the implementation of Public Law 94–142: the Education for All Handicapped Children Act.*

U. S. Department of Health, Education, and Welfare, Bureau of Education for the Handicapped. *Federal Register,* (1975). *40* (35).

U. S. Department of Health, Education, and Welfare/Office of Civil Rights. Statistical report: Enrollment in special education (Prepared for the Subcommittee on Select Education, Education and Labor Committee, House of Representatives), (October, 1979).

U. S. Department of Health, Education, and Welfare/Office of Education. Progress toward a free appropriate education: A report to Congress on the implementation of Public Law 94–142: the Education for All Handicapped Children Act, (1979). (HEW Publication No. OE-79-05003).

UZGIRIS, I. C. (1970). Sociocultural factors in cognitive development. In H. C. Haywood (Ed.). *Social-cultural aspects of mental retardation.* New York: Appleton-Century-Crofts.

UZGIRIS, I. C. & HUNT, J. McV. (1975). *Assessment in infancy: Ordinal scales of psychological development.* Urbana: University of Illinois Press.

VANDENBERG, S. G. (1971). What do we know today about the inheritance of intelligence and how do we know it? In R. Cancro (Ed.). *Intelligence: Genetic and environmental influences.* New York: Grune & Stratton.

VANDEVER, T. R. & STUBBS, J. C. (1977). Reading retention and transfer in TMR students. *American Journal of Mental Deficiency, 82,* 233–237.

VITELLO, S. J. (1976). Quantitative abilities of mentally retarded children. *Education and Training of the Mentally Retarded, 11,* 125–129.

WAISBREN, S. E. (1980). Parents' reactions after the birth of a developmentally disabled child. *American Journal of Mental Deficiency, 84,* 345–351.

WAITE, K. B. (1972). *The Trainable Mentally Retarded Child.* Springfield, Illinois: Charles C Thomas.

WALKER, V. S. (1974). The efficacy of the resource room for educating retarded children. *Exceptional Children, 40,* 288–289.

WALLIN, J. E. (1955). *Education of mentally handicapped children.* New York: Harper & Row.

WARBURG, M. (1970). Tracing and training of blind and partially sighted patients in institutions for the mentally retarded. *Danish Medical Bulletin, 17,* 148–152.

WECHSLER, D. (1974). *Manual for the Wechsler Intelligence Test for Children—Revised.* New York: Psychological Corp.

WECHSLER, D. (1958). *The measurement and appraisal of adult intelligence* (4th ed.). Baltimore: Williams & Wilkins.

WEHMAN, P. H. (1976). A leisure time activities curriculum for the developmentally disabled. *Education and Training of the Mentally Retarded, 11,* 309–313.

WEHMAN, P. H. (1976). Selection of play materials for the severely handicapped: A continuing dilemma, *Education and Training of the Mentally Retarded, 11,* 46–50.

WEHMAN, P. & HILL, J. W. (1981). Competitive employment for moderately and severely handicapped individuals. *Exceptional Children, 47,* 338–345.

WEHMAN, P. & HILL, J. (1980). *Instructional programming for severely handicapped youth: A community integration approach.* Richmond: Virginia Commonwealth University.

WEHMAN, P. & HILL, M. (1982). *Vocational training and placement of severely disabled persons: Project employability* (Vol. III). Richmond: Virginia Commonwealth University.

WEHMAN, P., HILL, M., GOODALL, P., CLEVELAND, P., BROOKE, V. & PENTECOST, J. H. (1982). Job placement and follow-up of moderately and severely handicapped individuals after three years. *Journal of the Association for the Severely Handicapped, 7*(2), 5–16.

WEHMAN, P., HILL, J. W. & KOEHLER, F. (1979). Placement of developmentally disabled individuals into competitive employment. *Education and Training of the Mentally Retarded, 14,* 269–276.

WEHMAN, P. & MCLAUGHLIN, P. J. (1981). *Program Development in Special Education.* New York: McGraw-Hill.

WEHMAN, P. & MCLAUGHLIN, P. J. (1980). *Vocational Curriculum for Developmentally Disabled Persons.* Baltimore: University Park Press.

WEHMAN, P. & SCHLEIEN, S. (1980). Assessment and selections of leisure skills for severely handicapped learners. *Education and Training of the Mentally Retarded, 15,* 50–57.

WEHMAN, P., SCHLEIEN, S. & KIERNAN, J. (1980). Age appropriate recreation programs for severely handicapped youth and adults. *Journal of the Association for the Severely Handicapped, 5,* 395–407.

WEINER, D., ANDERSON, R. J. & NIETUPSKI, J. (1982). Impact of community-based residential facilities for mentally retarded adults on surrounding property values using realtor analysis methods. *Education and Training of the Mentally Retarded, 17,* 278–282.

WEISBERG, P. (1971). Operant procedures with the retardate: An overview of laboratory research. In N. R. Ellis (Ed.). *International review of research in mental retardation* (Vol. 5). New York: Academic Press.

WHEELER, J., FORD, A., NIETUPSKI, J., LOOMIS, R. & BROWN, L. (1980). Teaching moderatly and severely handicapped adolescents to shop in supermarkets using pocket calculators. *Education and Training of the Mentally Retarded, 15,* 105–112.

WHITEHEAD, C. W. (1979). Sheltered workshops in the decade ahead: Work and wages, or welfare. In G. T. Bellamy, G. O'Connor and O. C. Karan (Eds.). *Vocational rehabilitation of severely handicapped persons.* Baltimore: University Park Press.

WHITMAN, T. L., MERCURIO, J. R. & CAPONIGRI, V. (1970). Development of social responses in two severely retarded children. *Journal of Applied Behavior Analysis, 3,* 133–138.

WHITMAN, T. L. & SCIBACK, V. W. (1979). Behavior modification research with the severely and profoundly retarded. In N. R. Ellis (Ed.). *Handbook of mental deficiency: Psychological theory and research* (2nd ed.). Hillsdale, New Jersey.

WIEGEL-CRUMP, C. A. (1981). The development of grammar in Down's syndrome children between the mental ages of 2–0 and 6–11. *Education and Training of the Mentally Retarded, 16,* 24–30.

WILCOX, B. & BELLAMY, G. T. (1982). *Design of high school programs for severely handicapped students.* Baltimore: Paul H. Brookes.

WILLER, B. S., INTAGLIATA, J. C. & ATKINSON, A. C. (1981). Deinstitutionalization as a crisis event for families of mentally retarded persons. *Mental Retardation, 19,* 28–29.

WILLIAMS, R. L. (1970). Danger: Testing and dehumanizing black children. *Clinical Child Psychology Newsletter, 9*(1), 5–6.

WILMARTH, A. (1906). To whom may the term, feeble-minded, be applied? *Journal of Psycho-Asthenics, 10,* 203–205.

WINDMILLER, M. (1977). An effective use of the public school version of the AAMD adaptive behavior scale. *Mental Retardation, 15*(3), 42–45.

WOHLHUETER, M. J. & SINDBERG, R. M. (1975). Longitudinal development of object permanence in mentally retarded children: An exploratory study. *American Journal of Mental Deficiency, 79,* 513–518.

WOLFENSBERGER, W. (1967). Counseling the parents of the retarded. In A. A. Baumeister (Ed.). *Mental retardation: Appraisal, education, and rehabilitation.* Chicago: Aldine Publishing Co.

WOLFENSBERGER, W. (1972). *The principle of normalization in human services.* Toronto, Canada: National Institute on Mental Retardation.

WOLFENSBERGER, W. (1967). Vocational preparation and occupation. In A. A. Baumeister (Ed.). *Mental retardation: Appraisal, education, and rehabilitation.* Chicago: Aldine Publishing Co.

WOLFENSBERGER, W. & GLENN, L. (1975). *PASS 3: A method for the quantitative evaluation of human services* (3rd ed.). Toronto, Canada: National Institute on Mental Retardation.

WOODWARD, W. M. (1962). The application of Piaget's theory to the training of the subnormal. *Journal of Mental Subnormality, 8,* 3–11.

WOODWARD, M. (1963). The application of Piaget's theory to research in mental deficiency. In N. R. Ellis (Ed.). *Handbook of mental deficiency: Psychological theory and research.* New York: McGraw-Hill.

WOODWARD, W. M. (1972). Problem-solving strategies of young children. *Journal of Child Psychology and Psychiatry, 13,* 11–24.

WOODWARD, W. M. (1979). Piaget's theory and the study of mental retardation. In N. R. Ellis (Ed.). *Handbook of mental deficiency: Psychological theory and research* (2nd ed.). Hillsdale, New Jersey: Erlbaum.

WOODWARD, W. M. & HUNT, M. R. (1972). Exploratory studies of early cognitive development. *British Journal of Educational Psychology, 42,* 248–259.

World Health Organization. *International classification of diseases,* (9th rev.). (ICD–9), 1978.

Wyatt v. Stickney. 325 F. Supp. 781 (M.D., Ala.), 1971.

Wyatt v. Stickey. 344 F. Supp. 387 (1972).

YODER, P. & FOREHAND, R. (1974). Effects of modeling and verbal cues upon concept acquisition of nonretarded and retarded children. *American Journal of Mental Deficiency, 78,* 566–570.

YOSHIDA, R. K., FENTON, K. S., KAUFMAN, M. J. & MAXWELL, J. P. (1978). Parent involvement in the special education pupil planning process: The schools' perspective. *Exceptional Children, 44,* 531–534.

YOSHIDA, R. K. & GOTTLIEB, J. (1977). A model of parental participation in the pupil planning process. *Mental Retardation, 15*(3), 17–20.

YOUNG, S., ALGOZZINE, B. & SCHMID, R. (1979). The effects of assigned attributes and labels on children's peer acceptance ratings. *Educational Training of the Mentally Retarded, 14,* 257–261.

ZEAMAN, D. & HOUSE, B. J. (1963). The role of attention in retardate discrimination learning. In N. R. Ellis (Ed.), *Handbook of mental deficiency: Psychological theory and research.* New York: McGraw-Hill.

ZEAMAN, D. & HOUSE, B. J. (1979). A review of attention theory. In N. R. Ellis (Ed.). *Handbook of mental deficiency: Psychological theory and research* (2nd ed.). Hillsdale, New Jersey: Erlbaum.

ZEDLER, E. P. (1953). Public opinion and public education for the exceptional child—Court decisions 1873–1950. *Exceptional Children, 19,* 187–198.

ZIDER, S. J. & GOLD, M. W. (1981). Behind the wheel training for individuals labeled moderately retarded. *Exceptional Children, 47,* 632–639.

ZIGLER, E. (1969). Developmental versus difference theories of mental retardation and the problem of motivation. *American Journal of Mental Deficiency, 73,* 536–556.

ZIGLER, E. (1967). Familial mental retardation: A continuing dilemma. *Science, 155,* 292–298.

ZIGLER, E. (1970). The nature-nurture issue reconsidered. In H. C. Haywood (Ed.). *Social-cultural aspects of mental retardation.* New York: Appleton-Century-Crofts.

ZIGLER, E. (1966). Research on personality structure in the retardate. In N. R. Ellis (Ed.). *International review of research in mental retardation* (Vol. 1). New York: Academic Press.

ZIGLER, E. & BALLA, D. (1977). Impact of institutional experience on the behavior and development of retarded persons. *American Journal of Mental Deficiency, 82,* 1–11.

ZIGLER, E. & CASCIONE, R. (1977). Headstart has little to do with mental retardation: A reply to Clarke and Clarke. *American Journal of Mental Deficiency, 82,* 246–249.

Author Index

MacMillan, D.L., 25, 58, 60, 180, 181, 185, 187, 288
Magid, D.F., 128–29
Magy, M.A., 140, 141
Mahoney, G., 125
Mahoney, K., 235
Malpass, L.F., 156, 157
Maney, A.C., 204
Margolis, J., 208
Marholin, D., 167, 264, 266, 268
Marolla, F., 85
Marozas, D., 32
Martin, A.S., 266, 267
Martin, G.L., 235
Martin, J.E., 165, 169
Martin, M.B., 234
Marwin, J.L., 115
Mascari, B.G., 187
Mason, J.M., 127
Matarazzo, J., 3, 6
Mattson, B.D., 293
Maurer, S., 182
Maxwell, J.A., 59
Maxwell, J.P., 290
May, D., 32
Mayeda, T., 209, 211
Mayer, G.R., 232n
Mayhall, W.F., 184
Mengel, W., 106
Menolascino, F.J., 192, 206
Mercer, C.D., 102, 117, 120–23,131
Mercer, J.R., 12–13, 24, 34, 35, 50, 51, 55, 56, 58, 203
Mercurio, J.R., 235
Merrill, M., 48
Mesibov, G.B., 178, 208
Messina, R., 182, 186, 191
Meyer, R.J., 207, 279
Meyers, C.F., 25, 49, 50, 60, 144, 180, 181, 187, 206, 282, 284
Meyerson, L., 120, 170, 172, 235
Milazzo, T.C., 180
Milgram, N.A., 113
Miller, C., 215, 216
Miller, C.K., 116
Miller, C.R., 27
Miller, J.O., 94, 95, 99, 100, 102
Millham, J., 51
Milunsky, A., 89
Mink, I.T., 144, 282, 284
Mitchell, L., 150
Mithaug, D.E., 120, 269, 270
Molloy, J.S., 240
Molnar, G.E., 157
Moore, W., 244
Morehead, A., 125
Morehead, D.M., 125
Moreno-Milne, N., 10–11
Morris, H.L., 150, 151
Morris, J.L., 266, 267
Morrison, D.F., 204
Morrison, G.M., 25, 60
Mosier, H.D., 155
Mulick, J.A., 144, 146
Muller, P., 255, 256, 257, 259
Muma, J., 11

Murphy, D.M., 282
Murphy, R., 235

Nagler, B., 12
Nakaji, M.J., 115
Nathan, M., 51
Nazzaro, J.N., 175
Neafsey, S.S., 247
Neef, N., 246
Neisworth, J., 26, 140, 172, 232n
Nelson, R., 235
Neman, R., 32
Nietupski, J., 182, 208, 235
Nihira, K., 4, 49–52, 144, 203, 204, 282, 284
Nirje, B., 205, 212
Nisbet, J., 182, 186, 191, 246

O'Brien, F., 235
O'Connell, C.Y., 229
O'Connor, G., 204, 211, 212, 213
O'Dell, S., 281, 287
Odom, S.L., 149
Olshansky, S., 277
Opper, S., 15
Opton, E., 56
Ora, J., 244
O'Reilly, C.D., 248
Orelove, F.P., 122
Orlando, C.P., 126, 127
Oseroff, A., 26

Paden, L.Y., 102
Page, E.B., 104
Page, R., 204
Page, T., 246
Palk, B.E., 206
Palmer, D.J., 59
Parsons, C.K., 112
Patrick, J.L., 36, 40, 47
Pavenstedt, E., 99
Payne, D., 161
Payne, J., 102, 207
Pearson, L.B., 115
Peck, C.A., 192
Peck, J.R., 191
Pennypacker, H.S., 234
Penrose, L., 12
Pentecost, J.H., 262, 264, 268–70
Peoples, A., 235
Perkins, S.A., 100, 101
Perlmutter, L., 235, 244
Perret, Y.M., 61, 71, 77, 80, 83, 86, 89
Perry, N., 240
Peterson, J., 255, 258, 264, 267
Pfaeffle, H.A., 180
Pfeiffer, S.J., 43, 46
Phillips, J.L., 126
Pierce, L., 235
Piper, T.J., 120
Polifka, J.C., 288
Pomerantz, D.J., 264, 266, 268
Porcella, A., 292
Porter, R.B., 180
Pratt, S.S., 248
Price, M., 229
Pumpian, I., 182, 186, 191, 245, 246

Woodward, M., 114–15
Woodward, W.M., 114, 115, 125
Wool, R., 204
Wright, S., 32, 34–35, 37, 38, 39
Wrobel, C., 238
Wunderlich, R.A., 235

Yanagi, G., 217
Yee, S., 217
Yoder, P., 121
York, B., 235
York, R., 244, 247

Yoshida, R.K., 187, 289, 290
Young, A., 239
Young, S., 59
Ysseldyke, J., 45, 48

Zeaman, D., 109, 110–12, 114, 116–17
Zetlin, A., 49, 50
Zia, B., 222, 223, 230
Zider, S.J., 246
Ziegler, E.W., 59
Zigler, E., 93, 97–98, 102, 112, 114, 120, 137, 138–42, 204–5

Subject Index

Intelligence
 development of, 94
 plasticity of, 101
 subaverage general, 3, 9
 tests, 6–8, 45, 47–49, 54–58, 65
Intelligence and Experience (Hunt), 98
Intelligence Quotient (IQ). *See* IQ
Interactionist position, 98
Internal locus of control, 137–38
Interpersonal functioning, 135–36. *See also* Social
  characteristics
Intervention, early, 98, 101–6, 246
Intrinsic mental retardation, 30
Intuition, 115–16
Inventory approach, vocational, 267–68
Involvement in education, parent, 286–93
Iowa Child Welfare Station, 102
IQ
 AAMD standard for retardation, 3
 adaptive behavior deficits and, 5
 attentional response and, 116
 calculation of, 109
 cerebral palsy and, 159
 changes in mental age and, 109–12
 classification by, 23–28, 30–31
 community placement and, 215, 216
 correlations between relatives', 94–97
 criticism of criterion, 9–11
 decision to institutionalize and, 203–4
 drug treatment and, 167
 early intervention and, 102, 104, 105
 employability and, 255, 256
 for evaluation, 16,45
 observational learning and, 121
 original use of term, 7
 prevalence according to, 32, 34–35, 37
 school programs and, 191
 socialization and, 148
 states' guidelines concerning, 18–19
 tests, 7, 48–49
Itard, J.M.G., 222
Itinerant instruction in classroom, 183

Jacksonian seizure, 160
Jobs. *See* Employment

Karyotyping, 76–78
Kennedy administration, 25
Kernicterus, 87
Ketogenic diet, 168
Kline v. *Armstrong*, 193

Labeling, effects of, 58–60
Language, 54, 62–63, 91–95, 100, 123–26
Larry P. v. *Riles*, 56
Laurence-Moon-Bied syndrome, 156
Law, normalization movement and, 206–7
Learning. *See also* Teaching approaches
 disability concept, general, 13–14
 goals or objectives, 221
 potential, 131
 process, 116–23, 145–46
 products, 123–31
Least restrictive environment, 175, 178–82,
  186–87, 191–92, 229
Leisure activities, 149–50, 212

Lesch-Nyhan syndrome, 75–76
Level I and II abilities, 94
Locus of control, 137–38
Logic, use of, 118–19
Logographic symbols, 128–29
Low-disclosure family, 283
LSD, 83–84

Mainstreaming, 180–82, 187–190, 194–95
Males, prevalence among, 39–40
Malnutrition, 84–85, 100–101
Maple syrup urine disease, 72
Maryland Association for Retarded Citizens v. *State of
  Maryland*, 178
Mattie T. v. *Holladay*, 56–57
Media, instructional, 230–32
Mediational strategies, 118
Medical classification, 28–30
Medical diagnosis, 61–64
Meiosis, 68, 69, 77
Mellaril, 166, 167, 168
Memory, 117–18
Mental age, 7, 27, 48–49, 109–14, 116, 121, 138
Mental retardation, defining. *See* Definitions
Metabolism, inborn errors of, 71
Microcomputers, 231–32
Mildly retarded
 adults, adjustment of, 251–58
 classification by IQ, 24–26
 competitive employment of, 267–70
 curriculum for, 236–40
 identification in schools of, 44–60
 learning, 126–28, 130
 play behavior of, 149
 programs for, 186–90
 reinforcers for, 120–21
 resource room approach to, 183–84
Milwaukee Project, 103, 104
Minorities
 classification of, 13, 14, 24–26
 identification and placement of, 54–58
 language development of, 125–26
 prevalence among, 40
 in special classes, 179, 180, 185
Mitosis, 68, 77
Mobility, community, 261
Modeling, 121–22
Models, educational, 186–92
Moderately retarded
 adults, adjustment of, 258–63
 classification, 23–24, 26
 competitive employment for, 270–71
 curriculum for, 240–46
 identification of, 60–66
 learning, 128–31
 play behavior of, 149
 programs for, 190–92
Mongolism, 77–80, 121, 124–25, 128, 156
Monitoring, prenatal, 88–89
Montessori, M., 223–24
Mortality rate, 101
Mosaicism, 79–80
Motivation, 99, 135
Motor skills, 62–63, 155–57, 237
Multistore memory model, 117